Diet Evaluation

Diet Evaluation

A Guide to Planning a Healthy Diet

G. Richard Jansen, Patricia A. Kendall,
and Coerene M. Jansen

Department of Food Science and Human Nutrition
Colorado State University
Fort Collins, Colorado

Academic Press, Inc.
Harcourt Brace Jovanovich, Publishers
San Diego New York Boston London Sydney Tokyo Boston

This book is printed on acid-free paper. ∞

Issued in furtherance of Cooperative Extension work, Acts of May 8 and June 30, 1914, in cooperation with the U.S. Department of Agriculture, Kenneth R. Bolen, director of Cooperative Extension, Colorado State University, Fort Collins, Colorado. Cooperative Extension programs are available to all without discrimination. To simplify technical terminology, trade names of products and equipment occasionally will be used. No endorsement of products named is intended nor is criticism implied of products not mentioned.

Academic Press, Inc.
San Diego, California 92101

United Kingdom Edition published by
Academic Press Limited
24–28 Oval Road, London NW1 7DX

Library of Congress Cataloging-in-Publication Data

Jansen, G. Richard.
Diet evaluation : a guide to planning a healthy diet / G. Richard Jansen, Patricia A. Kendall, and Coerene Jansen.
p. cm.
Includes bibliographical references.
ISBN 0-12-380215-6 (alk. paper)
1. Dietetics. I. Kendall, Patricia A. (Patricia Ann), Date.
II. Jansen, Coerene. III. Title.
[DNLM: 1. Diet--handbooks. 2. Nutritional Requirements--handbooks. QU 39 J35d]
RM216.J355 1990
613.2--dc20
DNLM/DLC
for Library of Congress

90-179
CIP

Printed in the United States of America
90 91 92 93 9 8 7 6 5 4 3 2 1

Contents

Introduction

Americans have a high degree of interest in nutrition, especially the role of nutrition in health promotion and disease prevention. Nutrition is a popular topic in newspapers, magazines, and on talk shows. Important government reports are coming out on a regular basis, and research papers on the subject often are reported on television before the scientific journal even arrives at college and university libraries around the country.

Unfortunately, much information provided to the public is unreliable and not based on scientific knowledge. Adding to the confusion are legitimate differences of opinion among well-informed scientists. The purpose of this Guide is to provide, in concise form, the current state of knowledge about diet and health along with an accurate and convenient way to assess the nutritional adequacy of individual and family diets.

There are two basic approaches to dietary guidance: Food groups and nutrients. A number of food group approaches have been recommended. The basic four food group plan, in which foods are grouped as meats and meat alternatives, dairy products, breads and cereals, and fruits and vegetables, is one such system. Consuming a variety of foods within all food groups is good advice. Recently a fifth group of foods of very low nutrient value, such as candy, soft drinks, and alcoholic beverages, has been added as a group of foods to restrict.

The food group approach is designed to assure nutritional adequacy, particularly for protein, vitamins, and minerals. It does not address nutritional excesses, especially of calories, fat, and cholesterol. In addition, many foods are mixtures of food ingredients and are not exclusively contained in one food group or another, making evaluation by food groups difficult.

This Diet Guide uses the "nutritional shares" concept which is a nutrient approach to diet evaluation and menu planning. This method, to be described below, helps individuals evaluate their diet in terms of individual nutrients and helps control nutritional excesses appropriately while assuring nutritional adequacy. In addition, it helps the reader better understand food composition and the nutritional value of individual foods.

Nutritional Standards and Guidelines

In order to use a nutrient approach in diet evaluation, an appropriate nutritional standard is needed. Since the 1940s, the Food and Nutrition Board of the National Academy of Sciences has published recommended dietary allowances (RDA) for key nutrients approximately every 5 years. According to the ninth edition published in 1980, "Recommended Dietary Allowances (RDA) are the levels of intake of essential nutrients considered, in the judgment of the Committee on Dietary Allowances of the Food and Nutrition Board on the basis of available scientific knowledge, to be adequate to meet the known nutritional needs of practically all healthy persons." The tenth edition, which should have been published in 1986, was held up for several years because of controversy within the scientific community and the National Academy of Sciences. It was released in 1989 and is used in this Diet Guide. Recommended dietary allowances which vary by age, sex, and reproductive status for women have been established for energy (calories), protein, 11 vitamins, and 7 minerals. In addition, estimated "safe and adequate" levels have been established for two vitamins and five trace elements. Estimated "minimum requirements" have been set for the electrolytes sodium, potassium, and chloride. The scientific information on which these "estimated" levels are based is not as complete as that for the RDA nutrients.

Not to be confused with the "RDAs" are the "U.S. RDAs." These are based on the 1968 version of the Recommended Dietary Allowances (seventh edition) and were established by the Food and Drug Administration (FDA) for nutritional labeling of food. Food labeling regulations are currently undergoing extensive review in Congress as well as within the FDA.

Since the 1977 report on "Dietary Goals for the United States" by the United States Senate Select Committee on Nutrition and Human Needs, increasing attention has been directed to the role of nutrition in health promotion and disease prevention. Current concerns are directed toward the role of all nutrients in growth and good health and the role of such nutrients as fat, cholesterol, carbohydrate, and dietary fiber in chronic diseases such as obesity, heart disease, diabetes, and cancer. These are nutrients for which no RDAs have been established or, in fact, can be established.

Both quantitative and nonquantitative approaches have been applied to dietary guidance to reduce risk of chronic disease. The "Dietary Guidelines for Americans," established collaboratively by the United States Department of Agriculture (USDA) and the United States Department of Health and Human Services (USDHHS) provide a nonquantitative approach to health promotion/disease prevention. The Dietary Guidelines recommend less consumption of fat, saturated fat, cholesterol, refined sugar, and salt, in the context of a varied diet balanced among the four food groups with increased emphasis on whole grain cereals, legumes, fruits, and vegetables to provide more dietary fiber. These guidelines do not indicate how much less fat or how much more fiber is desirable, primarily because the committee that established these guidelines either couldn't agree on quantitative guidelines or the need for such guidelines for the general public.

In contrast to the "Dietary Guidelines for Americans," the National Cholesterol Education Program, American Heart Association, American Diabetes Association, the Surgeon General, the National Cancer Institute, and the National Academy of Sciences all have established quantitative guidelines. For the most part, these guidelines all are consistent with the "Dietary Goals for the United States" established in 1977. They recommend consuming no more than 30% of calories as total fat with equal proportions of saturated, monounsaturated, and polyunsaturated fatty acids, less than 300 mg of dietary cholesterol per day, and approximately 5 g of salt per day. This Diet Guide provides a method for planning and evaluating menus to meet these quantitative goals and remain adequate in essential nutrients.

Who Are Guidelines For?

The major causes of death in the United States today are heart disease and cancer, with obesity, diabetes, and hypertension being important contributing factors. Since 1977 when the report "Dietary Goals for the United States" was issued by the United States Senate Select Committee on Nutrition and Human Needs, there have been many government and private reports that have made dietary recommendations to promote health and prevent disease. Although they vary slightly, there is general agreement on major recommendations. In food terms, it is generally recommended that the consumption of whole-grain breads and cereals, fruits, and vegetables be increased and that lower fat selections of dairy foods, meat, poultry, and fish be served.

A diet as described above often is referred to as a "prudent" diet. There is good agreement among most nutrition experts that individuals at increased risk of heart disease for whatever reason are advised to consume a prudent diet. What is not yet agreed on is whether everyone should follow these dietary recommendations. This is because our understanding of the causes of heart disease and cancer as well as our understanding of the role of diet in the initiation and development of these diseases is incomplete.

This Diet Guide is based on the concept that the purpose of nutrition education is to provide consumers with objective information so they can make better and more informed decisions. Food choices are a matter of individual choice. Individuals need to understand what is known and not known about the role of diet and other important risk factors related to health promotion and disease prevention, assess their own situation, and then act accordingly. One individual at low known risk of heart disease may elect to consume a prudent diet to reduce known and unknown risks even further. However, this same individual may as a matter of choice engage in technical rock climbing for challenge and personal enjoyment. Another individual, also at low known risk for heart disease, may not engage in rock climbing because the risk of injury is high, but not feel the need to consume a diet reduced in fat and cholesterol and high in dietary fiber to further reduce health risks.

This Diet Guide is thus designed to help consumers make better and more informed decisions on diet and to assist those interested in moving toward a prudent diet do so effectively without sacrificing nutritional quality.

Basis of Diet Guide

We have seen that nutritional guidelines are expressed in a variety of ways. Grams, international units, milligrams, and micrograms are used to express the daily need for essential nutrients such as protein, vitamins, and minerals. In contrast, quantitative guidelines for such nutrients as carbohydrate and fat are expressed as percentages of food energy consumed. In the face of this complexity, many individuals are content to follow the dietary guidelines in food terms, that is, use the time-tested food group approach.

This Diet Guide follows a nutrient approach and is designed for individuals that have a higher degree of interest in the relationship between nutrition and health and who are interested in learning more about the nutritional value of food. The Diet Guide reduces complexity in the expression of nutritional requirements and guidelines by expressing both in terms of "nutritional shares." This concept was developed over 60 years ago by Mary Swartz Rose, a very perceptive nutritionist. Very simply, her idea was to express nutritional content not as grams or milligrams, but rather in terms of the number of shares a food supplied of the daily need for a particular nutrient. At the time, daily requirements had been established for few nutrients, and little knowledge about nutrients in food was available. Today, however, the advent of the high-speed computer combined with our knowledge of nutritional requirements and food composition makes it possible to use the nutritional share concept in evaluating diets and planning menus.

In this Diet Guide, the nutritional values of over 2000 individual foods are expressed in nutritional shares, called nutri-units (See Table 1 and the table of Nutrient Nutri-Unit values for Foods and Beverages on page 61). Twenty nutri-units of each nutrient provide a 2000-kcal diet, rich in complex carbohydrates and dietary fiber, controlled in fat, saturated fat, sugar, cholesterol and sodium, and adequate in 8 indicator vitamins and minerals.

One nutri-unit of food energy equals 100 kcal. For those nutrients expressed as percentages of food energy, nutri-units are calculated such that when they equal calorie shares, the diet is suitably controlled in restricted nutrients. Thus, a 2700-kcal diet would meet the prudent diet guidelines if it supplied 27 calorie nutri-units and no more than 27 nutri-units of fat, saturated fat, polyunsaturated fat, and sugar. Similarly, the guideline for an 1800-kcal prudent diet would be 18-calorie nutri-units and 18 nutri-units of fat, saturated fat, polyunsaturated fat, and sugar.

Dietary fiber goals also are set equal to calorie goals, such that 10 g of

Table 1
Nutrient Standards for the Diet Guide

Nutrient	1 Nutri-unit	20 Nutri-units	Basis of standard
Kilocalories	100	2000	23- to 50-year-old woman
Protein	3.25 g	65 g	13% of total calories
Carbohydrates	14.25 g	285 g	57% of total calories
Dietary fiber	1 g	20 g	10 g/1000 kcal
Sugars	5 g	100 g	20% of total calories
Fats	3.3 g	66 g	30% of total calories
Saturated fat	1.1 g	22 g	10% of total calories
Polyunsaturated fat	1.1 g	22 g	10% of total calories
Cholesterol	15 mg	300 mg	Prudent guidelines
Sodium	100 mg	2000 mg	Prudent guidelines
Vitamin A	250 IU	5000 IU	100% of U.S. RDA
Vitamin C	3 mg	60 mg	100% of U.S. RDA
Thiamin	0.075 mg	1.5 mg	100% of U.S. RDA
Riboflavin	0.085 mg	1.7 mg	100% of U.S. RDA
Vitamin B_6	0.1 mg	2.0 mg	100% of U.S. RDA
Calcium	50 mg	1000 mg	100% of U.S. RDA
Iron	0.9 mg	18 mg	100% of U.S. RDA
Zinc	0.75 mg	15 mg	100% of U.S. RDA

dietary fiber is recommended per 1000 kcal. This allows for a diet generous in dietary fiber, but not so overly high that it interferes with mineral bioavailability.

Cholesterol and sodium standards are set independent of calorie level. Twenty nutri-units of cholesterol provides 300 mg cholesterol and 20 nutri-units of sodium, 2000 mg sodium. Consuming less than 20 nutri-units of each of these will meet the prudent diet guidelines for all diets.

Dietary evaluation of eight indicator vitamins and minerals (vitamin A, vitamin C, thiamin, riboflavin, vitamin B_6, calcium, iron, and zinc) is also included. These were chosen as representative of the 40 to 50 essential nutrients and the 4 major food groups. When these eight nutrients are provided through traditional nonfortified foods, other nutrients provided by the major food groups also are likely to be present. For example, vitamins A, C, and B_6 represent nutrients provided by the Fruit and Vegetable group; thiamin, vitamin B_6, iron, and zinc, the Meat, Poultry, Fish, and Beans group and the Bread and Cereal group; and calcium and riboflavin, the Milk and Cheese group. For each, 20 nutri-units provides 100% of the U.S. RDA. The U.S. RDAs were developed for use with nutrition labeling to represent the amounts of protein and certain vitamins and minerals needed to meet the daily needs of most healthy adults and children over age four. For most nutrients, the U.S. RDA is set equal to the amount recommended for those individuals with the greatest need. Thus, the recommendations frequently are higher than the needs of many people. Table 2 is a chart for setting nutri-unit goals for these nutrients according to recommendations for age and sex.

It is not intended that this quantitative approach to menu planning and evaluation be used routinely. However, it is suggested that if used occasionally but regularly, it would offer a number of advantages.

Table 2
Daily Nutri-Unit Goals for Individuals

Persons	Age	Kilocalories[a]	Nutri-units: Kilocalories[a]	Protein[b]	Carbohydrate[b]	Fiber[b]	Sugar[b]	Fat[b]	Saturated fatty acids[b]	Polyunsaturated fatty acids[b]	Cholesterol[c]	Sodium[c]	Vitamin A[a]	Vitamin C[a]	Thiamin[a]	Riboflavin[a]	Vitamin B_6[a]	Calcium[a]	Iron[a]	Zinc[a]
Children	4–6	1800	18	18	18	18	18	18	18	18	20	20	10	15	12	13	11	16	11	13
	7–10	2000	20	20	20	20	20	20	20	20	20	20	14	15	13	14	14	16	11	13
Males	11–14	2500	25	25	25	25	25	25	25	25	20	20	20	17	17	18	17	24	13	20
	15–18	3000	30	30	30	30	30	30	30	30	20	20	20	20	20	21	20	24	13	20
	19–24	2900	29	29	29	29	29	29	29	29	20	20	20	20	20	20	20	24	11	20
	25–50	2900	29	29	29	29	29	29	29	29	20	20	20	20	20	20	20	16	11	20
	51+	2300	23	23	23	23	23	23	23	23	20	20	20	20	16	16	20	16	11	20
Females	11–14	2200	22	22	22	22	22	22	22	22	20	20	16	17	15	15	14	24	17	16
	15–18	2200	22	22	22	22	22	22	22	22	20	20	16	20	15	15	15	24	17	16
	19–24	2200	22	22	22	22	22	22	22	22	20	20	16	20	15	15	16	24	17	16
	25–50	2200	22	22	22	22	22	22	22	22	20	20	16	20	15	15	16	16	17	16
	51+	1900	19	19	19	19	19	19	19	19	20	20	16	20	13	14	16	16	11	16
Pregnant	Second and third trimester	+300	+3	+3	+3	+3	+3	+3	+3	+3	20	20	16	23	20	19	22	24	30	20
Lactating	First 6 months	+500	+5	+5	+5	+5	+5	+5	+5	+5	20	20	26	32	21	21	21	24	17	25
	Second 6 months	+500	+5	+5	+5	+5	+5	+5	+5	+5	20	20	24	30	21	20	21	24	17	21

[a]Based on *Recommended Dietary Allowances*, 10th Ed., 1989, Food and Nutrition Board, Commission on Life Sciences, National Research Council, National Academy Press, Washington, D.C.
[b]One nutri-unit equals 13 kcal of protein, 57 kcal of total carbohydrates, 1 g of dietary fiber, 20 kcal of sugar, 30 kcal of total fat, 10 kcal of saturated fatty acids, and 10 kcal of polyunsaturated fatty acids.
[c]One nutri-unit equals 15 mg of cholesterol and 100 mg of sodium (0.26 g salt).

First, following the guidelines makes sure that a diet is suitably controlled in calories, fat, and cholesterol, and at the same time contains generous quantities of required nutrients such as protein, vitamins, and minerals. This is important since concern about controlling sodium could compromise calcium intake, and concern about saturated fat consumption could result in an inadequate intake of iron.

Another advantage of this nutrient approach is that it helps the user obtain a better understanding of food composition. This makes it possible to make better food choices in the future even without extensive dietary analysis.

In understanding the nutritional value of individual foods two aspects are important. One is the amounts of nutrients supplied by a food per serving. The other is the level of nutrients supplied by the food relative to food energy, the index of nutritional quality (INQ). The food composition information in this diet guide provides direct information on the nutrient levels per serving in all foods listed. In addition, the INQ can be simply calculated for each nutrient in each food by dividing the number of nutri-units for a given nutrient by the number of calorie nutri-units in the food.

The next section of this diet guide shows how to use this nutritional shares system to evaluate your diet and plan menus, and also how to incorporate information from food labels into the menu planning process.

How to Use This Guide

Materials Needed

Diet Guide Worksheet

The Diet Guide Worksheet (shown on page 10) is a simple tool to assist you in planning and evaluating meals using this Diet Guide and nutrition information labels. The Worksheet provides space to record the nutri-units in the foods eaten during the day. At the end of the day, the columns are totaled, and the differences between the totals and goals for each nutrient are recorded.

It is important to understand that for some nutrients it is desirable to be at or above the goal, while in others it is desirable to be at or below the goal. Goals for calories, sugar, total fats, saturated fat, polyunsaturated fat, cholesterol, and sodium are considered maximum goals. Goals for protein, total carbohydrates, fiber, vitamin A, vitamin C, thiamin, riboflavin, vitamin B_6, calcium, iron, and zinc are considered minimum goals.

Diet Guide

This Guide provides information on the kilocalorie (actual and nutri-unit), protein (PRO), carbohydrate (CAR), dietary fiber (FIB), sugar (SUG), total fat (FAT), saturated fat (SFA), polyunsaturated fat (PFA), cholesterol (CHL), sodium (SOD), vitamin A (A), vitamin C (C), thiamin (THI), riboflavin (RIB), vitamin B_6 (B_6), calcium (CA), iron (IRN), and zinc (ZN) content of foods. The foods are grouped into 14 main sections.

Most main sections are further divided into subsections. For example, the section on Appetizers and Snack Foods is subdivided into Chips and Crackers, Dips, Cheese and Meats, Nuts and Seeds, Popcorn and Pretzels, and Vegetables and Fruits.

Most foods are listed in the ready-to-eat form. The section on Cooking Ingredients and Sauces lists some ingredients widely used in food preparation, such as flour and shortening. Unless specified in the name, e.g., "popcorn with salt and butter," the nutrient composition of menu items does not account for condiments, such as butter, salt, and catsup, that may be added by the cook or at the table. If these are used, be sure to add them as a separate unit. Condiments often served with foods are listed at the end of most sections. In addition, many are listed in the section on Cooking Ingredients and Sauces.

Nutrients are listed across the top of each page in abbreviated form.

Diet Guide Worksheet

INSTRUCTIONS: Record the nutri-unit value for each food item from the Diet Guide manual. Total the nutri-units for each column and figure differences between totals and goals. Goals in CAL, SUG, FAT, SFA, PFA, CHL, and SOD are considered maximum goals. Therefore, it is desirable for totals to be at or below goals for these nutrients. Goals in PRO, CAR, FIB, Vit. A, Vit. C, THI, RIB, B_6, CA, IRON and ZN are minimum goals. Thus, it is desirable for totals to be at or above goals for these nutrients.

Food item and amount Item number	CAL	PRO	CAR	FIB	SUG	FAT	SFA	PFA	CHL	SOD	A	C	THI	RIB	B_6	CA	IRN	ZN

Total:																		
Goal:																		
Differences:																		

Nutri-unit information is provided to the nearest whole nutri-unit for easy addition. The portion sizes required to provide the nutrients specified are listed directly below each food item. The portion sizes given are considered average for one portion. They are listed in common household measures, e.g., tablespoons, cups, portions of a whole, and by weight in ounces. Note that in some cases, fluid ounces listed under portion size (e.g., one 8-oz. cup lemonade) differs from weight ounces given for the same product (in this case 8.7 oz.).

The serving size measurements and nutrient values listed in this Guide are approximations. The actual nutrient composition of certain foods or dishes will vary somewhat with brand, recipe, season, area, etc. However, the method is designed to allow for these small differences so that, on a varied diet, you may generally use values given in the Diet Guide for your favorite recipe or brand without great concern for substitution differences. For a more precise evaluation, you also may use nutrition information directly from the label of specific brands or calculate the nutri-unit value of recipe combinations using nutri-unit information for individual ingredients. Specific instructions on how to do this are given in the section on Expanding the Diet Guide.

Information on Food Labels

This method of diet evaluation is designed to incorporate information from nutrition labels. Instructions on using nutrition information labels in your dietary evaluations are found in the section on Expanding the Diet Guide. Table 3 shows how to convert nutrition information labels to nutri-units.

Step-by-Step Instructions for Evaluating Food Intake

1. Set nutri-unit goals and enter on goal line of diet guide worksheet.
   A. Basic Prudent Diet Plan
      Set all goals at 20, the basic recommended level. This allows for an intake of 2000 kcal, 300 mg cholesterol, 2000 mg sodium, 20 g dietary fiber, and 100% of the U.S. RDA for eight vitamins and minerals.
   B. Individual Prudent Diet Plan
      i. **Kilocalories (CAL):** Set goal so that ideal weight is achieved and maintained. To do this, first determine an ideal weight for your height and build. Table 4 lists desirable weights for men and women ages 25 and over.
      Next, estimate the number of calories needed to maintain your weight at this level with the help of two charts: (1) Daily Nutri-Unit Goals for Individuals (Table 2) and (2) Daily Calorie Nutri-Unit Goals for Specific Age, Weight, and Activity Levels (Table 5).
      If you need to lose weight to reach your "ideal" level, set calorie nutri-unit goals 5 to 10 nutri-units below that

(Text continues on p. 16)

Table 3
Converting Information on Nutrition Labels to Nutri-Units

Kilocalories		Protein		Carbohydrate		Dietary fiber		Sugar	
kcal	Nutri-units	g Protein	Nutri-units	g Carbohydrate	Nutri-units	g Fiber	Nutri-units	g Sugar	Nutri-units
0–50	0	0–1	0	0–7	0	0 –0.5	0	0–2	0
51–150	1	2–4	1	8–21	1	0.6–1.5	1	3–7	1
151–250	2	5–8	2	22–35	2	1.6–2.5	2	8–12	2
251–350	3	9–11	3	36–49	3	2.6–3.5	3	13–17	3
351–450	4	12–14	4	50–64	4	3.6–4.5	4	18–22	4
451–550	5	15–17	5	65–78	5	4.6–5.5	5	23–27	5
551–650	6	18–21	6	79–92	6	5.6–6.5	6	28–32	6
651–750	7	22–24	7	93–106	7	6.6–7.5	7	33–37	7
		25–27	8	107–121	8	7.6–8.5	8	38–42	8
		28–30	9	122–135	9	8.6–9.5	9	43–47	9
		31–34	10	136–149	10	9.6–10.5	10	48–52	10
		35–37	11			10.6–11.5	11		
		38–40	12			11.6–12.5	12		

Fat		Saturated or polyunsaturated fat		Cholesterol		Sodium		Percentage U.S. RDA	
g Fat	Nutri-units	g Saturated or polyunsaturated fat	Nutri-units	mg Cholesterol	Nutri-units	mg Sodium	Nutri-units	Percentage U.S. RDA[a]	Nutri-units
0–1	0	0	0	0–7	0	0–50	0	0–2	0
2–5	1	1	1	8–22	1	51–150	1	3–7	1
6–8	2	2	2	23–37	2	151–250	2	8–12	2
9–11	3	3	3	38–52	3	251–350	3	15	3
12–14	4	4	4	53–67	4	351–450	4	20	4
15–18	5	5–6	5	68–82	5	451–550	5	25	5
19–21	6	7	6	83–97	6	551–650	6	30	6
22–24	7	8	7	98–112	7	651–750	7	35	7
25–28	8	9	8	113–127	8	751–850	8	40	8
29–31	9	10	9	128–142	9	851–950	9	45	9
32–34	10	11	10	143–157	10	951–1050	10	50	10
				158–172	11			60	12
				173–187	12			70	14
				188–202	13			80	16
				203–217	14			90	18
				218–232	15			100	20
				233–247	16				
				248–262	17				
				263–277	18				
				278–292	19				
				293–307	20				

[a]Vitamin A, vitamin C, thiamin, riboflavin, vitamin B_6, calcium, iron, zinc.

Table 4
Desirable Weights for Adults 25 Years and Older[a,b]

Women[c]

Height (with shoes on; 2-in. heels) Feet	Inches	Small frame	Medium frame	Large frame
4	10	92– 98	96–107	104–119
4	11	94–101	98–110	106–122
5	0	96–104	101–113	109–125
5	1	99–107	104–116	112–128
5	2	102–110	107–119	115–131
5	3	105–113	110–122	118–134
5	4	108–116	113–126	121–138
5	5	111–119	116–130	125–142
5	6	114–123	120–135	129–146
5	7	118–127	124–139	133–150
5	8	122–131	128–143	137–154
5	9	126–135	132–147	141–158
5	10	130–140	136–151	145–163
5	11	134–144	140–155	149–168
6	0	138–148	144–159	153–173

Men

Height (with shoes on; 1-in. heels) Feet	Inches	Small frame	Medium frame	Large frame
5	2	112–120	118–129	126–141
5	3	115–123	121–133	129–144
5	4	118–126	124–136	132–148
5	5	121–129	127–139	135–152
5	6	124–133	130–143	138–156
5	7	128–137	134–147	142–161
5	8	132–141	138–152	147–166
5	9	136–145	142–156	151–170
5	10	140–150	146–160	155–174
5	11	144–154	150–165	159–179
6	0	148–158	154–170	164–184
6	1	152–162	158–175	168–189
6	2	156–167	162–180	173–194
6	3	160–171	167–185	178–199
6	4	164–175	172–190	182–204

[a]Courtesy of Metropolitan Life Insurance Company, 1959.
[b]Weight in pounds according to frame (in indoor clothing).
[c]For girls between 18 and 25, subtract 1 lb for each year under 25.

Table 5
Daily Calorie Nutri-Unit Goals for Specific Age, Weight, and Activity Levels[a]

Weight (lb)	Activity level[b]	Age 19–30	31–60	>60
Males				
150	Sedentary	24	23	19
	Light	27	26	22
	Moderate	32	30	25
	Active	35	34	29
	Strenuous	39	38	32
175	Sedentary	26	25	21
	Light	30	29	25
	Moderate	34	33	28
	Active	38	37	32
	Strenuous	43	41	35
200	Sedentary	28	17	16
	Light	33	31	27
	Moderate	37	35	31
	Active	42	39	35
	Strenuous	47	43	39
Females				
115	Sedentary	17	17	16
	Light	20	20	18
	Moderate	23	23	21
	Active	26	26	23
	Strenuous	28	28	26
140	Sedentary	20	19	17
	Light	23	22	20
	Moderate	26	25	23
	Active	29	28	26
	Strenuous	32	31	28
165	Sedentary	22	20	19
	Light	25	24	22
	Moderate	29	27	25
	Active	32	30	28
	Strenuous	36	33	31

[a]Derived from tables in *Recommended Dietary Allowance*, 10th ed., 1989, Food and Nutrition Board, Commission of Life Sciences, National Research Council, National Academy Press, Washington, D.C.

[b]Sedentary activity: 8 hr sleeping, resting; 15 hr seated and standing activities; 1 hr walking lightly (2.5–3 mph).

Light Activity: 8 hr sleeping, resting; 10 hr seated and standing activities; 6 hr walking lightly (2.5–3 mph).

Moderate Activity: 8 hr sleeping, resting; 9 hr seated and standing activities; 5 hr walking lightly (2.5–3 mph); 2 hr walking rapidly (3.5–4 mph).

Active Activity: 8 hr sleeping, resting; 7 hr seated and standing activities; 5 hr walking lightly (2.5–3 mph); 2 hr walking rapidly (3.5–4 mph); 1 hr walking uphill with load.

Strenuous Activity: 8 hr sleeping, resting; 6 hr seated and standing activities; 4 hr walking lightly (2.5–3 mph); 4 hr walking rapidly (3.5–4 mph); 1 hr walking uphill with load.

Table 6
Daily Nutri-Unit Goals for Special Diet Needs

Recommended kcal	kcal Nutri-units[a]	Recommended cholesterol (mg)	Cholesterol nutri-units	Recommended sodium (mg)	Sodium nutri-units	Recommended Dietary Fiber (gm)	Fiber nutri-units
1000	10	150	10	Severe restriction	200......2	8	8
1100	11	200	13		500......5	12	12
1200	12	250	17	Moderate restriction	1000....10	16	16
1300	13	300	20		1200....12	20	20
1400	14	350	23		1500....15	24	24
1500	15	400	27	Mild restriction	2000....20	28	28
1600	16	450	30		2500....25	32	32
1700	17	500	33		3000....30	36	36
1800	18	550	37		3500....35	40	40
1900	19	600	40		4000....40		
2000	20						
2100	21						
2200	22						
2300	23						
2400	24						
2500	25						
2600	26						
2700	27						
2800	28						
2900	29						
3000	30						

[a]Set protein, carbohydrate, sugar, fat, saturated fatty acid, and polyunsaturated fatty acid goals all equal to kilocalorie nutri-unit goals.

recommended for your ideal weight, but no lower than 9 nutri-units per day. This should result in a 1- to 2-lb weight loss per week. Adding 20 min of exercise per day will help assure these results. Any faster weight loss generally is not recommended without the supervision of a physician or dietitian.

Kilocalorie goals also may be set according to recommendations from a physician or dietitian using Table 6, "Daily Nutri-Unit Goals for Special Diet Needs."

ii. **Protein (PRO); total carbohydrates (CAR); dietary fiber (FIB); sugars (SUG); total fats (FAT); saturated fat (SFA); polyunsaturated fat (PFA):** With the possible exception of protein, set nutri-unit goals for each of these equal to the kilocalorie (CAL) nutri-unit goal as shown in Table 2. Since protein needs are a function more of body weight than of calorie intake, do not set protein goals any lower than 20 nutri-units for men and 15 for women.

iii. **Cholesterol (CHL); sodium (SOD):** Set nutri-unit goals for these at 20 as recommended for all age and sex groups in Table 2. Nutri-unit goals also may be set according to levels recommended by a physician or dietitian using Table 6.

iv. **Vitamin A (A); vitamin C (C); thiamin (THI); riboflavin (RIB); vitamin B_6 (B_6); calcium (CA); iron (IRON); zinc (ZN):** Set nutri-unit goals for these at 20, the U.S. RDA, or according to recommendations for your age and sex group in Table 2.

Below is a sample set of nutri-unit goals for a normal-weight 25- to 50-year-old female set according to recommendations in Table 2.

	CAL	PRO	CAR	FIB	SUG	FAT	SFA	PFA	CHL	SOD	A	C	THI	RIB	B_6	CA	IRON	ZN
Goal	22	22	22	22	22	22	22	22	20	20	16	20	15	15	16	16	17	16

2. Record the names and portion sizes of all foods consumed or planned in the "Food Item and Amount" column.

   Be sure to include all beverages except water and any condiments such as extra butter, salt, or sauces that are added by the cook or at the table. Do not forget snacks and sneaks to the refrigerator or cupboard.
3. Look up each food item in the food sections of the diet guide and record the nutri-units for the portion size used.

   When recording nutri-units be sure to adjust for portion sizes different from those listed in the Guide. For example, if a half-portion is served, divide all nutri-units by two; if a double portion is served, multiply nutri-unit values by two. Round fractions to the nearest whole nutri-unit. Round half-nutri-units to the nearest even nutri-unit. For example, round 0.5 nutri-units to 0 and 1.5 nutri-units to 2. If more precision is desired, nutri-units also may be rounded off to the nearest half-nutri-unit. Rounding to any portion smaller than a half-nutri-unit is not recommended, as it makes calculations more tedious than necessary, especially considering the approximate nature of the original nutri-unit values.

   Use the index of foods in the back of the Guide to help locate hard-to-find items. If the exact recipe or food item consumed is not listed for the Guide, e.g., hot chicken sandwich and gravy, look for a similar item, e.g., turkey sandwich with gravy, and record the nutri-units listed for that item.

   When a recipe does not fit the description of any of those listed in the Diet Guide, you may need to figure nutri-units from individual ingredients. See the section on Expanding the Diet Guide with Recipe Evaluation and Information from Food Labels for instructions.
4. Total columns and figure differences between totals and goals.

   Once the nutri-units in each food item have been recorded, total each column and subtract the total from the goal for each nutrient. Enter the difference, noting whether it is positive or negative, in the Differences row. A sample diet illustrating steps 1 through 4 for an adult female, using the basic nutri-unit goals of 20 for each nutrient, is shown on page 19.

5. Evaluate the diet.

Kilocalories: The example diet just meets the kilocalorie nutri-unit goal. How well your individual calorie totals compare with the calorie goal you have set is best determined by the bathroom scale (when daily activity level and calorie consumption remain fairly constant).

If you are maintaining weight, your calorie intake is in balance with your needs at this time. If you are gaining or losing weight, you are consuming more or fewer calories than you are burning, respectively.

Actual kilocalorie needs can be estimated from the fact that it takes 35 calorie nutri-units (3500 kcal) above or below body needs to gain or lose a pound of body fat. For example, suppose during the last 5 weeks you gained two unwanted pounds on a daily intake of approximately 25 calorie nutri-units (2500 kcal). This means that in a period of 35 days you consumed 70 calorie nutri-units (35 for each pound gain) above your body needs, or two nutri-units above needs per day. At 100 kcal per nutri-unit, your actual calorie needs are approximately 2300 (23 nutri-units) rather than the 2500 (25 nutri-units) you were consuming per day.

Protein, carbohydrates, sugars, fats, saturated fat, polyunsaturated fat: The method evaluates energy nutri-units as a percentage of total calories. When energy nutri-units equal calorie nutri-units, kilocalories are distributed as shown below. It is recommended that total protein nutri-units equal or be above calorie nutri-units, carbohydrate nutri-units be within 10 nutri-units of calorie nutri-units and that sugar, fat, saturated fat, and polyunsaturated fat nutri-units be at or below calorie nutri-units.

Nutrient	Percentage of total calories at goal	Diet recommendation
Protein	13	At or above goals
Carbohydrates	57	Range of ± 10 nutri-units above or below goals
Sugars	20	At or below goals
Fats	30	At or below goals
Saturated fat	10	At or below goals
Polyunsaturated fat	10	At or below goals

You may find adapting your current eating patterns to meet these goals a bit difficult at first. It is important to remember that these goals are not absolute requirements that must be attained, but ideals for which to strive.

The example diet is within these recommendations, as the

Sample Diet Guide Worksheet

INSTRUCTIONS: Record the nutri-unit value for each food item from the Diet Guide manual. Total the nutri-units for each column and figure differences between totals and goals. Goals in CAL, SUG, FAT, SFA, PFA, CHL, and SOD are considered maximum goals. Therefore, it is desirable for totals to be at or below goals for these nutrients. Goals in PRO, CAR, FIB, Vit. A, Vit. C, THI, RIB, Vit. B_6, CA, IRON, and ZN are minimum goals. Thus, it is desirable for totals to be at or above goals for these nutrients.

Food item and amount	Item number	CAL	PRO	CAR	FIB	SUG	FAT	SFA	PFA	CHL	SOD	A	C	THI	RIB	B_6	CA	IRN	ZN
Orange juice, 6-oz. glass	348	1	0	1	0	4	0	0	0	0	0	1	24	2	0	1	0	0	0
40% bran flakes, 2/3 c.	394	1	1	2	5	1	0	0	0	0	2	5	0	5	5	5	0	5	5
Skim milk, 1/2 c.	340	0	1	0	0	1	0	0	0	0	1	1	0	1	2	0	3	0	1
Whole wheat toast, 2 slices	383	1	2	2	3	1	0	0	0	0	3	0	0	1	1	1	1	2	1
Margarine, soft, 2 tsp	506	1	0	0	0	0	2	1	3	0	1	1	0	0	0	0	0	0	0
Skim milk, 8-oz. glass	339	1	3	1	0	2	0	0	0	0	1	2	1	1	4	1	6	0	1
Coffee, 1 c., black	335	0	0	0	0	0	0	0	0	0	0	0	0	0	0	0	0	0	0
Quiche, cheese, 1/8 of 8-in. pie	1658	2	2	1	1	1	4	4	2	7	3	1	0	1	2	1	3	1	1
Tossed salad, vinegar/oil, 1 c.	1709	1	0	0	1	1	3	1	4	0	0	3	4	0	0	1	1	1	0
Bread sticks, 2	203	1	0	1	1	0	0	0	0	0	1	0	0	1	1	0	0	0	0
Fruit cocktail,canned,light syrup,1/2 c.	1211	1	0	1	1	4	0	0	0	0	0	1	1	0	0	1	0	0	0
Iced tea, 8-oz. glass	144	0	0	0	0	0	0	0	0	0	0	0	0	0	0	0	0	0	0
Carrot strips, 6 strips	88	0	0	0	1	0	0	0	0	0	0	32	1	0	0	0	0	0	0
Swiss cheese, 1 oz.	650	1	2	0	0	0	2	4	0	2	1	1	0	0	1	0	5	0	1
Wheat crackers, 5 pieces	17	1	1	1	2	0	1	1	0	0	1	0	0	1	1	0	0	1	0
Pork loin roast,lean,3-oz. slice	1516	2	7	0	0	0	4	4	1	5	1	0	0	9	4	4	0	1	3
Lima beans, frozen, boiled,1/2 c.	1986	1	2	1	5	0	0	0	0	0	0	1	3	2	1	2	1	2	1
Coleslaw w apples,cream dressing,1/2c.	1690	1	0	0	2	1	2	1	3	0	0	0	6	0	0	1	0	0	0
Hard roll, 1	233	2	2	2	1	1	0	0	0	0	3	0	0	3	1	0	0	2	1
Margarine, soft, 2 tsp	309	1	0	0	0	0	2	1	3	0	1	1	0	0	0	0	0	0	0
Wine, red, 4-oz. glass	136	1	0	0	0	1	0	0	0	0	0	0	0	0	0	0	0	1	0
	Total:	20	23	13	23	18	20	17	16	14	19	50	40	27	23	18	20	16	15
	Goal:	20	20	20	20	20	20	20	20	20	20	20	20	20	20	20	20	20	20
	Difference:	0	+3	−7	+3	−2	0	−3	−4	−6	−1	+30	+20	+7	+3	−2	0	−4	−5

protein total is three nutri-units higher than goal and the carbohydrate total is seven nutri-units under the goal. Also, nutri-unit totals for sugar, fat, saturated fat and polyunsaturated fat are all at or below goals.

Fiber: The fiber nutri-unit goal also is set equal to the calorie nutri-unit goal. For the 25- to 50-year-old woman with a calorie goal of 2200, 22 nutri-units of fiber provides 22 g of dietary fiber. For a 25- to 50-year-old adult male with a calorie goal of 29 (2900 kcal), the fiber goal would be 29 (29 g of dietary fiber). The American Cancer Institute recommends a daily intake of 20 to 30 g of dietary fiber with an upper limit of 35 g. The Diet Guide goals are in line with these recommendations. The sample diet is three units above the fiber nutri-unit goal. The appendix includes a table listing especially good sources of fiber.

Cholesterol: Twenty nutri-units provides 300 mg of cholesterol, the upper amount recommended by the American Heart Association for persons prone to heart disease. Therefore, 20 is considered a maximum goal, with any total less than this also considered desirable. The sample diet provides 14 nutri-units of cholesterol, well below the upper recommended goal.

Sodium: Twenty nutri-units provides 2000 mg (2 g) of sodium. This is equivalent to 5 g, or approximately 1 teaspoon (tsp), of table salt (sodium chloride). Because most Americans consume far more than this amount of sodium per day, this is considered a mild level of restriction. However, there is good evidence that an excessive intake of sodium may predispose at least 20% of the population to hypertension and subsequently to heart disease. Diabetics and others at risk of hypertension and heart disease are especially advised to lower their intake of sodium to reach the 20 nutri-unit goal as closely as possible.

The sample diet provides 19 nutri-units of sodium, just below the upper limit recommended. If you find yourself consistently having trouble staying within your sodium goal, you may need to alter some of your food preparation and selection practices. The Appendix includes a table listing menu items that are highest in sodium content. You may need to eliminate or lower your intake of some of these items or make lower sodium substitutes.

Indicator vitamins and minerals: For each of the five indicator vitamins (vitamin A, vitamin C, thiamin, riboflavin, and vitamin B_6) and three indicator minerals (calcium, iron, and zinc), 20 nutri-units provide 100% of the U.S. RDA. Since the U.S. RDA for each nutrient is designed to meet the needs of most healthy Americans over age four, 20 nutri-units may provide more than is needed by many people. For a closer approximation to your own needs, nutri-unit goals also may be set according to Table 2, Daily Nutri-Unit Goals for Individuals.

All eight indicator vitamins and minerals are considered goals to achieve, with excesses more desirable than deficiencies. The sample diet meets or exceeds the 20 nutri-unit goal for each nutrient except for vitamin B_6, iron, and zinc. It is 2 nutri-units below the goal for vitamin B_6, 4 nutri-units below the goal for iron, and 5 nutri-units below the goal for zinc.

If your evaluations consistently show deficiencies of more than 20% for any vitamin or mineral, you should consider ways to improve your intake of that nutrient. The Appendix lists good sources of each of the indicator vitamins and minerals.

Expanding the Diet Guide with Recipe Evaluation and Information from Food Labels

Occasionally you may not be able to find a listing in the Diet Guide that appears to come close to the recipe or combination of foods you served or plan to serve. If it is a commercially processed food with a nutrition information label, you may convert the information on the label to nutri-units. In other cases, you may be able to figure the nutri-unit contribution from individual ingredients.

Converting Information on Nutrition Labels to Nutri-Units

Use Table 3, Converting Information on Nutrition Labels to Nutri-Units, found on p. 13. Nutrition information labels may not list information for every nutrient in the Diet Guide. When this happens, draw a dash through the space provided for the nutrient on the Diet Guide Worksheet to indicate a lack of information rather than an absence of nutri-units. The example on page 22 illustrates how to use Table 3 to translate nutrition information labels to nutri-units.

Note that the Shredded Wheat biscuit label does not provide information on the grams of saturated fat and polyunsaturated fat or the milligrams of cholesterol per serving. These would need to be entered as dashes on the Diet Guide Worksheet to indicate a lack of information. However, since the cereal is 100% whole wheat, you can assume that it contains no cholesterol. Also, since it provides no total fat nutri-units, it is not likely to provide any saturated or polyunsaturated fat nutri-units.

Also note that protein information is taken from the top of the nutrition information label listing the grams of protein per serving rather than from the lower part of the label listing percentage of the U.S. RDA. According to Table 3, 3 g of protein translates to 1 nutri-unit of protein. If this product is commonly served, you may also want to add the nutrient information between one of the lines in the ready-to-eat cereals subsection on Breakfast, All Items.

Recipe Evaluation

Two example recipe evaluations are given on page 23. To figure the nutri-unit contribution of a special recipe or combination of foods, list

Example Conversion of Nutrition Information Labels to Nutri-Units

SHREDDED WHEAT BISCUITS
Nutrition Information
Per Serving

Serving size 2/3c. (1 oz.)

Servings per container 18

	1 oz.	with 1/2 c. whole milk
Calories	110	190
Protein	3 g	7 g
Carbohydr.	23 g	29 g
Fat	1 g	5 g
Sucrose & other sugars	0 g	6 g
Fiber	0.7 g	0.7 g
Sodium	**	60 mg

**Not more than 10 mg/100 g

Percentage of U.S. Recommended Daily Allowances (U.S. RDA)

Protein	4%	15%
Vitamin A	*	2%
Vitamin C	*	*
Thiamin	4%	8%
Riboflavin	*	10%
Niacin	8%	8%
Calcium	*	15%
Iron	6%	6%

*Contains less than 2% of the U.S. RDA of these nutrients.

Shredded Wheat Biscuits with and without Milk: Conversion to Nutri-Units

	One oz. Cereal		One oz. Cereal with 1/2 cup whole milk	
Nutrient	Label Information	Nutri-Units	Label Information	Nutri-Units
Calories	110	.1	190	.2
Protein	3 g.	.1	7 g.	.2
Carbohydrates (total)	23 g.	.2	29 g.	.2
Fiber (dietary)	0.7 g	.1	0.7 g	.1
Sugars	0 g.	.0	6 g.	.1
Fat (total)	1 g.	.0	5 g.	.1
Saturated fat		—		—
Polyunsaturated fat		—		—
Cholesterol		—		—
Sodium	<10 mg	.0	60 mg.	.1
Vitamin A	< 2%	.0	< 2%	.0
Vitamin C	< 2%	.0	< 2%	.0
Thiamin	4%	.1	8%	.2
Riboflavin	<2%	.0	10%	.2
Vitamin B_6		—		—
Calcium	<2%	.0	15%	.3
Iron	6%	.1	6%	.1
Zinc		—		—

The example above would appear as shown below on the Diet Guide Worksheet:

Food item and amount	CAL	PRO	CAR	FIB	SUG	FAT	SFA	PFA	CHL	SOD	Vit. A	Vit. C	THI	RIB	Vit. B_6	CA	IRON	ZN
2/3 c. shredded wheat biscuits	1	1	2	1	0	0	—	—	—	0	0	0	1	0	—	0	1	—
2/3 c. shredded wheat bisuits with 1/2 c. whole milk	2	2	2	1	1	1	—	—	—	1	0	0	2	2	—	3	1	—

Example 1:

Example Recipe Evaluations Low-sodium chicken sprout sandwich

Food item and amount	Item number	CAL	PRO	CAR	FIB	SUG	FAT	SFA	PFA	CHL	SOD	A	C	THI	RIB	B_6	CA	IRN	ZN
Low-sodium bread, 2 slices	1830	2	2	2	1	1	1	0	0	0	0	0	0	2	2	0	1	2	0
Mayo-type salad dressing, low calorie,low sodium,1 T	1898	0	0	0	0	0	1	0	1	0	0	0	0	0	0	0	0	0	0
Beef slice,no salt, 1-oz.piece	1841	1	3	0	0	0	1	1	0	2	0	0	0	0	1	1	0	1	2
Tomato slices, 1/4c.	1762	0	0	0	1	0	0	0	0	0	0	2	4	0	0	0	0	0	0
Alfalfa sprouts, 1 oz.	1741	0	0	0	0	0	0	0	0	0	0	1	1	0	0	0	0	0	0
	Total:	3	5	2	2	1	3	1	1	2	0	3	5	2	3	1	1	3	2

Example 2:

Raisin nut loaf

Food item and amount	Item number	CAL	PRO	CAR	FIB	SUG	FAT	SFA	PFA	CHL	SOD	A	C	THI	RIB	B_6	CA	IRN	ZN
Sugar, 3/4 c.	607	6	0	10	0	30	0	0	0	0	0	0	0	0	0	0	0	0	0
Margarine, soft, 1/4 c.	527	4	0	0	0	0	14	7	16	0	6	8	0	0	0	0	0	0	0
Egg, 1	663	1	2	0	0	0	2	2	1	14	1	1	0	0	2	1	1	1	1
Orange rind, 1 T	1244	0	0	0	0	0	0	0	0	0	0	0	3	0	0	0	0	0	N
Flour, all purpose, 2 c.	565	10	8	14	8	2	0	0	0	0	0	0	0	22	12	2	0	12	2
Baking powder, 1 tsp	609	0	0	0	0	0	0	0	0	0	3	0	0	0	0	0	1	0	0
Baking soda, 1/2 tsp	610	0	0	0	0	0	0	0	0	0	4	0	0	0	0	0	0	0	0
Salt, 1/2 tsp	612	0	0	0	0	0	0	0	0	0	12	0	0	0	0	0	0	0	0
Milk, skim, 1 c.	690	1	3	1	0	2	0	0	0	0	1	2	1	1	4	1	6	0	1
Raisins, 1/2 c.	596	2	1	4	5	10	0	0	0	0	0	0	1	1	1	2	1	2	0
Walnuts, 1/4 c., chopped	598	2	2	0	1	0	6	1	11	0	0	0	0	1	0	2	0	2	1
	Total:	26	16	29	14	44	22	10	28	14	27	11	5	25	19	8	9	17	5
18 = one 1/2-in. slice		1	1	2	1	2	1	1	2	1	2	1	0	2	1	0	0	1	0

the amount of each ingredient contained in the entire recipe or one unit of the food (e.g., one sandwich) on a separate Diet Guide Worksheet. Then, record the nutri-units for each ingredient in the recipe or food combination and total each column. The section on Cooking Ingredients and Sauces lists several common recipe ingredients, such as flour and shortening.

Next, divide your individual totals by the number of portions served, rounding off to the nearest whole nutri-unit. Round half-nutri-units to the nearest even nutri-unit. Transfer this information to the Diet Guide Worksheet you are compiling for your day's intake. If the recipe or food combination is one you often enjoy, you also may want to add it to the page listing similar items in the Diet Guide.

Summary

Steps for Evaluating Diets

1. Set Nutri-Unit goals
   - A. Basic Prudent Diet Plan
     Set all goals at 20 nutri-units
   - B. Individual Prudent Diet Plan
     - i. Calories — Set goal at level needed to reach and maintain ideal weight, but no lower than 9 nutri-units.
     - ii. Protein — Set goals at calorie goal, but no lower than 20 for men and 15 for women.
       Carbohydrates, Dietary Fiber, Fats, Saturated fat, Polyunsaturated fat — Set goals at calorie nutri-unit goal.
     - iii. Cholesterol, Sodium — Set goals at 20 or according to special diet recommendations.
     - iv. Vitamin A, Vitamin C, Thiamin, Riboflavin, Vitamin B_6, Calcium, Iron, Zinc — Set goals at age–sex recommendations.
2. Record food items and amounts consumed during day on Diet Guide Worksheet.
3. Record nutri-units on Diet Guide Worksheet to credit nutrient contributions of each food item in your day's diet.
4. Total each column on the Diet Guide Worksheet, then calculate and record the differences (+ or −) between your totals and goals for each nutrient.

5. Evaluate the diet according to the following guidelines:

Calories	Total at the goal needed to attain desired weight
Protein	Total at or above the goal
Total carbohydrate	Total within a range of ±10 nutri-units on either side of goal
Dietary fiber	Total at or above the goal (maximum 35 nutri-units)
Sugars Total fats Saturated fat Polyunsaturated fat Cholesterol Sodium	Totals at or below goals, with saturated fat supplying no more nutri-units than polyunsaturated fat
Vitamin A Vitamin C Thiamin Riboflavin Vitamin B_6 Calcium Iron Zinc	Totals at or above goals

Health Promotion and Disease Prevention

That the public has a high degree of interest in the role of nutrition in health is apparent from the many articles on the subject in national news magazines and newspapers as well as in traditionally women's magazines. In 1988–1989 alone, there were three major reports published on the subject, two by the National Academy of Sciences and one by the Surgeon General of the United States.

Maintaining good health is clearly a broader and more positive goal than preventing disease. Although many things could be discussed under this heading, the major issue centers around the role of diet in heart disease and cancer. Obesity, hypertension, and diabetes also are important, on their own and as contributors to heart disease and stroke. Because much public attention has also been directed to the role of an adequate supply of calcium in bone health and in reducing the incidence of osteoporosis, attention needs to be directed toward obtaining an adequate supply of this essential nutrient.

Although this discussion will be directed toward the role of nutrition in reducing the incidence of obesity, heart disease, diabetes, hypertension, cancer, and osteoporosis, it needs to be remembered that nutrition has a much broader role to play in health promotion. An optimal intake of protein, vitamins, and minerals is needed to provide for growth of children, successful pregnancies and breast feeding experiences, and good health and well being for all adults, including senior citizens.

Obesity

Maintaining an ideal weight throughout life has been called the single most important nutritional challenge facing many Americans today. It has been shown that maintaining a normal body weight reduces the risks of illness and death from coronary heart disease, diabetes, and other diseases. In addition, complications associated with degenerative arthritis and gout are more serious when one is overweight, and the hazards of surgery, pregnancy, and childbirth are also higher in the obese.

Various epidemiological studies have shown a higher incidence of cancer among obese persons, particularly cancer of the gall bladder and kidney. Furthermore, some studies have shown an increased incidence of breast and uterus cancer in obese than in lean women and increased incidence of prostate and colon cancer in obese than in lean men. Although most researchers do not favor severely restricting calories as a method of reducing the risk of cancer in humans, achieving and maintaining an ideal body weight is well advised.

In addition to health reasons, many formerly overweight individuals cite increased self-confidence, reduced fatigue, improved physical appearance, and greater ease of movement as sufficient reasons for taking off and keeping off extra pounds.

Prevalence

Estimates on the percentage of people who are considered to be obese or overweight vary considerably for several reasons. Different measures for measuring fatness produce variable results. Also, there is disagreement on what the appropriate weight standards should be.

Height–weight charts are the most common method of estimating desirable body weight. In some cases, height–weight charts may be misleading. Obesity means having an excess proportion of fat tissue in the body, not just being overweight for one's height and body build. For example, football linemen are always overweight but rarely overfat. On the other hand, it is quite possible for sedentary persons to be overfat but not overweight for their height. For most individuals, however, being overweight implies being overfat and hence obese.

A variety of appropriate height/weight standards are used to assess the incidence of obesity or overweight. This Diet Guide uses the widely accepted 1959 Metropolitan Life Insurance Company standard. The more recent 1983 Metropolitan Life standard established desirable weights higher than those for 1959, but these somewhat more generous standards are controversial and not generally accepted.

The most recent National Health and Nutrition Examination Study (NHANES II) reported that 26% of Americans, ages 20–74, were overweight. Overweight was defined as meeting or exceeding the eighty-fifth percentile of the body mass index (weight in kilograms divided by height in meters squared for men, or meters to the 1.5 power for women). The overweight prevalence rates for white and black males, 24% and 26%, respectively, were about the same. However, the 45% prevalence rate of overweight for black females was almost twice the 25% prevalence of overweight in white women.

Recent studies indicate that the health risk of obesity varies with the location of fat distribution. Specifically, excessive fat deposited in the abdominal region is more likely to be a risk for subsequent heart disease than is fat deposited in the upper arms or thighs. The former pattern of fat deposition is typical of middle-aged men and is commonly referred to as "executive spread" or a "beer belly." It is an important reason overweight men are at higher risk of heart disease than are women with the same level of overweight. In fact, a high waist-to-hip ratio predicts an increased risk of heart disease and diabetes in both sexes. In still another study, subscapular skinfold thickness, i.e., fat deposited over the shoulder blades, was shown to be a predictor of coronary heart disease in men, independent of body weight or body mass index.

Factors Involved in the Development of Obesity

Obesity results when the consumption of food exceeds the body's need for energy. To say that obesity is caused by overeating and inactivity, however, is an oversimplification of a much more complex problem. After years of research, scientists still do not know exactly why some people seem to have no trouble with weight control while others must continually "battle the bulge." Many complex factors are involved. These include heredity, metabolic function, efficiency of energy utilization, hormonal function, appetite regulation, eating behavior, dietary patterns, lack of exercise, life style, and possible personality and emotional problems.

Familial factors are known to be very important in relation to the occurrence of obesity. For example, children of two obese parents are three times as likely to be fat as children of two nonobese parents. This familial influence could either be environmental and related to eating habits and dietary patterns in the family, or genetic in origin.

Studies with identical twins raised apart demonstrate that fatness is highly heritable. A recent widely reported adoption study confirmed the importance of these genetic factors. Over 500 adult Danish adoptees were classified as thin, medium weight, overweight, or obese. Across the entire range of body fatness evaluated, i.e., thin to obese, a strong relationship was seen between the body mass index of biologic parents and adoptees, but not between adoptive parents and adoptees.

What causes this similarity? One cause is our inherited body type or shape. Body shape may be divided into three classifications: endomorphic (plump and round), mesomorphic (muscular), and ectomorphic (thin and bony). Most of us are a blend of all three types with a tendency toward one or two types. Because the soft tissues of endomorphs have a greater fat storage capacity, these types tend to gain weight much more easily than their ectomorphic friends, whose stringy tissues have a low fat storage capacity. The fat storage capacity of the mesomorph is greater than that of the ectomorph, but less and more evenly distributed over the body than that of the endomorph.

A factor that may have both genetic and environmental roots is our capacity for storing fat. Obesity can result either from too many fat cells or a normal number of oversized fat cells. Although recent evidence indicates that the fat cells of some people may divide and multiply at any time throughout life, the most critical periods of fat cell multiplication appear to be the third trimester of pregnancy, the first 2 to 3 years of life, and adolescence. For this reason, persons who become obese during childhood often have an overabundance of fat cells whereas those who gain most of their excess weight later in life have a normal number of extra-large fat cells. Unfortunately, one does not lose fat cells during weight loss, but merely depletes their size.

Although there is some evidence that obesity starting in childhood is more difficult to treat, this has not yet been established. It is not true that fat babies will necessarily become fat adults, nor that formula-fed infants are more likely than breast-fed infants to become obese in later life. It is important that parents do not overreact to concern about obesity in feeding their children. Growth retardation due to malnutrition has been reported to occur in the United States as a result of a self-imposed calorie restriction on young children arising out of a fear of future obesity. In addition, eating disorders such as anorexia or bulimia, especially in young women, appear in part to develop secondary to a preoccupation with thinness.

Efficiency of energy utilization is another factor which plays an important role in the development of obesity. Energy expenditure may be somewhat arbitrarily divided into three components: (1) basal metabolism, that is, calories expended at rest and in a fasted state, (2) additional calories required to metabolize food, and (3) calories burned during physical activity, ranging from sedentary activity to highly vigorous exercise.

For many of us, basal metabolism and sedentary activity account for most of our energy needs. The number of calories spent per day for these needs appears to vary widely, depending on such factors as the shape and composition of our body, our gender, and the amount of food we eat. For example, basal metabolic rate is 10% higher for men than women. It is also higher for lean people and for larger people with more surface area of either sex.

Diet also appears to cause differences in energy expenditure among people. Unfortunately, calorie restriction has been shown to produce decreases in basal metabolic rate of 15 to 30%, decreases in spontaneous activity, and decreases in the energy cost of a particular task.

This lowering of metabolic rate is generally seen as an adaptive response to food restriction, as a way to conserve energy. Its effects are compounded by the fact that recovery to the original higher metabolic rate once calorie consumption is increased is slow, thus leading to weight regain. Also, there is good evidence that with each successive diet change, metabolic rate drops more rapidly with underfeeding and returns to normal more slowly with refeeding. As a result, repeated cycles of dieting followed by regaining lost weight makes keeping unwanted pounds off more difficult.

On the other side of the coin, people vary in their response to overeating in that some "burn off" a larger percentage of the extra calories they consume than do others. This phenomenon, called "diet-induced thermogenesis," is caused by an increase in metabolic rate following food ingestion. However, the increase in conversion of dietary energy to heat accounts for only 10% of total energy expended. It has not yet been established whether or not obese individuals have defects in diet-induced thermogenesis.

Several recent studies have suggested strongly that differences in energy utilization are related to the development of obesity in families and that genetic factors are involved.

In one study, energy intake and expenditure were measured in infants born to lean and overweight mothers. Half of the infants born to overweight mothers became overweight during the course of study. In contrast, no infants born to lean mothers became overweight during this time. Most interestingly, the infants who did become overweight showed lowered rates of energy expenditure, primarily because of lowered physical activity. This study suggests a strong familial or genetic component in childhood obesity, as does the Danish adoption study already mentioned.

Another interesting study was carried out in adult southwestern American Indians known, for genetic reasons, to be predisposed to obesity. Those subjects, most overweight, also exhibited significantly lower rates of energy utilization, again confirming an important genetic component in obesity.

The weight of most people remains quite stable over time, leading to the concept of a "setpoint" at which body weight will tend to be controlled. Such setpoints have been demonstrated in animal experiments and although the concept appears to have validity for humans, controlling mechanisms have not yet been demonstrated. Control of energy utilization is likely involved, as is control of energy stores, i.e., body fat. Also of known importance is the control of appetite, the desire for food.

Controlling Appetite

In theory, tipping the energy balance so the body loses some of its fat reserves is very simple. One has only to achieve some mix of increased energy expenditure and decreased food intake. Further, the amount of increased energy expenditure over food intake need not be large, if it is continual. For example, a consistent intake of 100 cal *less* than daily expenditure will result in a 10-lb loss in 1 year.

Increasing energy output is a fairly obvious matter. Once an appropriate activity is chosen—usually one such as jogging, swimming, bicycling, or walking that can be done on a regular schedule and involves moving weight over a long distance—the problem is largely one of persistence.

But, unless food intake is also effectively controlled, the effort to spend more energy may not accomplish enough. In this respect, we must confront and somehow deal with appetite.

One encouraging fact about appetite which surprises many people is that a moderate increase in activity by an otherwise sedentary person can actually help curb appetite. This phenomenon was discovered in animal studies and has since been seen in human studies. For example, in one study using obese children, the group put on a daily 1-hr exercise program actually consumed less or at least no more than their sedentary counterparts.

Also, experimental evidence indicates that overweight people do not necessarily have an unusually active appetite, nor find taste extremely stimulating. Rather, they seem more responsive to external or environment-related food cues than their leaner friends. A variety of experimental designs have demonstrated this phenomenon, including speeding clocks, slowed clocks, and the amount of food within easy reach during meal or snack time.

Appetite appears to be controlled by a number of physical and emotional factors, many of which are not well understood. Both short-term controls sensitive to blood glucose and/or liver glycogen as well as long-term controls sensitive to the total amount of body fat seem to be involved. A variety of receptors located in the mouth, throat, and gastrointestinal tract are also involved. These send messages to the brain which are perceived as a feeling of fullness or hunger.

Because of the complex nature of internal appetite regulation, it becomes attractive for overweight individuals to blame their obesity on some malfunction within their system and to seek some sort of miracle drug or cure-all for their problem. Although billions of dollars have been spent on dietary aids designed to depress appetite, long-term successful weight control seldom occurs. Any weight reduction that does occur often is short term. Once the person eliminates the aid, he or she usually regains or exceeds his or her original weight within a short period of time. For results to be long lasting, a permanent change in eating and activity habits must occur. This is true whether or not an inherited tendency for excess weight and body fat is present, or whether the problem is primarily poor eating habits combined with physical inactivity.

"Permanent change" is probably one of the most important concepts in weight loss and control. One can lose weight on just about any diet if calories consumed are less than calories expended. Unfortunately, many diets designed to take pounds off quickly are unappetizing, monotonous, and nutritionally unbalanced. As a result, one does not, and in many cases, should not stay on such diets for long periods of time.

Once off the diet, old eating habits return and weight is regained, often more quickly and to a greater extent than was gained originally. This is because our bodies are very efficient organisms and respond to a lower calorie intake by becoming more efficient in the way they utilize food for energy and store excess calories as fat. While this was no doubt essential to the survival of our early ancestors living in a food-short environment, it does not help the chronic dieter. Not only does it eventually cause a reduction in the rate of weight loss, but the improved metabolic efficiency remains for some time *after* reverting back to a higher calorie intake. As a result, there are more calories available for conversion to fat on the same calorie intake after, than before, dieting. This leads to a tendency to quickly put on lost and perhaps even new fat while the body adapts to the new level of calorie consumption.

A more reasonable and long-term solution to the problem is to approach weight loss a little more calmly and with more patience and perseverance. The key lies in modifying behavior and adopting a new lifestyle that places less emphasis on eating as a pacifier or reward.

Achieving Long-Term Weight Control

Although prevention is, no doubt, the most promising answer to long-term control of obesity, weight reduction programs can yield long-term results when undertaken with motivation, a working knowledge of the nutrients and calories in food, self-discipline, and increased physical activity.

A good place to start is to keep a record of all foods eaten for a day or preferably a week. This can be done on the Diet Guide Worksheets included with this Guide. Note when, where, why, and with whom each food was eaten on a separate sheet or diary. Next, use the food sections of the Guide to look up and record the calories (or more precisely kilocalories) and nutrients in each of the foods consumed. Use this information to identify how many calories you are taking in and which foods are high in calories and low in nutrients.

The next step is to make plans to effectively reduce your calorie intake. Assuming your food record provides a reasonably accurate estimate of your usual calorie intake, reducing your usual intake by 500 to 1000 cal/day theoretically should result in a weight loss of 1 to 2 lb/week. (There are 3500 cal in a pound of body fat.) Adding 20 to 30 min of exercise per day will help assure these results.

Once you have decided how many calories to cut out each day, look for those foods which have a higher number of calorie nutri-units than protein, fiber, vitamin A, vitamin C, thiamine, riboflavin, vitamin B_6, calcium, iron, and zinc nutri-units as ideal candidates to cut down or eliminate first. Such foods have a low "nutrient density." The greater the number of these 10 nutrients with nutri-unit values equal to or greater than the calorie nutri-unit value for the food, the better the overall nutrient density of the food.

When cutting down or eliminating high-calorie foods, think when, where, and why these foods are eaten and plan alternate activities or a lower calorie menu to take their place. For example, if the first place you go when you get home from work is to the refrigerator for a beer or piece of cake, do not stock these items in the refrigerator. It may also help to plan another activity such as taking the dog for a walk, working in the yard, or playing tennis after work to help keep the refrigerator out of sight and mind.

Below are a few examples of behavioral changes that have been found helpful in restructuring fattening eating habits:

1. Eat more slowly. Put less food on your fork or spoon; chew it longer, and put down your eating utensil between bites.
2. Use a smaller plate to feel less deprived by "skimpy" servings.
3. Do not place serving dishes on the table. If you are still hungry after your first serving, wait at least 20 min before getting up for seconds. It takes this long for the satiety signal to register in your brain.
4. Restrict all your eating to one or two places in your home, i.e., the kitchen and dining room table. Always sit down with a plate, napkin, and utensils at one of these places to eat, regardless of whether it is a three-course dinner or a cracker with peanut butter. This helps reduce the chances of sneaking in extra calories "on the run."
5. Do not do anything else, i.e., read, watch television, etc., while you eat. This will help make you more conscious of the amount of food you are eating. If you like to nibble while watching television, take up some handy work such as knitting, rug hooking, or doodling to keep your hands busy and out of the cookie jar or bag of chips. If this does not work, you may need to avoid the television and take up an activity in another room or outdoors to break the habit.

While these changes will help restructure eating behavior, much can also be done to reduce the number of calories in the foods that are eaten. This involves modifying recipes and substituting lower calorie ingredients and menu items for higher calorie ones.

For example, many recipes call for more fat and sugar than is needed to cook the food properly, particularly at elevations above 2000 feet. Depending on the recipe, fat and sugar can often be reduced by one-quarter to one-half without adversely affecting the product. At approximately 100 cal/tablespoon (T) of fat and 40 cal/T of sugar, any reduction that can be made does add up.

Another way to help cut calories is to substitute lower calorie items for higher calorie ones on the menu. For example, yogurt provides approximately one-fourth as many calories as sour cream, yet works just as well as a base in dips and in many other recipes calling for sour cream. Banana splits and chocolate sundaes are both favorites at the ice cream store, yet a banana split provides 540 cal compared with 300 in a medium-sized chocolate sundae. A small soft-serve ice cream cone, at 110 cal, is an even better choice for the calorie counter.

These are just a few of the many different ways to lower the number of calories in your foods. By looking through the food sections of this Guide and using a little imagination, you may be amazed at how easy it is to reduce calories without reducing variety or even the bulk amount of food eaten per day.

Coronary Heart Disease

Prevalence

Both public and scientific interest in the role of nutrition in health promotion and disease prevention is highest as related to diet and coronary heart disease. This is understandable, since heart disease is still the leading cause of death in the United States, accounting for ≈ one-third of all deaths. Contrary to some perceptions, age-adjusted death rates from heart disease in the United States have been coming down for at least 25 years and probably longer. The reasons for the declining death rates from heart disease are not understood. Improved and earlier diagnosis, health care, lifestyle, and diet changes are all thought to play a role, but since the fundamental causes of heart disease are not well understood, it is not possible to determine exactly why heart disease is declining in the United States population.

It is important when comparing death rates that they be adjusted to reflect the fact the people are living longer and thus there is an increasing proportion of older persons in the general population. Nevertheless, as other causes of death have been eliminated, especially infectious diseases, it is natural that most attention is focused on the leading cause of death.

The following table from the National Center for Health Statistics provides information on the prevalence of coronary heart disease in the United States in 1985 as related to age, race, and sex.

Prevalence per 1000 Persons in 1985

Age (years)	Men	Women	White	Black
Total	32.9	24.7	31.8	11.3[a]
Under 45	0.9[a]	1.6[a]	1.3[a]	1.1[a]
45–64	80.9	44.4	65.1	46.3
65–74	175.6	107.0	143.9	62.2
75 and over	169.0	124.6	154.7	[a]

[a]Figure does not meet standards of reliability or precision.

These data illustrate what most people already know, namely heart disease rates increase with age and are higher for men than for women. The prevalence of heart disease appears to be higher for whites than blacks. As shown by the following table, also from the National Center for Health Statistics, death rates from heart disease in 1985 for men and women over 65 were higher for whites than for blacks.

Death Rates in 1985 per 100,000 Population[a]

Age (years)	White men	Black men	White women	Black women
Total	180.8	164.9	82.9	100.8
Under 45	8.2	13.2	1.7	4.3
45–64	294.5	317.8	85.1	161.1
65–74	1132.6	990.6	506.0	645.9
75 and over	3071.8	2205.0	2010.2	1717.5

[a]Age adjusted to the age structure of the United States population, 1940.

The average age at death from heart attacks in men increased from 66 years old in 1931 to 72 years old in 1980. For women during the same period, the average age at death from this cause increased from 70 to 79 years old. The general health of the United States public has never been better. This point is sometimes overlooked by those who advocate marked dietary changes for the general population.

What Is Coronary Heart Disease?

Coronary heart disease (CHD) is a condition that results from an inadequate supply of blood to the heart muscle. When this happens the heart can no longer function effectively and a heart attack results. The important underlying cause is atherosclerosis.

Atherosclerosis is a process by which lesions develop in the inner lining of the arterial wall, thus narrowing the opening through which blood flows. The lesion starts as a fatty streak, quite often in childhood. These lesions under some conditions become larger and more fibrous in nature. As the lesions progressively narrow the lumen in the artery, symptoms of angina pectoris may occur, along with shortness of breath. In other cases, the disease may progress silently for decades before symptoms occur. Often, a blood clot will form in the narrowed lumen, cutting off the oxygen supply to the affected area. When this occurs in the coronary arteries supplying the heart, a myocardial infarction (heart attack) occurs. If it occurs in the cerebral arteries supplying the brain, what results is a stroke.

What causes the development of atherosclerosis is still somewhat of a mystery. Unlike infectious diseases such as measles, it does not have a single cause, nor does it develop overnight. One theory regarding the direct cause of atherosclerosis is the "response to injury" hypothesis. According to this hypothesis, an injury occurs to the cells lining the arteries. The injury could be the result of numerous factors, including hyperlipidemia (an excessive amount of fatty substances in the blood), improper functioning of hormones, and/or increased stress from hypertension. The arterial wall quickly responds by making more smooth muscle cells and connective tissue to patch the injured wall lining. The patch, however, like that on a tire, forms an extra bump on the lining of the arterial wall. Eventually the bump regresses. But, if injury happens repeatedly or if the tissues lose their ability to respond quickly to injury, the lining of the arterial wall will eventually become heavy and irregular and display a thick deposit called plaque. Not only does this narrow the channel through which the blood must flow, but it also affects the ability of the artery to expand and contract. This may lead to a condition known as angina pectoris, in which a sudden pain occurs in the chest. Angina results when the heart cells do not get enough oxygen. Although it is not thought that angina causes permanent heart damage, it is a warning sign of a possible heart attack and should not be neglected.

Risk Factors

Extensive studies over a number of years have identified a number of factors that contribute to an increased risk of having a heart attack. It needs to be understood that risk is an expression of probability and should not be confused with cause and effect. For example, if person A has a serum cholesterol level of 200 mg/dl and person B a level of 300 mg/dl, it does not mean that person B will have a heart attack and person A will not. In fact, it is quite possible that the opposite would be true. However, if we compared 1000 individuals with cholesterol levels of 200 mg/dl with 1000 with levels of 300 mg/dl, we would expect over time to see twice as many heart attacks in the second as compared to the first group.

For convenience, we can group risk factors into two categories: Diet or nondiet related.

Non-Diet-Related Risk Factors

Some of the most important risk factors for CHD unfortunately cannot be changed. These include family history, sex, and age. There is no doubt that one's genetic heritage is an important risk factor; early heart attacks are more common in some families than others. Coronary heart disease is more common in men than in women. Although the risk of CHD increases in women after menopause, it does not appear to reach the level in men and, as discussed earlier, the average age of death for women from CHD is 8 years older than for men. Although genetic factors or one's sex cannot be changed, they both interact with diet. Individuals at increased risk of CHD for these reasons are advised to make appropriate dietary changes as discussed later in this section.

Age is an obvious risk factor for CHD, and it is one that cannot be avoided. Interestingly, the increased relative risk of CHD associated with an elevated serum cholesterol level becomes less pronounced with age and, above the age of 50, may no longer be predictive of increased risk.

Diet-Related Risk Factors

The most important diet-related risk factors are circulating levels of blood lipids, specifically serum cholesterol and serum triglycerides. In addition, certain disease states also are included in this category because they have diet components. These are obesity, diabetes, and hypertension. Obesity has already been discussed. Diabetes and hypertension will be considered later in this chapter.

Serum Cholesterol

Cholesterol, a fatty-like material, is an important body constituent found in most membranes. In the brain, it acts as an insulator. It is found in all foods of animal origin and is made in the body, with most synthesis taking place in the liver and intestines. Because cholesterol is not soluble in water, it is carried in the blood in the form of lipoproteins, which are complexes of lipids and protein. There are two major classes of lipoproteins, namely low density (LDL) and high density (HDL). Cholesterol carried in low-density lipoprotein is referred to as LDL-cholesterol. Conversely, HDL-cholesterol is cholesterol carried in high-density lipoproteins. Total *serum* cholesterol is the total amount of cholesterol circulating in the *blood*.

Many studies have demonstrated that individuals with higher levels of blood cholesterol are at higher risk of death from CHD. According to a 30-year follow-up of men in a long-term study in Framingham, Massachusetts, overall mortality increased 5% and CHD mortality 9% for every 10 mg/dl increase in serum cholesterol in men under 50 years of age at entry. Thus, CHD mortality would be roughly twice as high in individuals with serum cholesterol levels of 300 mg/dl as compared to 200 mg/dl. Other studies suggest that there is little increase in risk of death in the serum cholesterol range of 180–240 mg/dl with death rates increasing more sharply above 240 mg/dl. The 30-year follow-up data from Framingham also suggest that above the age of 50, total serum cholesterol may no longer be a risk factor for CHD. The reason is not known.

Of the two types of lipoproteins, LDL-cholesterol increases and HDL-cholesterol decreases the risk of CHD. The much-studied and validated risk of CHD associated with total serum cholesterol is believed to be attributable to a corresponding increase in LDL-cholesterol. High levels of HDL-cholesterol are believed to be protective by facilitating the removal of cholesterol from tissues, including from the arterial wall. The long-term Framingham study indicates that in individuals with total cholesterol levels above 260 mg/dl the incidence of CHD was three times higher if HDL-cholesterol levels were less than 40 mg/dl than if they were greater than 60 mg/dl. At lower serum cholesterol levels, the data suggest that the increased relative risk from low HDL-cholesterol levels may be even greater.

The National Cholesterol Education Program (NCEP) has proposed that individuals with total cholesterol levels greater than 200 mg/dl are at moderate increased risk of CHD and should make appropriate dietary changes as discussed later in this Diet Guide. This has led to a considerably increased interest in and availability of cholesterol screening sites. Although it is desirable that adults know their own risk profile for CHD, including their serum cholesterol levels, there are several cautions that need to be observed. First, there are measurement errors that are likely to be greater at a health fair or in a discount store than if the measurement were made in a reputable and accredited clinical laboratory. If a cholesterol measurement indicates moderate risk, it is desirable to confirm the measurement at a clinical laboratory. Cholesterol levels go up with age, and a serum cholesterol level of 200 mg/dl is more of a risk factor for someone in his or her 30s than in his or her 50s. Also, less information is available for women than for men as to what the risk of CHD is at any cholesterol level.

Recent information suggests that the HDL-cholesterol level can modify the CHD risk of total serum cholesterol level considerably. For example, an individual with total and HDL-cholesterol levels of 190 mg/dl and 35 mg/dl, respectively, may be at higher risk of CHD than another individual with a total cholesterol level of 260 mg/dl but HDL-cholesterol at 60 mg/dl.

Serum Triglycerides

Serum triglycerides are fatty substances transported in the blood in the form of lipoproteins since they, like cholesterol, are not soluble in water. High levels of serum triglycerides are associated with increased risk of CHD, but since serum cholesterol levels usually are increased along with triglycerides, it is not completely clear whether serum triglycerides represent an independent risk factor for heart disease. However, increased serum triglyceride levels result from increased levels of very low density lipoproteins, and these are associated with decreased levels of HDL-cholesterol. Therefore, it is prudent to monitor changes in triglyceride as well as cholesterol levels. This is the case especially for patients with diabetes, many of whom show greater elevations of triglycerides than cholesterol in their serum.

Role of Diet

What is the role of diet in heart disease? This is a question that has intrigued and baffled scientists and practioners alike for most of this century. The most recent report from the National Academy of Sciences, entitled "Diet and Health," is useful as a summary of the state of our knowledge on this important issue today. Although there is much we know, there remain many questions still to be answered.

The dietary constituents most important in regard to CHD are fat, cholesterol, and fiber. They are not themselves risk factors, but they affect the level of serum cholesterol, acknowledged to be an important CHD risk factor.

Dietary Fat

By far the most important dietary factor affecting serum cholesterol levels is dietary fat. Fats, or more accurately the fatty acids they contain, are divided into three major categories, saturated, monounsaturated and polyunsaturated. Polyunsaturated fatty acids are further divided into the omega-3 and omega-6 categories (see below).

A fatty acid is a long chain of carbon atoms ending in an acid function. When the carbon atoms are attached to as many hydrogen atoms as they will hold, the fatty acid is referred to as saturated, i.e., saturated with hydrogen. In some cases two hydrogen atoms are removed, resulting in a double bond. Such fatty acids are referred to as monounsaturated, i.e., they contain one double bond. If the fatty acid contains two or more such double bonds, it is referred to as polyunsaturated. Finally, if the double bond furthest from the acid function is three carbon atoms away from the other end of the molecule, the result is an omega-3 fatty acid. If this double bond is six carbon atoms from the end of the molecule, an omega-6 fatty acid results. Fatty acids are also distinguished by their chain length, with dietary fatty acids usually ranging from 12 to 22 carbon atoms in length.

Saturated fatty acids in food range from 12 to 18 carbon atoms in length. They generally raise serum cholesterol levels and in fact are twice as potent in raising serum cholesterol as polyunsaturated fatty acids are in lowering serum cholesterol. For unknown reasons, the saturated fatty acid with 18 carbon atoms known as stearic acid neither raises nor lowers cholesterol levels. As a practical matter, this exception to the general rule is not of great practical significance since the shorter chain saturated fatty acids which do raise serum cholesterol are present in the same foods that contain stearic acid.

The most prevalent monounsaturated fatty acids in the diet are 16–18 carbons in length. Until recently, they were believed to have no effect on serum cholesterol levels. Within the last several years, data have been published indicating that monounsaturated fatty acids such as oleic acid found in olive oil or peanuts lower serum cholesterol. This is not yet well established, however.

Polyunsaturated fatty acids generally lower serum cholesterol levels, whether they are of the omega-3 or omega-6 variety. However, they are less effective in lowering serum cholesterol than saturated fatty acids are in raising it. Also, some evidence suggests that omega-6 polyunsaturated fatty acids lower both LDL- and HDL-cholesterol. Therefore, more emphasis is placed on reducing the amount of saturated fat than in raising the amount of polyunsaturated fat in the diet.

Some generalizations can be made about the sources of fat in food. Liquid oils are typically unsaturated and solid fat saturated. Most vegetable oils, such as corn, soybean, or cottonseed oil, are highly polyunsaturated and are of the omega-6 type. Tropical oils, such as coconut, are the exception to this general rule. These oils contain significant amounts of saturated fatty acids. They are oils because they contain short-chain fatty acids, not because they are highly polyunsaturated.

Most animal fats contain high proportions of saturated fatty acids; this is why they are solid at room temperature. In contrast, fish oils are liquid at room temperature because they contain large amounts of long-chain polyunsaturated fatty acids of the omega-3 type.

It is possible to convert a highly polyunsaturated oil such as corn or soybean oil into a solid fat at refrigerator temperature by chemically adding hydrogen, i.e., by hydrogenation. This is commonly done in making margarine, and results in still another type of fatty acid referred to as a trans-fatty acid. These are not believed to either raise or lower serum cholesterol.

It is apparent that the issue of how fat affects serum cholesterol is highly technical and complex. The dietary recommendations discussed in the next section do not go beyond lowering the intake of saturated fatty acids and raising, modestly but not excessively, the level of polyunsaturated fatty acids. This Diet Guide provides extensive information on the amounts of saturated and polyunsaturated fat in food, but does not attempt to further divide polyunsaturated fatty acids into the omega-3 and omega-6 varieties, nor does it provide information on monounsaturated or trans fatty acids.

Dietary Cholesterol

One of the most commonly exploited misconceptions among consumers is that dietary and serum cholesterol are synonymous. Advertisers reinforce this misunderstanding when they claim their product "contains no cholesterol." This means no dietary cholesterol, but seems to be understood by at least some of the public as referring to serum cholesterol.

Serum cholesterol, not *dietary* cholesterol, is an acknowledged risk factor for heart disease. Cholesterol is an important body constituent that is made in the body. Generally, the less cholesterol that is consumed the more that is made. Saturated fat is a much more important dietary factor in raising serum cholesterol than is dietary cholesterol. The reason for this is that about two-thirds of us compensate very well for consuming dietary cholesterol by reducing synthesis in the body. Thus, most people can consume the equivalent of one or two eggs a day with little effect on serum cholesterol. However, about a third of the population do not compensate well in this way and are referred to as "cholesterol responders," i.e., they respond to consumption of cholesterol with increases in their serum cholesterol levels. Such individuals can best be identified by greatly restricting consumption of dietary cholesterol and measuring the change in serum cholesterol. If serum cholesterol goes down significantly, such an individual is likely to be a cholesterol responder and would benefit from a reduction in intake of dietary cholesterol.

Dietary Fiber

Dietary fiber is, for the most part, the remnants of plant cell walls found in food consisting of cellulose, hemicellulose, and lignin. It also includes such soluble polysaccharides as pectin and plant gums. From a structural standpoint fiber is very complex and not yet well characterized. Fiber is found in fruits, vegetables, whole grain cereals, and legumes. We generally divide fiber into two main types, namely soluble and insoluble fiber. It appears that soluble fiber has the greater ability to lower serum cholesterol. Insoluble fiber is effective in reducing constipation, but seems to have little effect on serum cholesterol. Such foods as oat or rice bran, which have significant amounts of soluble fiber, have been shown to be more effective in lowering serum cholesterol than wheat bran. In practice, it is desirable to consume a variety of different types of fiber. Dietary recommendations from the government or other authoritative agencies do not attempt to make distinction between types of fiber, but recommend increased consumption of fruits, vegetables, whole grain cereals, and legumes, which are good sources of all types of dietary fiber.

Diabetes Mellitus

Prevalence

Diabetes mellitus is considered to be a major health problem in the United States. It has been estimated by the Surgeon General that it currently affects 11 million Americans. Further, the number of diabetics has been increasing at a rate of around 6% per year. At this rate, the incidence of diabetes can be expected to double every 15 years. As a result, the National Commission on Diabetes estimates that the average American born today has a greater than one in five chance of developing diabetes, unless a method of prevention is found.

Major Complications

Among the complications of poorly controlled diabetes are cataracts and retina damage leading to blindness, kidney disease, coronary heart disease, hypertension, and damage to the small blood vessels and nervous system. Blindness occurs 25 times more frequently, kidney disease 17 times more often, and gangrene 5 times more often among diabetics than nondiabetics. Coronary heart disease occurs twice as frequently among diabetics as nondiabetics, accounting for an estimated 75% of all deaths among known diabetics.

What Is Diabetes?

Diabetes mellitus is the most common form of diabetes and is what is generally meant when one uses the term diabetes. The other type, diabetes insipidus, results from an inability to retain water and is unrelated to diabetes mellitus.

Diabetes mellitus, itself, is characterized by abnormal carbohydrate metabolism, with protein and fat metabolism also affected. In diabetes, glucose formed from carbohydrates or protein has difficulty entering muscle and fat cells and is not converted to glycogen in the liver in amounts needed for storage and energy. Rather, it builds up in excessive quantities in the blood and is excreted in the urine.

A key controlling factor in diabetes is the hormone insulin. It is produced by beta cells located in the pancreas within a cluster of cells known as the islets of Langerhans. After a meal, the level of glucose in the blood rises. This triggers the production of insulin to help facilitate the transport of glucose from the blood to target body cells, thus lowering the level of glucose in the blood. When insulin is not functioning properly, because of a deficiency in insulin production or a resistance to the action of insulin on muscle and fat cells, high blood sugar, or hyperglycemia, results.

Persons with the first type of defect, a deficiency of insulin production, are classified as "type 1" or "insulin dependent"; they account for approximately 10% of the total diabetic population. Of these, approximately one-half are juveniles. Persons with the other type of defect, a resistance to the action of insulin on target cells, often have normal or even elevated levels of circulating insulin. They are classified as "type 2" or "noninsulin dependent." This is by far the more common type of defect, accounting for 90% of the known cases of diabetes. In some diabetics, both defects may be present or may develop over time.

Type 2 (Non-Insulin-Dependent) Diabetes

Occurrence and Cause

Type 2 diabetes most often occurs among people over 40 who are also overweight. In fact, it has been shown that one's chances of getting this form of diabetes more than doubles for every 20% increase in excess weight and doubles for every decade of life. Thus, it is often referred to as "adult," or "maturity-onset," diabetes.

Persons with type 2 diabetes may, but do not necessarily have, a family history of diabetes. Onset is usually gradual and often mild in nature. In many cases, diagnosis of the disease is not made until years after onset first begins. In some cases, the diabetic becomes aware of the disease only as the result of a routine blood or urine test. In other cases, one or more of the classical symptoms (excessive thirst, frequent urination, extreme fatigue, unexplained weight loss and/or blurred vision from time to time) may be present.

The exact cause or causes of the problem are not well understood. One hypothesis is that genetic factors cause insulin target cells to produce defective insulin receptors or a serious deficiency of such receptors. Another hypothesis is that increased food intake associated with obesity leads to the secretion of an excessive amount of insulin in the blood. This causes a negative feedback of some kind, which results in a reduction in the number of receptors on target cells that accept insulin. Eventually the cells become less responsive to insulin and less capable of utilizing glucose.

Regardless of the mechanism involved, reducing weight to a normal level usually results in an improvement in the action of insulin and in a reduction in complications associated with diabetes. Thus, proper control of diet and body weight is considered the most important and often the only necessary treatment for noninsulin-dependent diabetics.

Dietary Management of Type 2 Diabetes

Before 1970, the diet most often prescribed for diabetics was a low-carbohydrate, high-fat diet, eliminating sugar as much as possible. If the person was overweight, the diet was also restricted in calories.

Calorie restriction has continued to be a primary goal of diet therapy for overweight diabetics. However, concepts regarding the proportion of calories from carbohydrate and fat have changed dramatically.

In recent years, it has become increasingly evident that a high-fat, especially a high-saturated fat, diet may be a contributing factor in the development of atherosclerosis. This is important because individuals with diabetes are at increased risk of atherosclerosis and resulting coronary heart disease. As a result, the Committee on Food and Nutrition of the American Diabetes Association began recommending in 1971 that diabetics not restrict carbohydrates, provided they were not prone to hypertriglyceridemia (a high level of triglycerides in the blood).

In 1979, the recommendations of the Committee were expanded to suggest that carbohydrates account for 50 to 60% of total calories, protein for 12 to 20%, saturated fats for less than 10%, polyunsaturated fats for up to 10% and monounsaturated fats for the rest of 30% of total energy intake that was suggested to come from fat. Advantages reported for using a high-carbohydrate, low-fat, especially low-saturated fat, diet include decreased blood glucose levels, presumably because of enhanced insulin sensitivity, reduced blood cholesterol levels, even in the absence of weight loss, and reduced risk of cardiovascular disease. Although questions still remain, these 1979 recommendations remain as the current guidelines from the American Diabetes Association.

In recent years, the concept of "glycemic index" has been introduced as a way of expressing the rapidity with which a carbohydrate source is digested, absorbed, and gets into the bloodstream. Foods with high glycemic indexes generally are absorbed faster and raise blood sugar to a greater extent than foods with a low glycemic index. Thus, it has been found that some starchy foods, such as rice, are digested faster and have a higher glycemic index than other sugar-containing foods that also contain fat which slow stomach emptying.

It is too early to assess the value of the glycemic index as an educational tool for patients with diabetes. It does seem to blur the distinction between complex and simple carbohydrates. A recent conference on diabetes at the National Institutes of Health concluded that much more work is needed before the glycemic index becomes practical. We need to know more about how combinations of foods affect the glycemic index, and also how an individual's race, sex, age, body weight, and other factors affect the blood sugar response.

Other current dietary recommendations of the Committee on Food and Nutrition of the American Diabetes Association include a modest restriction of salt for well-controlled diabetics, especially those with, or prone to, high blood pressure (hypertension), and the substitution of foods containing unrefined carbohydrates with fiber for highly refined carbohydrates low in fiber. However, those diabetic patients identified by their physicians as prone to an increase in triglycerides in the blood should not be advised to increase consumption of carbohydrates.

In addition, persons using oral hypoglycemic agents must space their meals properly to avoid hypoglycemic reaction. It is usually recommended either that calories be evenly divided among the morning, noon, and evening meals or that two-sevenths of the calories be consumed each at the morning and noon meals and three-sevenths at the evening meal.

It has been found repeatedly that diabetics who follow the diet recommendations given above are able to reduce or eliminate their need for insulin or oral glucose-lowering agents to control blood glucose levels. This is considered desirable, since in treating long-term health problems, it is generally considered good medical practice to reduce dependence on medication to the greatest extent consistent with a desirable outcome.

Type 1 (Insulin-Dependent) Diabetes

Occurrence and Cause

Persons who do not produce insulin are classified as insulin-dependent diabetics. Since this type of diabetes is often first seen in children during the growing years, it has also been called "growth onset" or "juvenile" diabetes. However, it may also develop in adults.

In contrast to type 2 diabetes, onset is usually sudden and acute in nature. The patient is often in a state of ketoacidosis at the time of diagnosis. This is an acute condition resulting from a chain of events in which a deficiency of insulin accelerates breakdown of the body's reserve of fat, eventually leading to the accumulation of ketone bodies and organic acids in the blood plasma, increasing the acidity of the blood. If the person is not treated immediately with insulin, water, and electrolytes, coma and death can result.

The majority of patients are average to below average in weight at the time of diagnosis. Otherwise, symptoms at onset are similar to those seen in type 2 diabetics. Many have recently lost weight because of an inability to use glucose (the primary body fuel) and a subsequent loss of it in the urine (glucosuria).

As with type 2 diabetes, the cause or causes of type 1 diabetes are not well understood. In other cases they may involve a genetic vulnerability of the insulin-producing cells of the pancreas to destruction or impairment by certain viruses or drugs. In other cases, an autoimmune response, in which the body attacks its own tissues, may be involved. In any case, the person can no longer produce insulin and becomes dependent on daily injections of the hormone to keep his or her blood sugar in the proper range.

Dietary Management of Type 1 Diabetes

In addition to daily injections of insulin, adherence to a regular eating and exercise pattern are key components in the treatment of type 1 diabetes. Meals should be eaten at about the same time each day. Also, the amounts and types of food eaten at each meal and snacks should be about the same from day to day. Regularity is important, as a change in either eating or exercise habits will cause a change in the amount of insulin needed. If insulin dosage is not changed, the level of sugar in the blood may rise too high (hyperglycemia) or dip too low (hypoglycemia).

At the core of the diabetic's diet is a "diet prescription" outlining the types of food to be eaten. The dietitian works with the patient to convert this prescription into a diet plan that works for their own lifestyle. In planning the diet, it is best if calories are distributed evenly over the day. It is also recommended that carbohydrates, protein, and fat also be distributed so that some of each are included at each meal or snack. For example, a bedtime snack might consist of an apple and milk or cheese, not just an apple or other food that is primarily carbohydrate.

The recommended proportion of calories from protein, carbohydrates, and fats is the same for type 1 as it is for type 2 diabetics. Approximately 50–60% of total calories should come from carbohydrates, 12 to 20% from protein, less than 10% from saturated fats, and up to 10% from polyunsaturated fats. In addition, it is recommended that salt intake be modestly restricted and that the majority of carbohydrates come from unrefined sources high in fiber.

Since the majority of insulin-dependent diabetics are thin when first diagnosed, calories usually are not restricted. Rather it is recommended that the energy level of the diet be adequate for normal growth and development in children and the maintenance of a desirable to slightly below normal-weight in adults.

Hypertension

What Is Hypertension?

Hypertension, or high blood pressure, is not a disease per se but an indication of an underlying condition that is generally considered unhealthy.

Blood pressure (the pressure in the arteries as blood passes through them) is expressed numerically as two numbers that refer to two types of pressure. The first, systolic pressure, is the maximum amount of pressure generated by the systole (contraction) of the heart as it pumps blood through the vessels. The second, diastolic pressure, is the lowest pressure in the arteries at diastole, the resting period between beats, when the heart is refilling with blood. Both are measured in units of millimeters of mercury (mmHg). For example, a reading of 120/80 means a systolic pressure of 120 mmHg and a diastolic pressure of 80 mmHg.

It is entirely normal for blood pressure to vary, going down during rest and sleep and up during physical exertion or excitement. In some individuals, the procedure of measuring blood pressure in a doctor's office can cause blood pressure to temporarily rise above normal. Also, the normal range is wide, from 90/60 to 140/90.

But, when blood pressure goes up and stays above 160/90, the person is considered hypertensive. Persons with blood pressures between 140/90 and 160/90 are borderline hypertensive. Moderate hypertension is also present if diastolic pressure is greater than 105 mmHg.

Prevalence

Hypertension is one of the most common chronic disorders in the United States. Approximately 58 million Americans have high blood pressure (140/90 or higher), with 39 million of these under the age of 65. The prevalence of hypertension increases with age and is higher for black than for white Americans.

Reasons for Concern

For most people, consistently high blood pressure is cause for concern for a number of reasons. Hypertension speeds up the development of atherosclerosis (hardening of the arteries). In atherosclerosis, fatty plaques (deposits) harden in the walls of the arteries and the walls thicken, even in mild hypertension. As a result, blood flow to important organs such as the heart, brain, eye, and kidney is decreased, and functioning becomes impaired.

It has been shown that heart attacks and strokes are more common among hypertensive patients. Hypertension also is associated with an increased risk of kidney failure and blindness. The higher the pressure, the greater the risk. But even mild hypertension, left untreated, may shorten life by several years.

Development and Treatment of Hypertension

High blood pressure may result from a heart that pumps too much blood and/or a heart with normal output but with narrowed blood vessels, causing an increased resistance to the forward flow of blood. One theory is that elevated blood pressure may initially be caused by an increase in cardiac output. As time passes, the body attempts to slow down this increased output by narrowing the passageway through the blood vessels. This, however, also affects blood pressure and eventually may be what is responsible for maintaining blood pressure at the high level.

The development of hypertension can be attributed to a specific disease or condition in only about 10% of the cases. Disorders associated with increased blood pressure include blood vessel abnormalities, certain tumors, and the abnormal release of hormones from the kidneys, adrenals, thyroid, or pituitary glands. Since many of these disorders can be improved or cured with surgery, such persons are said to have secondary, or nonessential, hypertension. Treatment is generally directed toward the underlying condition.

Approximately 90% of the cases of hypertension, however, cannot be attributed to a specific treatable disorder and thus are classified as primary, or essential, hypertension. While the specific cause or causes of essential hypertension are not known and thus not curable, several factors are thought to contribute to the development of the disorder. These include heredity, increasing age, male sex, black race, tense or stressed emotional status, weight, smoking, and eating habits.

Role of Diet

Little can be done about risk factors related to one's heredity, gender, or increasing age. Risk factor related to lifestyle, including diet, smoking, and emotional status, however, can be affected.

Risk factors related to nutrition, specifically overweight or obesity and dietary intake of sodium, potassium, and calcium, will be discussed here.

Obesity

Obesity is often a contributing factor in the development of high blood pressure. Every pound of extra weight represents body tissues (usually fat tissue), and that tissue requires extra blood vessels for nourishment. This means that the heart of an overweight person must work harder to pump blood through the extra miles of blood vessels. The extra burden does not appear to be a problem for all overweight individuals, as not all overweight persons become hypertensive. However, it is for many. And for those individuals who do become hypertensive, weight reduction to an ideal level usually is effective in bringing down blood pressure, often to the point that the level of drug therapy can be reduced. In some cases, effective weight loss can even eliminate the need for drug therapy. In addition, maintaining weight at an ideal level can help persons with a family history of high blood pressure reduce their risk of developing hypertension.

Sodium Intake

In terms of specific nutrients, more attention has been focused on dietary sodium in the development and control of hypertension than on any other nutrient. Sodium works with potassium to regulate body fluids. Every cell in the body is surrounded by water containing nutrients and other substances essential for proper functioning. For water to move in and out of the cells as it should, the number of sodium and chloride ions outside the cells needs to be in proper balance with the number of potassium ions inside the cells. Normally, the kidney adjusts for any imbalances. For example, if excess sodium is present, the kidneys will retain water and excrete the excess sodium in the urine.

Sodium and potassium also play an important role in the buffering systems of the body which help regulate the acidity of body fluids. In addition, they work together with calcium in transmitting nerve impulses across cell membranes for proper muscle function.

Although sodium is an essential nutrient, most Americans consume much more than their minimum needs, except under heavy sweating conditions in individuals not acclimated to the heat. For some this does not appear to present a problem, but for around 20% of the population, excessive sodium consumption causes an increase in blood pressure. Such persons are considered genetically sensitive to salt. The condition appears to affect the kidney, altering its ability to effectively excrete excess sodium. When a person has this condition or has heart or kidney disease and cannot get rid of extra sodium, sodium stays in the body's tissues and holds water. As a result, blood volume increases, causing the heart to work harder and blood pressure to rise.

Persons who are sensitive to salt or who have heart disease, kidney disease, or high blood pressure are generally advised to reduce their sodium intake. In so doing they are usually able to lower their blood pressure and thus the amount of diuretic agents (agents that reduce water retention) needed to help control blood pressure.

Potassium Intake

In contrast to excessive dietary sodium, recent evidence indicates that a low potassium intake, particularly when sodium consumption is high, may contribute to high blood pressure. The mechanism of potassium's antihypertensive effect is undefined, although potassium has a diuretic effect on the kidneys, resulting in an increase in sodium excretion.

The Food and Nutrition Board recently concluded that the current average intake of potassium be consumed in a 1:1 ratio with sodium (on an equivalent basis). This recommendation was made for all age groups except young infants. In early infancy, a higher intake ratio of potassium to sodium, such as that in human milk, was suggested.

For most people, this puts greater emphasis on decreasing sodium intake than on increasing intake of potassium. Excessively high intake of potassium, especially in a person with chronic kidney failure, can be potentially toxic. On the other hand, for those on medications such as certain diuretics, which are "potassium losing," potassium depletion may occur if efforts are not made to replace potassium in the diet. For these people, increasing intake of potassium and decreasing intake of sodium provide the best means of maintaining potassium balance.

Foods high in potassium and low in sodium include fruits, fruit juices, and vegetables, especially when served raw rather than canned, and unsalted meats, poultry, and fish. Milk products are generally good sources of potassium and contain low to moderate levels of sodium. On the other hand, many highly processed foods are high in sodium and relatively low in potassium.

Calcium Intake

Another nutrient that has recently received considerable attention in relation to the development and control of essential hypertension is calcium.

Several lines of investigation suggest that insufficient dietary calcium, either alone or in combination with other factors such as excessive sodium intake, may promote the development of high blood pressure. While such an association is still suggestive, persons prone to hypertension would probably be wise not to neglect calcium in their diets. Milk and dairy products are considered the best sources of calcium, but dark green leafy vegetables such as kale, collards, and mustard greens also provide some calcium, as do salmon and sardines (when the tiny bones are eaten). As is the case for sodium, not all individuals with hypertension will respond to increased calcium intake with a reduction in blood pressure.

Cancer

Cancer is an umbrella term that refers to a group of diseases in which uncontrolled growth of cells occurs. Cells in most tissues in the body are constantly dividing. During growth, this process results in both more cells (hyperplasia) as well as larger cells (hypertrophy). In cancer, normal controlled growth becomes uncontrolled growth, also referred to as malignant growth. The cells of origin can be from any tissue in the body. Often as the malignant tumor grows, some cells break off and are carried to other sites in the body where new growths or tumors result. This process is referred to as metastasis.

Prevalence

The Surgeon General estimates that about a fifth of all deaths in the United States are caused by cancer and that an individual born today has about a 30% chance of dying of cancer. Although the number of cancer deaths in the United States keeps increasing, the population is also getting older and other than for lung cancer, which is strongly related to smoking, most age-adjusted cancer rates have been relatively stable for the last 40 years. Rates are higher for blacks than for whites, however. Cancers at 10 sites—lung, colon–rectum, breast, prostate, pancreas, leukemia, stomach, ovary, bladder, and liver—account for three-quarters of all cancer deaths in the United States.

Causes of Cancer

Since the factors controlling normal growth are not well understood, it is not surprising that we do not understand why in cancer the growth of certain cells becomes uncontrolled. This process is called carcinogenesis and is generally divided into three phases; initiation, promotion, and progression. In the initiation phase, an event occurs that results in an alteration of the genetic information (i.e., DNA) of the cell. This could be from ionizing radiation, a chemical carcinogen, or a still unknown cause. In the promotion and progression phases, the altered cells divide in an uncontrolled manner, become dedifferentiated, i.e., unlike their tissue of origin, and ultimately become malignant.

What Is the Role of Diet?

The role of diet in cancer prevention is much less well established than is the case for diet related to heart disease. A widely quoted estimate by two epidemiologists is that 35% of all cancer is diet related. What is often ignored is that these workers estimated the range as from 10 to 70%. This gives a better understanding of the uncertainties surrounding this question.

There are basically two times that diet can affect the development of cancer. One is during the initiation phase and the other during promotion and/or progression phases.

Cancer Initiation

The food we eat may contain carcinogenic, i.e., cancer-causing chemical compounds. These compounds may occur naturally in food, may be added inadvertently through contamination, may be added deliberately as food additives, or may be formed in cooking or food processing. The artificial sweeteners, cyclamate and saccharin, in years past received considerable attention in this regard with cyclamate banned and saccharin restricted in uses. More recent studies have shown these compounds at most to be weak carcinogens, and epidemiologic studies have been unable to confirm a link between increased evidence of cancer and the heavy use of either compounds.

The carcinogenic effects of nitrates and nitrites also have been highly debated. Nitrates and nitrites have been used to cure foods, particularly meat, for thousands of years. Under certain conditions, nitrites can combine with naturally occurring substances known as amines to form nitrosamines. These have been identified as potent carcinogens in laboratory animals. In 1973, it was shown that some bacon products developed small quantities of nitrosamines after severe frying. As a result, the level of nitrite allowed in the curing of bacon has since been reduced to the point that most nitrite-cured products do not form nitrosamines at confirmable levels. However, the United States Department of Agriculture continues to monitor nitrite-cured bacon and other meats to be sure no unexpected problems develop.

More recently, public concern about the safety of the use of the growth regulator Alar on apples prompted manufacturers to voluntarily withdraw the chemical from the market. Alar provides a good illustration of a chemical with known benefits and exceedingly small, but known, risks. Scientists, policy makers, industry spokespersons, and consumer advocates differ on how to best regulate such food components.

Adding to the confusion is the fact that chemicals produced naturally by plants to help them fight off invaders and many other natural toxicants that may occur as a result of microbial contamination, for example patulin in apples, are not regulated in the United States.

Cancer Promotion and/or Progression

The other mechanism by which diet may affect cancer incidence may occur during the promotion and/or progression phases. Several dietary patterns and factors have been associated with an increased incidence of cancer either through epidemiological and/or laboratory studies. These have been summarized in a report by the Committee on Diet, Nutrition, and Cancer of the National Research Council. Nutritional factors that have been linked from time to time with certain types of cancers include excessive calorie intake with resultant obesity, high-fat diets, low-fiber diets, diets high in animal protein, deficiencies of vitamins A and C, or excesses of certain heavy metals such as lead and cadmium.

High-Fat Diet

Statistical studies comparing different groups of people often, but not always, link high-fat diets with increased incidence of colon and breast cancer. Prostate cancer in men also may be related to high-fat diets. Several possible explanations have been proposed for the relationship between high-fat diets and cancer, but none has been clearly established. In the case of colon cancer, one theory is that digestion of a high-fat diet causes an increase in the formation of bile salts in the colon, which may be carcinogenic themselves or may encourage the growth of intestinal bacteria which produce cancer-causing substances.

As for breast cancer, a current theory is that high-fat diets increase the secretion of the hormone prolactin and the ratio of prolactin to estrogen in the blood. This, in turn, is thought to alter the body's biochemical balance so that the breasts and other female organs are less immune to disease and more prone to the development of cancerous tumors.

Still another theory on the role of high-fat diets in the development of various cancers is simply that the high fat is the major component of a cancer-causing, high-calorie diet. The relative importance of excessive consumption of fat compared to excess calorie consumption has not yet been determined.

The role of saturated and polyunsaturated fats in the etiology of various types of cancer is even less clear than that of total fat. Current evidence suggests that both types of fat may promote the development of cancer. Therefore, a diet in which total fat is reduced to 30% of calories seems prudent for persons interested in reducing their risk of cancer. This is particularly the case for persons with a family history of breast, prostate, or colon cancer.

Dietary Fiber

Fiber has received wide publicity in recent years in the claimed prevention of a number of disease conditions, including cancer of the colon.

These claims are based on comparative studies that show very low rates of colon cancer and certain other conditions among people, particularly Africans, who eat high-fiber foods. Most claims have not been substantiated.

In the case of colon cancer, several theories have been proposed to explain how dietary fiber may reduce the incidence of colon cancer. First, fiber increases fecal bulk, thereby reducing the concentration of possible carcinogens in the intestinal tract. Second, fiber increases the speed at which wastes move through the intestinal tract, reducing the length of time during which potentially harmful substances can be absorbed. Third, certain fibers, such as lignin and pectin, may bind potentially carcinogenic substances, thereby preventing or impairing their absorption. Fourth, fiber may change the type of bacteria in the intestine, resulting in an increased concentration of potentially carcinogenic substances.

These are just a few of the dietary factors which have been implicated from time to time in the development of various types of cancer. While each study has provided some clue to the mystery of cancer causation and prevention, they have not collectively nor singly proved any one dietary element to be the answer. On the other hand, persons with a family history of breast or colon cancer would be wise to reevaluate their eating habits in light of what is currently proposed about the effects of diet on cancer.

Osteoporosis

Osteoporosis is a condition characterized by loss of bone mass, resulting ultimately in bone deformities and fractures. One type of osteoporosis is age related and occurs both in men and women. Another type occurs in postmenopausal women secondary to a reduction in circulating estrogen. Because of this and the fact that women live longer than men, the prevalence of hip fractures is more than twice as high in women as in men. The Surgeon General states that osteoporosis has become the most important bone disease in the United States.

Many nutrients are needed to ensure adequate bone mass during the growing years, including calcium, phosphorus, magnesium, fluoride, and protein. Since all individuals lose calcium from their skeleton to a greater or lesser extent in their later years, it is believed important to build up a peak bone mass during the growing years. This means that the diet should be adequate in all known nutrients including but not limited to those listed above.

It is not clear whether or not dietary calcium, whether in food or in supplements, can in later years reduce the occurrence or severity of osteoporosis. Estrogen is more important than calcium in this regard. Nevertheless, the best advice that can be given at the present time is to consume a diet that over time meets the recommended levels of all essential nutrients, including calcium. This Diet Guide helps make it possible to do this.

Dietary Recommendations

The overall food supply of the United States is of high quality and Americans are living longer than ever. Nevertheless, there is still room for improvement, especially in the quality of health. The Dietary Guidelines for Americans" jointly issued by the United States Departments of Health and Human Services and of Agriculture (1980, rev. 1985) are designed to help individuals make food choices that promote rather than adversely affect good health and well being. Some of the guidelines are of obvious importance to all; others are of greater importance to high-risk individuals.

Foods cannot be classed into categories of "good foods" and "bad foods." Rather it is the nutritional quality of the overall diet that is important. Foods also are important in providing pleasure to people as well in providing nutrients. Below is a general discussion of the seven dietary guidelines for Americans.

Guideline 1: Eat a Variety of Food

This is an important general guideline and is applicable to all people. There are over 40 essential nutrients, and these are found in greater or lesser amounts in a whole variety of foods. These essential nutrients are all needed for growth, good health, and well being. The best way to make sure that a nutritionally superior diet is consumed is to eat a variety of foods within a variety of different food groups; and to eat all foods in moderation.

Guideline 2: Maintain Desirable Weight

This guideline also is applicable to all people. Exactly what constitutes desirable weight is still a matter of some debate. We recommend the 1959 Metropolitan Desirable Weight Table as described in this Diet Guide as a point of reference. This guideline is of increased relevance for those individuals who are moderately to severely overweight according to these standards.

Guideline 3: Avoid Too Much Fat, Saturated Fat, and Cholesterol

This guideline is probably the most controversial of the seven dietary guidelines. Some feel it should be more specific in stating numerical goals for fat and cholesterol consumption. Others feel that the data are not compelling enough to make this recommendation to the general public. Individuals who are moderately or severely obese, are diagnosed with diabetes or hypertension, or are at increased risk of CHD or cancer should follow a prudent diet reduced in fat and cholesterol. This Diet Guide recommends that not more than 10 and 30% of calories be supplied by saturated and total fat, and that cholesterol intake be kept below 300 mg/day. As 70% of all deaths in the United States population are due to cardiovascular diseases and cancer, the Surgeon General of the United States and the Diet and Health Committee of the National Academy of Sciences recommend that the general public alter their eating habits in this direction.

Guidelines 4 and 5: Eat Foods with Adequate Starch and Fiber, and Avoid Too Much Sugar

These two guidelines go together and represent sound nutritional advice. Adequate intakes of complex carbohydrates such as starch and fiber are desirable to reduce symptoms of chronic constipation and diverticular disease. Diets high in carbohydrates and fiber are likely to be useful in weight reduction diets because of their lower caloric density. Maintaining adequate starch and fiber intake can best be accomplished by reducing consumption of sugar and fat. Excessive sugar consumption is a potential problem because it often is associated with reducing the nutrient density of the diet and also promoting tooth decay, especially when consumed in sticky foods between meals. It is important to note that consumption of sugar is not known to be a dietary risk for heart disease, diabetes, or cancer for most individuals, although serum triglycerides are elevated by high sugar intake in susceptible individuals. In this Diet Guide, it is recommended that carbohydrate supply 55–60% of dietary energy, that simple carbohydrates supply no more than 20% of dietary energy, and that 10 g of dietary fiber be consumed per 1000 kcal of dietary energy.

Guideline 6: Avoid Too Much Sodium

Most sodium is consumed in the form of salt present in food with smaller amounts added at the table. Since most Americans typically consume far more sodium than is needed to meet physiological needs, moderating salt consumption is generally sound advice. However, only about 20% of the population respond to salt consumption with increased blood pressure. Individuals even mildly hypertensive should reduce salt consumption and monitor the blood pressure response. Normotensive individuals with no history of CHD or stroke in the family have no strong reason to be particularly concerned about salt intake. All individuals need to be sure to maintain adequate calcium intake. This is particularly the case when sodium is being restricted, since many dairy foods are high in both sodium and calcium.

Guideline 7: If You Drink Alcoholic Beverages, Do So in Moderation

This guideline is not an admonition to drink alcoholic beverages. Heavy drinking clearly leads to health problems, including nutritional deficiencies. Moderate drinking can add significantly to calorie intake, thus promoting obesity, and can raise blood pressure. However, consuming one or two drinks daily does not appear to pose a health risk for most nonpregnant adults. Alcohol does adversely affect fetal development and growth. Pregnant women are therefore advised to abstain from alcohol consumption for the duration of their pregnancy.

Summary of Diet Recommendations

Individuals who are obese, have been diagnosed with CHD, breast or colon cancer, diabetes, hypertension, or are at increased risk of these conditions are best advised to follow a prudent diet reduced in fat and cholesterol and increased in complex carbohydrates and fiber. Specifically in food terms, a prudent diet means consuming lean cuts of meat and low-fat dairy products, and increasing consumption of fruits, vegetables, and whole-grain cereals and legumes. In nutrient terms, it means reducing saturated and total fat consumption to 10 and 30% of calories, respectively, reducing consumption of cholesterol to 300 mg/day, sodium to 2000 mg/day (5 g salt), and increasing consumption of dietary fiber to 10 g/1000 kcal/day.

It is increasingly important that educational programs and diagnostic technologies be developed and implemented that assist interested individuals in assessing their own health risk profile and to make appropriate changes in their diet and life style. This Diet Guide has been developed to assist in this process.

Diet Guide Nutrient Nutri-Unit Tables

Nutrient Nutri-Unit Values for Foods and Beverages

Appetizers and Snack Foods

Chips and Crackers

No.	Name/Portion Size		KCAL	CAL	PRO	CAR	FIB	SUG	FAT	SFA	PFA	CHL	SOD	A	C	THI	RIB	B6	CA	IRN	ZN
									NUTRI–UNITS												
1	Animal crackers 10 crackers	.9 oz	110	1	1	1	0	1	1	1	0	0	1	0	0	1	1	0	0	1	0
2	Butter crackers 6 (1 7/8 in dia × 3/16)	.6 oz	80	1	0	1	0	0	1	1	0	0	2	0	0	1	1	0	1	1	0
3	Cheese crackers 6 (1 7/8 in dia × 3/16)	.6 oz	90	1	1	1	0	0	1	1	0	0	2	0	0	1	1	0	1	1	0
4	Cheese straws made w butter 5 (5 × 3/8 in dia)	1.1 oz	140	1	1	1	1	0	3	4	1	1	2	0	0	1	1	0	2	1	0
5	Cheese straws made w veg fat 5 (5 × 3/8 in dia)	1.1 oz	140	1	1	1	1	0	3	3	1	1	2	0	0	1	1	0	2	1	0
6	Cheese puffs 1 oz	1.0 oz	160	2	1	1	1	0	3	N*	N	0	4	0	0	1	1	0	0	1	0
7	Corn chips 3/4 cup	1.0 oz	160	2	1	1	3	0	3	2	2	0	2	0	0	0	0	1	1	0	1
8	Lo sodium crackers (saltine type 2 cx (2 × 3 × 3/16 in)	.5 oz	60	1	0	1	1	0	1	0	0	0	0	0	0	1	1	0	0	1	0
9	Melba toast 5 small pieces	.5 oz	50	0	1	1	0	0	0	0	0	0	1	0	0	1	0	0	0	0	0
10	Peanut-butr cheese sandw ckrs 3 (1 5/8 in sq × 3/8)	.7 oz	100	1	1	1	1	0	2	1	1	0	2	0	0	3	1	0	0	1	0
11	Potato chips 10 chips (2 1/2 × 1 3/4)	.7 oz	110	1	0	1	2	0	2	2	4	0	1	0	1	1	0	0	0	0	0
12	Potato sticks 1/2 cup	.6 oz	100	1	0	1	2	0	2	1	3	0	1	0	2	1	0	0	0	0	0
13	Rice cakes 2 cakes (2 1/2 in diam)	.6 oz	70	1	0	1	1	0	0	0	0	0	1	0	0	2	0	0	0	1	0

continued

*N, no value.

Appetizers and Snack Foods

No.	Name/Portion Size		KCAL	CAL	PRO	CAR	FIB	SUG	FAT	SFA	PFA	CHL	SOD	A	C	THI	RIB	B6	CA	IRN	ZN
			NUTRI–UNITS																		
14	Rye wafers 3 wafers (3½ × 2 in)	.6 oz	60	1	1	1	2	N	0	0	0	0	2	0	0	1	1	0	0	1	1
15	Snack crackers (ritz type) 5 crackers	.6 oz	90	1	0	1	1	N	1	1	1	0	2	0	0	1	1	0	1	1	0
16	Soda crackers or saltines 6 pc (1⅞ in sq)	.6 oz	80	1	1	1	1	0	1	1	1	0	2	0	0	1	1	0	0	1	0
17	Stoned wheat crackers 5 (1½ in sq × ⅛ in)	.7 oz	80	1	1	1	2	0	1	1	0	0	1	0	0	1	1	0	0	1	0
18	Stoned wheat crackers,less salt 5 (1½ in sq × ⅛ in)	.7 oz	80	1	1	1	2	0	1	1	0	0	0	0	0	0	0	0	0	0	0
19	Tortilla chips 1 oz (¾ cup)	1.0 oz	140	1	1	1	3	0	2	3	0	1	2	0	0	0	0	0	1	1	1
20	Wheat cake,puffed 2 cakes (2½ in diam)	.6 oz	70	1	1	1	1	0	0	0	0	0	1	0	0	1	1	0	0	1	0
21	Wheat,rye,onion,or sesame toasts 6 crackers	.7 oz	90	1	1	1	1	0	1	1	0	0	1	0	0	1	1	0	0	1	0
22	Whole wheat biscuit crackers 4 (1½ in sq × ⅛ in)	.6 oz	80	1	0	1	1	0	1	1	0	0	1	0	0	1	1	0	0	1	0
23	Whole wheat thin crackers 10 (1 in sq)	.6 oz	90	1	0	1	1	0	1	1	0	0	1	0	0	1	1	0	0	1	0
Dips																					
24	Clam dip w sour cream 2 tablespoons	1.1 oz	50	1	0	0	0	0	1	3	0	0	0	1	0	0	1	0	1	1	0
25	Cottage cheese dip 2 tablespoons	1.1 oz	30	0	1	0	0	0	0	1	0	0	2	0	0	0	1	0	1	0	0
26	Onion dip 2 tablespoons	1.1 oz	60	1	0	0	0	1	2	3	0	1	1	1	0	0	0	0	1	0	0
Cheeses and Meats																					
27	Caviar 1 tablespoon	.6 oz	50	1	2	0	0	0	1	0	0	4	4	0	0	0	0	1	1	2	N

28 Cheese,brie 1 oz	1.0 oz	90	1	2	0	0	0	2	4	0	2	2	1	0	0	2	1	1	0	1
29 Cheese,cheddar 1/2 oz(1 × 1 × 1/2 in pc)	.5 oz	60	1	1	0	0	0	1	3	0	1	1	1	0	0	1	0	2	0	1
30 Cheese,ched,swiss,montjack,lofat 1/2 oz(1 × 1 × 1/2 in pc)	.5 oz	40	0	1	0	0	0	1	1	0	1	1	0	0	0	1	0	2	0	1
31 Cheese,swiss 1/2 oz(1 3/4 in sq × 1/8)	.5 oz	50	1	1	0	0	0	1	2	0	1	0	0	0	0	1	0	3	0	1
32 Clams,cnd 2–3 clams	1.1 oz	30	0	1	0	0	0	0	0	0	1	0	0	0	0	0	0	0	1	0
33 Crab,steamed 1/4 cup	1.4 oz	40	0	2	0	0	0	0	0	0	3	1	3	0	1	0	1	0	0	2
34 Egg roll,chicken 2 (1 1/2 oz rolls)	3.0 oz	180	2	2	1	1	0	2	2	1	1	5	0	0	1	1	1	0	1	1
35 Egg roll,meat and shrimp 2 (2 1/2 oz rolls)	4.9 oz	270	3	3	1	1	0	2	1	1	2	7	1	0	2	1	1	1	1	2
36 Franks 2 small (2 in long)	1.4 oz	120	1	2	0	0	0	3	4	0	2	4	0	0	1	1	1	0	1	1
37 Ham, baked, lean 1/2 oz sl(4 × 3 × 1/16 in	.5 oz	20	0	1	0	0	0	0	0	0	1	2	0	1	2	0	1	0	0	0
38 Pate de foie gras 1 tablespoon	.5 oz	70	1	1	0	0	0	2	2	0	1	1	2	0	0	1	0	0	1	1
39 Shrimp,cnd 1/4 c small,6 lg(3 1/4 in	1.1 oz	40	0	2	0	0	0	0	0	0	3	0	0	0	0	0	0	1	1	1
40 Quiche,cheese 1 pc,1 3/4 in square	1.8 oz	100	1	1	0	1	0	2	2	1	4	1	1	0	1	1	1	1	0	1
41 Quiche,lorraine 1 pc,1 3/4 in square	1.8 oz	140	1	2	0	1	0	3	4	1	4	2	1	0	1	1	1	1	1	1
42 Quiche,swiss cheese + crab 1 pc,1 3/4 in square	1.8 oz	140	1	2	0	1	0	3	4	1	5	3	2	0	1	1	1	2	1	1
Nuts and Seeds (no salt unless specified)																				
43 Almonds,roasted w salt 22 almonds	1.0 oz	160	2	1	0	N	N	4	1	3	0	2	0	0	0	2	0	2	1	2

continued

Appetizers and Snack Foods

No.	Name/Portion Size		KCAL	CAL	PRO	CAR	FIB	SUG	FAT	SFA	PFA	CHL	SOD	A	C	THI	RIB	B6	CA	IRN	ZN
									NUTRI–UNITS												
44	Beechnuts 1 oz	1.0 oz	160	2	1	1	2	0	4	1	5	0	0	0	1	1	1	2	0	1	0
45	Brazilnuts 8 medium nuts	1.0 oz	180	2	1	0	2	0	6	4	6	0	0	0	0	4	0	1	1	1	2
46	Butternuts 8–10 nuts	1.0 oz	170	2	2	0	2	0	5	0	11	0	0	0	0	1	0	2	0	1	1
47	Cashew nuts,dry rst,w salt 18 medium nuts	1.0 oz	160	2	1	1	2	0	4	2	2	0	2	0	0	1	1	1	0	2	2
48	Cashew nuts,oil rst,w salt 18 medium nuts	1.0 oz	160	2	1	1	2	0	4	2	2	0	2	0	0	2	1	1	0	1	2
49	Cashew nuts,dry rst,no salt 18 medium nuts	1.0 oz	160	2	1	1	2	0	4	2	2	0	0	0	0	1	1	1	0	2	2
50	Chestnuts,fresh 1 oz (3 tablespoons)	1.0 oz	60	1	0	1	2	1	0	0	0	0	0	0	3	1	1	1	0	0	0
51	Chestnuts,dried 1 oz (1/4 cup)	1.0 oz	100	1	1	2	3	1	0	0	0	0	0	0	5	1	1	2	0	1	1
52	Filberts (hazel nuts) 20–25 nuts	1.0 oz	180	2	1	0	2	0	5	1	2	0	0	0	0	2	0	2	1	1	1
53	Hickorynuts 30 small nuts	1.0 oz	180	2	1	0	2	0	5	2	6	0	0	0	0	3	0	1	0	1	2
54	Macadamia nuts 1 oz (12 nuts)	1.0 oz	200	2	1	0	2	0	6	3	0	0	0	0	0	1	0	1	0	1	1
55	Mixed nuts,dry roasted,w salt 1 oz (3 tablespoons)	1.0 oz	170	2	1	0	2	0	4	2	3	0	2	0	0	1	1	1	0	1	1
56	Mixed nuts,oil roasted,w salt 1 oz (3 tablespoons)	1.0 oz	170	2	1	0	2	0	5	2	3	0	2	0	0	2	1	1	1	1	2
57	Mixed nuts,oil roasted,no salt 1 oz (3 tablespoons)	1.0 oz	170	2	1	0	2	0	5	2	3	0	0	0	0	2	1	1	1	1	2
58	Nuts'n stuff, no salt 1 ounce	1.0 oz	150	1	1	1	4	0	3	1	4	0	0	0	0	3	1	3	1	2	1

59 Peanuts,boiled,w salt 3 tablespoons	1.0 oz	90	1	1	0	2	0	2	1	2	0	2	0	0	1	0	0	0	0	1
60 Peanuts,dry roasted,w salt 3 tablespoons	1.0 oz	160	2	2	0	2	0	4	2	4	0	2	0	0	2	0	1	0	1	1
61 Peanuts,roasted + salted 3 tablespoons	1.0 oz	170	2	2	0	2	0	4	2	4	0	2	0	0	0	1	1	0	1	1
62 Peanuts,roasted,no salt 3 tablespoons	1.0 oz	170	2	2	0	2	0	4	2	4	0	0	0	0	0	1	1	0	1	1
63 Pecans dried 24 halves (4 tablespoons)	1.0 oz	190	2	1	0	2	0	6	1	4	0	0	0	0	3	0	1	0	1	2
64 Pecans dry roasted 24 halves (4 tablespoons)	1.0 oz	190	2	1	0	2	0	5	1	4	0	0	0	0	1	0	1	0	1	2
65 Pinenuts,pinon 4 tablespoons	1.0 oz	160	2	1	0	2	0	5	2	6	0	0	0	0	5	1	0	0	1	2
66 Pistachio nuts dried 60 nuts	1.1 oz	170	2	2	1	3	0	4	2	2	0	0	0	1	3	1	1	1	2	1
67 Pistachio nuts dry roasted 1 oz (60 nuts)	1.0 oz	170	2	1	1	3	0	4	2	2	0	0	0	1	2	1	1	0	1	1
68 Pop't wheat,seasoned 1 ounce	1.0 oz	150	1	1	1	3	0	2	1	6	0	1	0	0	1	0	3	0	1	1
69 Pop't wheat,no salt 1 ounce	1.0 oz	150	1	1	1	3	0	2	1	6	0	0	0	0	1	0	3	0	1	1
70 Pumpkin or squash kernels 3 tablespoons	1.0 oz	130	1	2	1	10	0	2	1	2	0	0	0	0	0	0	0	0	1	4
71 Soy nuts no salt 1/3 cup	1.3 oz	160	2	4	1	4	1	3	1	4	0	0	0	0	0	1	1	1	2	2
72 Soy nuts with salt 1/3 cup	1.3 oz	160	2	4	1	4	N	3	1	4	0	1	0	0	0	1	1	1	2	2
73 Sunflower seed,oil rst,salt 3 tablespoons	1.0 oz	170	2	2	0	2	0	5	2	10	0	2	0	0	1	1	2	0	2	2
74 Sunflower seed,dry rst,salt 3 tablespoons	1.0 oz	160	2	2	0	2	0	4	1	8	0	2	0	0	0	1	2	0	1	2

continued

Appetizers and Snack Foods

No.	Name/Portion Size		KCAL	CAL	PRO	CAR	FIB	SUG	FAT	SFA	PFA	CHL	SOD	A	C	THI	RIB	B6	CA	IRN	ZN
											NUTRI–UNITS										
75	Sunflower seed,dry rst,nosalt 3 tablespoons	1.0 oz	160	2	2	0	2	0	4	1	8	0	0	0	0	0	1	2	0	1	2
76	Trail mix (fruits+nuts+seeds) 1 ounce,unsalted	1.0 oz	120	1	1	1	3	2	2	2	2	0	0	0	0	2	0	1	1	1	0
77	Walnuts,black 20 halves (4 tablespoons)	1.0 oz	170	2	2	0	2	0	5	1	9	0	0	0	0	1	0	2	0	1	1
78	Walnuts,english 20 halves (4 tablespoons)	1.0 oz	180	2	1	0	2	0	5	1	10	0	0	0	0	1	0	2	1	1	1
Popcorn, Pretzels, etc.																					
79	Popcorn, air popped 2 cups	.4 oz	50	0	0	1	2	N	0	0	0	0	0	0	0	1	0	0	0	0	1
80	Popcorn,w salt+butter 2 cups w 1 tsp butter	.6 oz	80	1	1	1	2	N	1	2	0	1	3	0	0	1	0	0	0	0	1
81	Popcorn,w salt+margarine 2 cups w 1 tsp marg	.6 oz	80	1	1	1	2	N	1	2	0	1	3	0	0	1	0	0	0	0	1
82	Popcorn,w salt+coconut oil 2 cups	.6 oz	80	1	1	1	2	N	1	3	0	0	3	0	0	1	0	0	0	0	1
83	Popcorn,sugar coated, no salt 1 cup	1.2 oz	130	1	1	2	2	2	0	0	0	0	0	0	0	2	0	1	0	1	0
84	Pretzels 10 sticks ($3^1/_8 \times {}^1/_8$ in)	1.1 oz	120	1	1	2	1	0	0	0	0	0	5	0	0	0	0	0	0	1	0
85	Pretzels,dutch 1 ($2^3/_4 \times 2^5/_8 \times {}^5/_8$ in)	.6 oz	60	1	0	1	1	0	0	0	0	0	3	0	0	0	0	0	0	0	0
Vegetables and Fruits																					
86	Apple, unpared 1 apple ($2^3/_4$ in dia)	4.9 oz	80	1	0	1	3	3	0	0	0	0	0	0	3	0	0	1	0	0	0
87	Banana 1 banana (9 in long)	4.2 oz	110	1	0	2	4	4	0	0	0	0	0	0	4	1	1	7	0	0	0
88	Carrot sticks 6 strips ($3 \times {}^3/_8$ in)	1.0 oz	10	0	0	0	1	0	0	0	0	0	0	32	1	0	0	0	0	0	0

89 Cauliflower ¼ cup florets	.8 oz	10	0	0	0	1	0	0	0	0	0	0	0	5	0	0	1	0	0	0
90 Celery sticks 4 pc (4 × ¾ in)	1.4 oz	10	0	0	0	1	0	0	0	0	0	0	0	1	0	0	0	0	0	0
91 Grapes ½ cup	2.6 oz	50	1	0	1	1	3	0	0	0	0	0	0	3	1	0	1	0	0	0
92 Kiwi fruit,raw 1 medium	2.7 oz	50	0	0	1	1	1	0	0	0	0	0	1	25	0	0	N	0	0	N
93 Olives,canned green 5 large	.6 oz	20	0	0	0	1	0	1	0	0	0	4	0	0	0	0	0	0	0	0
94 Olives,canned,ripe mission 5 medium	.6 oz	30	0	0	0	1	0	1	0	0	0	1	0	0	0	0	0	0	0	0
95 Orange,raw Half of 2.6 in orange	2.3 oz	30	0	0	1	2	1	0	0	0	0	0	0	12	1	0	0	1	0	0
96 Pear,raw Half of 2.5×3.5 in pear	2.9 oz	50	0	0	1	2	2	0	0	0	0	0	0	1	0	0	0	0	0	0
97 Pineapple,raw ½ cup,diced	2.8 oz	40	0	0	1	1	2	0	0	0	0	0	0	4	1	0	1	0	0	0
98 Stuffed celery sticks 1 pc 5×¾ in,1 tsp pnutb	1.4 oz	70	1	1	0	1	0	2	1	1	0	1	0	1	0	0	0	0	0	0

Beverages

Cocktails

99 Bloody Mary 1 5 oz glass	5.2 oz	120	1	0	0	N	N	0	0	0	0	3	2	7	1	0	1	0	1	0
100 Daiquiri 1 3.5 oz glass	3.5 oz	190	2	0	0	N	N	0	0	0	0	0	0	1	0	0	0	0	0	0
101 Egg nog 1 4 oz glass	4.3 oz	320	3	2	1	0	3	3	4	0	4	1	2	1	0	3	1	3	0	1
102 Gin and tonic 1 7.5 oz glass	7.9 oz	170	2	0	1	0	N	0	0	0	0	0	0	0	0	0	0	0	0	0
103 Manhattan 1 3.5 oz glass	3.5 oz	220	2	0	0	0	N	0	0	0	0	0	0	0	0	0	0	0	0	0

continued

Beverages

No.	Name/Portion Size		KCAL	CAL	PRO	CAR	FIB	SUG	FAT	SFA	PFA	CHL	SOD	A	C	THI	RIB	B6	CA	IRN	ZN
										NUTRI–UNITS											
104	Martini 1 3.5 oz glass	3.5 oz	220	2	0	0	0	N	0	0	0	0	0	0	0	0	0	0	0	0	0
105	Pina colada 1 4.5 oz glass	5.0 oz	260	3	0	3	0	N	1	1	0	0	0	0	2	1	0	1	0	0	0
106	Screwdriver 1 7 oz glass	7.5 oz	180	2	0	1	0	N	0	0	0	0	0	1	22	2	0	1	0	0	0
107	Tequilla sunrise 1 5.5 oz glass	6.1 oz	190	2	0	1	0	N	0	0	0	0	0	1	11	1	0	1	0	1	0
108	Tom Collins 1 7.5 oz glass	7.8 oz	120	1	0	0	0	N	0	0	0	0	0	0	1	0	0	0	0	0	0
109	Whiskey sour 1 3.5 oz glass	3.7 oz	160	2	0	1	0	N	0	0	0	0	1	0	1	0	0	0	0	0	0
Distilled Spirits and Liqueurs																					
110	Anisette 2/3 oz (cordial glass)	.7 oz	80	1	0	0	0	1	0	0	0	0	0	0	0	0	0	0	0	0	0
111	Apricot brandy 2/3 oz (cordial glass)	.7 oz	70	1	0	0	0	1	0	0	0	0	0	0	0	0	0	0	0	0	0
112	Benedictine 2/3 oz (cordial glass)	.7 oz	70	1	0	0	0	1	0	0	0	0	0	0	0	0	0	0	0	0	0
113	Brandy 1 oz shot glass	1.0 oz	70	1	0	0	0	0	0	0	0	0	0	0	0	0	0	0	0	0	0
114	Creme de menthe 2/3 oz (cordial glass)	.7 oz	70	1	0	0	0	1	0	0	0	0	0	0	0	0	0	0	0	0	0
115	Curacao 2/3 oz (cordial glass)	.7 oz	60	1	0	0	0	1	0	0	0	0	0	0	0	0	0	0	0	0	0
116	Gin, 80 proof 1 1/2 oz (1 jigger)	1.6 oz	100	1	0	0	0	0	0	0	0	0	0	0	0	0	0	0	0	0	0
117	Gin, 90 proof 1 1/2 oz (1 jigger)	1.6 oz	120	1	0	0	0	0	0	0	0	0	0	0	0	0	0	0	0	0	0
118	Gin, 100 proof 1 1/2 oz (1 jigger)	1.6 oz	130	1	0	0	0	0	0	0	0	0	0	0	0	0	0	0	0	0	0

119 Gin, dry 1½ oz (1 jigger)	1.6 oz	100	1	0	0	0	0	0	0	0	0	0	0	0	0	0	0	0	0	0
120 Rum 1½ oz (1 jigger)	1.6 oz	100	1	0	0	0	0	0	0	0	0	0	0	0	0	0	0	0	0	0
121 Vodka, 80 proof 1½ oz (1 jigger)	1.6 oz	100	1	0	0	0	0	0	0	0	0	0	0	0	0	0	0	0	0	0
122 Whiskey, rye 1½ oz (1 jigger)	1.6 oz	120	1	0	0	0	0	0	0	0	0	0	0	0	0	0	0	0	0	0
123 Whiskey, scotch 1½ oz (1 jigger)	1.6 oz	100	1	0	0	0	0	0	0	0	0	0	0	0	0	0	0	0	0	0
Malt Liquors																				
124 Ale, mild 1 12 oz bottle/can	12.2 oz	150	1	0	1	0	1	0	0	0	0	0	0	0	0	1	2	0	0	0
125 Beer, 3.6 percent alcohol 1 12 oz bottle/can	12.7 oz	150	1	0	1	0	N	0	0	0	0	0	0	0	0	1	2	0	0	0
126 Beer, 4.2 percent alcohol 1 12 oz bottle/can	12.7 oz	180	2	0	1	0	1	0	0	0	0	0	0	0	0	1	2	0	0	0
127 Beer, light 1 12 oz bottle/can	12.7 oz	100	1	0	0	0	0	0	0	0	0	0	0	0	0	1	1	0	0	0
Wines																				
128 Champagne, domestic 1 4 oz glass	4.2 oz	90	1	0	0	0	0	0	0	0	0	0	0	0	0	0	0	0	1	0
129 Madeira 1 4 oz glass	4.0 oz	120	1	0	0	0	0	0	0	0	0	0	0	0	0	0	0	0	1	0
130 Muscatel or port 1 4 oz glass	4.0 oz	180	2	0	1	0	3	0	0	0	0	0	0	0	0	0	0	0	0	0
131 Sherry, dry, domestic 1 2 oz glass	2.1 oz	80	1	0	0	0	0	0	0	0	0	0	0	0	0	0	0	0	0	0
132 Vermouth, dry 1 4 oz glass	3.7 oz	110	1	0	0	0	0	0	0	0	0	0	0	0	0	0	0	0	0	0
133 Vermouth, sweet 1 4 oz glass	3.7 oz	180	2	0	1	0	2	0	0	0	0	0	0	0	0	0	0	0	0	0
134 Wine,10 percent alcohol 1 4 oz glass	4.2 oz	100	1	0	0	0	1	0	0	0	0	0	0	0	0	0	0	0	1	0

continued

Beverages

No.	Name/Portion Size		KCAL	CAL	PRO	CAR	FIB	SUG	FAT	SFA	PFA	CHL	SOD	A	C	THI	RIB	B6	CA	IRN	ZN
										NUTRI–UNITS											
135	Wine, dessert,15 percent alcohol 1 4 oz glass	4.2 oz	160	2	0	1	0	2	0	0	0	0	0	0	0	0	0	0	0	0	0
136	Wine, red 1 4 oz glass	4.0 oz	100	1	0	0	0	1	0	0	0	0	0	0	0	0	0	0	0	1	0
137	Wine, sauterne 1 4 oz glass	4.0 oz	100	1	0	0	0	1	0	0	0	0	0	0	0	0	0	0	0	1	0
Coffee, Tea, or Bouillon																					
138	Bouillon,beef or chicken,hot 1 8-oz cup	8.4 oz	0	0	0	0	0	0	0	0	0	0	4	0	0	0	1	0	0	0	0
139	Coffee,black,reg,instnt or decaf 1 8-oz cup	8.5 oz	0	0	0	0	0	0	0	0	0	0	0	0	0	0	0	0	0	0	0
140	Coffee beverage w grain 1 8-oz cup	8.5 oz	10	0	0	0	0	0	0	0	0	0	0	0	0	0	0	0	0	0	0
141	Coffee, almond or cafe mocha 1 8-oz cup	8.5 oz	80	1	0	1	0	2	0	0	0	0	0	0	0	0	0	0	0	0	0
142	Coffee, cafe capri or c viennese 1 8-oz cup	8.5 oz	60	1	0	1	0	2	0	0	0	0	0	0	0	0	0	0	0	0	0
143	Postum 1 8-oz cup	8.4 oz	20	0	0	0	0	0	0	0	0	0	0	0	0	1	0	0	0	1	0
144	Tea, instant or reg, hot or iced 1 8-oz cup	8.5 oz	10	0	0	0	0	0	0	0	0	0	0	0	0	0	0	0	0	0	0
145	Tea, iced w sugar, cnd $1^1/_2$ cup or 12 oz	12.7 oz	140	1	0	3	0	7	0	0	0	0	0	0	0	0	0	0	0	0	0
Coffee Sweeteners and Whiteners																					
146	Cream, half + half 1 tablespoon	.5 oz	20	0	0	0	0	0	0	1	0	0	0	0	0	0	0	0	0	0	0
147	Cream, light coffee 1 tablespoon	.5 oz	30	0	0	0	0	0	1	2	0	1	0	0	0	0	0	0	0	0	0
148	Cream subst,liq,veg and coc oil 1 tablespoon	.5 oz	20	0	0	0	0	N	0	0	0	0	0	0	0	0	0	0	0	0	0

149 Cream subst,powder,w coc oil 1 teaspoon	.1 oz	10	0	0	0	0	N	0	1	0	0	0	0	0	0	0	0	0	0	0
150 Cream substitute, polyrich 1 tablespoon	.5 oz	20	0	0	0	0	0	0	0	1	0	0	0	0	0	0	0	0	0	0
151 Milk,evaporated skim,cnd,unswnd 1 tablespoon	.5 oz	10	0	0	0	0	0	0	0	0	0	0	0	0	0	1	0	1	0	0
152 Milk, whole 1 tablespoon	.5 oz	10	0	0	0	0	0	0	0	0	0	0	0	0	0	0	0	0	0	0
153 Honey 1 teaspoon	.2 oz	20	0	0	0	0	1	0	0	0	0	0	0	0	0	0	0	0	0	0
154 Sugar 1 teaspoon	.1 oz	20	0	0	0	0	1	0	0	0	0	0	0	0	0	0	0	0	0	0
155 Sugar substitute 2½ teaspoon	.0 oz	0	0	0	0	N	0	0	0	0	0	0	0	0	0	0	0	0	0	0
Carbonated Beverages																				
156 Cola soft drinks 1½ cup or 12 oz can	13.0 oz	140	1	0	3	0	7	0	0	0	0	0	0	0	0	0	0	0	0	0
157 Unsweetened club soda 1½ cup or 12 oz can	12.5 oz	0	0	0	0	0	0	0	0	0	0	0	0	0	0	0	0	0	0	0
158 Sugar free soft drinks 1½ cup or 12 oz can	12.5 oz	0	0	0	0	0	0	0	0	0	0	0	0	0	0	0	0	0	0	0
159 Fruit flavored soft drinks 1½ cup or 12 oz can	13.1 oz	170	2	0	3	0	9	0	0	0	0	0	0	0	0	0	0	0	0	0
160 Ginger ale or swt quinine soda 1½ cup or 12 oz can	12.9 oz	110	1	0	2	0	6	0	0	0	0	0	0	0	0	0	0	0	0	0
Fruit-Flavored Drinks																				
161 Cherry flav drink, w vit c 1 8-oz cup	8.8 oz	120	1	0	2	0	6	0	0	0	0	0	0	3	0	0	0	0	0	0
162 Cranberry jc cocktail w vit c ½ cup or 4 oz	4.3 oz	90	1	0	2	0	4	0	0	0	0	0	0	10	0	0	0	0	1	0
163 Fruit flav drnk,powd,dil,w vitc 1 8-oz cup	8.8 oz	120	1	0	2	0	6	0	0	0	0	0	0	3	0	0	0	0	0	0

continued

Beverages

No.	Name/Portion Size		KCAL	CAL	PRO	CAR	FIB	SUG	FAT	SFA	PFA	CHL	SOD	A	C	THI	RIB	B6	CA	IRN	ZN
										NUTRI–UNITS											
164	Gatorade, citrus flavored 1 8-oz cup	8.1 oz	40	0	0	1	0	2	0	0	0	0	1	0	0	0	0	0	0	0	0
165	Grape drink, canned, w vit c 1 8-oz cup	8.8 oz	140	1	0	2	0	7	0	0	0	0	0	0	10	0	0	2	0	0	0
166	Lemonade,from conc.,diluted 1 8-oz cup	8.7 oz	110	1	0	2	0	5	0	0	0	0	0	0	6	0	0	0	0	0	0
167	Lemonade, artificial swtnr 1 8-oz cup	8.7 oz	10	0	0	0	0	0	0	0	0	0	0	0	2	0	0	0	1	0	0
168	Limeade,from conc., diluted 1 8-oz cup	8.7 oz	100	1	0	2	0	5	0	0	0	0	0	0	2	0	0	0	0	0	0
169	Orange instant breakfast drink 1/2 cup (vit c added)	4.4 oz	60	1	0	1	0	3	0	0	0	0	0	4	22	0	0	0	1	0	0
170	Orange+apricot jc drink,cnd 1/2 cup	4.4 oz	60	1	0	1	0	3	0	0	0	0	0	3	7	0	0	0	0	0	0
171	Pineapl+grapefrt jc drink,cnd 1/2 cup	4.4 oz	70	1	0	1	0	3	0	0	0	0	0	0	7	0	0	0	0	0	0
172	Pineapl+orange jc drink,cnd 1/2 cup	4.4 oz	70	1	0	1	0	3	0	0	0	0	0	0	7	0	0	0	0	0	0
Vegetable Juices																					
173	Carrot juice 1/2 cup	4.3 oz	30	0	0	1	2	1	0	0	0	0	1	54	3	1	1	1	1	0	0
174	Tomato juice,cnd 1/2 cup	4.3 oz	20	0	0	0	0	1	0	0	0	0	2	4	7	1	0	1	0	1	0
175	Vegetable juice cocktail 1/2 cup	4.3 oz	20	0	0	0	0	0	0	0	0	0	2	3	4	1	0	1	0	1	0
Milk and Milk Drinks																					
176	Buttermilk, cultured 1 8-oz glass	8.5 oz	100	1	2	1	0	2	1	1	0	1	3	0	1	1	4	1	6	0	1
177	Cocoa or hot choc w whole milk 1 8-oz cup	8.8 oz	240	2	3	2	0	5	4	6	0	2	1	1	1	1	5	N	5	1	1

178 Cocoa,made from mix + skim milk 1 8-oz cup	9.3 oz	160	2	3	2	0	5	1	1	0	0	2	0	1	1	6	N	7	0	1
179 Egg nog, non-alcoholic 1 8-oz glass	8.7 oz	340	3	3	2	0	6	6	9	0	10	1	3	2	1	6	1	6	1	2
180 Ice cream float 1 14-oz serving	14.0 oz	330	3	2	4	0	12	2	4	0	1	4	0	0	3	2	0	4	0	0
181 Malt, chocolate, small 1 8-oz serving	8.5 oz	340	3	3	4	0	8	4	7	0	2	2	2	1	1	4	1	6	2	2
182 Malt, chocolate, medium 1 15-oz serving	14.7 oz	600	6	5	6	0	13	6	11	0	3	4	3	1	1	6	2	10	4	4
183 Malt, chocolate, large 1 21-oz serving	20.7 oz	840	8	7	9	0	19	9	16	0	4	5	3	2	2	9	3	12	6	5
184 Milk, chocolate, 2 percent fat 1 8-oz glass	8.8 oz	180	2	2	2	0	5	2	3	0	1	2	2	1	1	5	1	6	1	1
185 Milk,chocolate,3.5 percent fat 1 8-oz glass	8.8 oz	210	2	2	2	0	5	3	5	0	2	1	1	1	1	5	1	6	1	1
186 Milk, malted, beverage 1 8-oz glass	8.3 oz	210	2	3	2	0	3	3	5	0	2	2	1	1	2	6	2	6	0	1
187 Milk, skim 1 8-oz glass	8.6 oz	90	1	3	1	0	2	0	0	0	0	1	2	1	1	4	1	6	0	1
188 Milk, 1 percent fat, a+d fort 1 8-oz glass	8.7 oz	110	1	3	1	0	2	1	1	0	1	1	2	1	1	5	1	6	0	1
189 Milk, 2 percent fat, a+d fort 1 8-oz glass	8.7 oz	130	1	3	1	0	2	1	3	0	1	1	2	1	1	5	1	6	0	1
190 Milk, whole, 3.5 percent fat 1 8-oz glass	8.6 oz	150	1	2	1	0	2	2	5	0	2	1	1	1	1	5	1	6	0	1
191 Milk, whole, low sodium 1 cup	8.6 oz	150	1	2	1	0	2	3	5	0	2	0	1	1	1	3	1	5	0	1
192 Ovaltine mix,dry 1 serving package	.7 oz	80	1	0	0	N	1	1	1	1	0	2	9	9	9	9	0	2	3	0
193 Soybean milk, fluid 1 cup	9.3 oz	90	1	3	0	0	0	1	0	0	0	0	0	0	3	1	1	1	2	1
194 Shake,chocolate 1 10-oz serving	10.2 oz	370	4	3	4	0	10	3	5	0	2	3	1	1	2	5	1	7	1	2

continued

Breads, Pastas, and Grain Products

No.	Name/Portion Size		KCAL	CAL	PRO	CAR	FIB	SUG	FAT	SFA	PFA	CHL	SOD	A	C	THI	RIB	B6	CA	IRN	ZN
195	Shake, strawberry 1 10-oz serving	10.3 oz	350	3	3	4	0	10	3	5	0	2	3	1	1	2	5	1	7	0	2
196	Shake, vanilla 1 10-oz serving	10.2 oz	320	3	3	4	0	10	3	5	0	2	3	1	1	2	8	1	7	0	1

Breads, Pastas, and Grain Products

Breads and Biscuits

No.	Name/Portion Size		KCAL	CAL	PRO	CAR	FIB	SUG	FAT	SFA	PFA	CHL	SOD	A	C	THI	RIB	B6	CA	IRN	ZN
197	Banana bread 1 slice (3 × 5 × 1/2 in)	2.0 oz	170	2	1	2	2	3	2	2	1	2	2	1	0	1	1	1	0	1	0
198	Biscuit,enriched,w lard 1 (2 in diam × 1 in)	1.0 oz	100	1	1	1	1	0	1	2	0	0	2	0	0	1	1	0	1	1	0
199	Biscuit,enriched,w veg fat 1 (2 in diam × 1 in)	1.0 oz	100	1	1	1	1	0	1	1	1	0	2	0	0	1	1	0	1	1	0
200	Biscuit,in can,veg fat 1 biscuit (3/4 oz)	.7 oz	60	1	0	1	1	0	0	0	0	0	2	0	0	1	1	0	0	1	0
201	Biscuit from mix,w milk 1 (2 in diam × 1 in)	1.0 oz	90	1	1	1	1	0	1	1	1	0	3	0	0	1	1	0	0	1	0
202	Boston brown bread 1 (3 in diam × 3/4 in)	1.6 oz	90	1	1	1	2	2	0	0	0	0	1	0	0	1	0	0	1	1	1
203	Bread sticks 2 (4 × 1/2 in diam)	.7 oz	50	1	0	1	1	0	0	0	0	0	1	0	0	1	1	0	0	0	0
204	Cracked wheat/wheat berry bread 2 slices (18 per lb)	1.8 oz	130	1	1	2	4	1	0	0	0	0	3	0	0	2	1	0	1	2	0
205	Cracked wheat toast 2 slices (18 per lb)	1.5 oz	130	1	1	2	4	1	0	0	0	0	3	0	0	2	1	0	1	2	0
206	French bread 1 slice(5 × 21/2 × 1 in)	1.2 oz	100	1	1	1	1	0	0	0	0	0	2	0	0	2	1	0	0	1	0
207	French bread, toasted 1 slice(5 × 21/2 × 1 in)	1.1 oz	100	1	1	1	1	0	0	0	0	0	2	0	0	1	1	0	0	1	0
208	Garlic toast w 1 tsp butter 1 slice(5 × 21/2 × 1 in)	1.1 oz	110	1	1	1	1	0	2	3	0	1	2	1	0	1	0	0	0	1	0

NUTRI–UNITS: CAL through ZN

209 Italian bread 1 slice(5 × 2½ × 1 in)	1.2 oz	100	1	1	1	1	0	0	0	0	0	2	0	0	2	1	0	0	1	0
210 Lo sodium bread 2 slices (18 per lb)	1.8 oz	160	2	2	2	1	1	1	0	0	0	0	0	0	2	2	0	1	2	0
211 Pita bread (pocket bread) ½ of 2½ oz pita	1.2 oz	100	1	1	1	1	0	0	0	0	0	1	0	0	4	2	0	1	1	0
212 Pumpernickel 1 sl (4½ × 3½ × 3/8	1.1 oz	80	1	1	1	2	1	0	0	0	0	2	0	0	1	1	1	1	1	0
213 Raisin bread 2 slices (18 per lb)	1.8 oz	130	1	1	2	2	2	0	0	0	0	2	0	0	3	1	0	1	2	0
214 Raisin bread,toasted 2 slices (18 per lb)	1.5 oz	130	1	1	2	2	2	0	0	0	0	2	0	0	2	1	0	1	2	0
215 Rice cake 2 cakes (2½ in diam)	.6 oz	70	1	0	1	1	0	0	0	0	0	1	0	0	2	0	0	0	1	0
216 Rye bread 2 slices (18 per lb)	1.8 oz	120	1	1	2	2	1	0	0	0	0	3	0	0	2	1	0	1	1	1
217 Rye bread,snack slice 2 slices(30 per 8 oz loaf	.5 oz	30	0	0	1	1	0	0	0	0	0	1	0	0	1	0	0	0	0	0
218 Rye bread,toasted 2 slices (18 per lb)	1.5 oz	120	1	1	2	2	1	0	0	0	0	3	0	0	2	1	1	1	1	1
219 Scones 2 oz	2.0 oz	140	1	1	2	2	0	0	1	0	0	1	0	0	3	2	0	2	2	0
220 Wheat cake,puffed 2 cakes (2½ in diam)	.6 oz	70	1	1	1	1	0	0	0	0	0	1	0	0	1	1	0	0	1	0
221 White bread,enriched 2 slices (18 per lb)	1.8 oz	140	1	1	2	1	1	0	0	0	0	3	0	0	3	1	0	1	2	0
222 White bread,thin sl, enr 2 slices (30 per lb)	1.1 oz	80	1	1	1	1	0	0	0	0	0	1	0	0	2	1	0	1	1	0
223 White bread,toasted 2 slices (18 per lb)	1.5 oz	140	1	1	2	1	1	0	0	0	0	3	0	0	2	1	0	1	2	0
224 White bread,unenriched 2 slices (18 per lb)	1.8 oz	140	1	1	2	1	1	0	0	0	0	3	0	0	0	1	0	1	0	0
225 Whole wheat bread 2 slices (18 per lb)	1.8 oz	120	1	2	2	3	1	0	0	0	0	3	0	0	2	1	1	1	2	1

continued

Breads, Pastas, and Grain Products

No.	Name/Portion Size		KCAL	CAL	PRO	CAR	FIB	SUG	FAT	SFA	PFA	CHL	SOD	A	C	THI	RIB	B6	CA	IRN	ZN
										NUTRI–UNITS											
226	Whole wheat bread,toasted 2 slices (18 per lb)	1.5 oz	120	1	2	2	3	1	0	0	0	0	3	0	0	1	1	1	1	2	1
Buns and Rolls																					
227	Bagel 1 bagel (3 in diam)	1.9 oz	170	2	2	2	2	0	0	0	0	1	2	0	0	3	2	0	0	2	0
228	Brown and serve roll,baked 1 roll (2½ in diam)	.9 oz	90	1	1	1	1	0	1	0	0	0	1	0	0	1	1	0	0	1	0
229	Croissant 1 medium,	2.0 oz	220	2	1	2	1	1	4	4	4	1	3	0	0	4	2	0	0	1	1
230	Cheese danish roll 1 roll,4 in diam × 1 in	2.0 oz	240	2	1	2	1	2	4	3	1	2	2	1	0	0	0	0	1	1	1
231	Cinnamon roll 1 roll,3.8 in dia × 2 in	4.0 oz	370	4	2	4	3	4	3	2	2	0	4	1	0	4	3	0	1	2	1
232	Hamburger bun 1 bun	1.6 oz	130	1	1	2	1	1	1	0	0	0	2	0	0	3	2	0	1	1	0
233	Hard roll,enriched 1 roll,3.8 in dia × 2 in	1.8 oz	160	2	2	2	1	1	0	0	0	0	3	0	0	3	1	0	0	2	1
234	Homemade roll with egg 1 roll,2.5 in dia × 2 in	1.2 oz	120	1	1	1	1	0	1	1	1	1	1	0	0	2	1	0	0	1	0
235	Hot dog bun 1 bun	1.4 oz	110	1	1	1	1	0	1	0	0	0	2	0	0	3	2	0	1	1	0
236	Pan roll,enriched 1 roll,2 × 2 × 2 in	1.0 oz	80	1	1	1	1	0	0	0	0	0	1	0	0	1	1	0	0	1	0
237	Raisin roll,enriched 1 roll,2 × 2 × 2 in	1.0 oz	80	1	1	1	1	1	0	0	0	0	1	0	0	0	0	0	0	0	0
238	Sweet roll,enriched 1 roll,3.8 in dia × 1 in	1.9 oz	170	2	1	2	2	2	2	1	0	0	2	0	0	1	1	0	1	0	0
239	Whole wheat roll 1 roll,2 × 2 × 2 in	1.0 oz	70	1	1	1	2	0	0	0	0	0	2	0	0	1	0	0	1	1	0

Cornbread																				
240 Cornbread,whole ground 1 piece(2.5 in sq × 1.5)	2.8 oz	160	2	2	2	4	2	2	1	1	4	5	0	0	1	2	1	2	1	1
241 Cornbread,degermed,enriched 1 piece(2.5 in sq × 1.5)	2.9 oz	190	2	2	2	3	2	1	1	1	4	5	0	0	2	2	1	2	1	1
242 Cornbread,johnny cake 1 piece(2 × 2 × 2 in)	1.4 oz	110	1	1	1	2	1	1	0	0	2	3	1	0	1	1	1	1	1	0
243 Corn pone 1/8 of 9 in pone	2.1 oz	120	1	1	2	4	2	1	1	1	0	2	0	0	1	0	0	1	1	0
244 Hushpuppies 1 1/2 oz	1.6 oz	150	2	1	1	1	0	2	1	4	0	2	0	0	1	1	0	0	1	0
245 Spoon bread 1/2 cup	4.2 oz	230	2	2	1	5	0	4	4	2	10	6	1	0	1	3	1	2	1	0
Crackers and Chips																				
246 Animal crackers 5 crackers	.5 oz	60	1	0	1	0	1	0	0	0	0	0	0	0	0	0	0	0	0	0
247 Butter crackers 5 crackers (1.8 in diam)	.5 oz	70	1	0	1	0	0	1	1	0	0	2	0	0	1	1	0	0	1	0
248 Cheese crackers 5 crackers (1.8 in diam)	.5 oz	70	1	1	1	0	0	1	1	0	0	2	0	0	1	1	0	1	1	0
249 Graham crackers,choc coated 2 (2.5 × 2 × 1/4 in)	.9 oz	120	1	0	1	2	1	2	2	0	0	1	0	0	0	2	0	1	1	0
250 Graham crackers,plain 2 (2.5 × 5 × 3/16 in)	1.0 oz	110	1	1	1	3	2	1	1	1	0	2	0	0	0	2	0	0	1	0
251 Graham crackers,sug/honey coated 2 (2.5 × 5 × 1/4 in)	1.0 oz	120	1	1	2	2	2	1	1	1	0	1	0	0	0	1	0	0	1	0
252 Lo sodium crackers (saltine type 2 crackers 2 × 3 × 3/16 in	.5 oz	60	1	0	1	1	0	1	0	0	0	0	0	0	1	1	0	0	1	0
253 Melba toast 5 pieces	.5 oz	50	0	1	1	0	1	0	0	0	0	1	0	0	1	0	0	0	0	0
254 Peanut butter-cheese sandwich 3 sandw (1.6 in sq × 3/8)	.7 oz	100	1	1	1	1	0	2	1	1	0	2	0	0	3	1	0	0	1	0

continued

Breads, Pastas, and Grain Products

No.	Name/Portion Size		KCAL	CAL	PRO	CAR	FIB	SUG	FAT	SFA	PFA	CHL	SOD	A	C	THI	RIB	B6	CA	IRN	ZN
										NUTRI–UNITS											
255	Potato chips 10 chips (2.5 × 1.8 in)	.7 oz	110	1	0	1	2	0	2	2	4	0	1	0	1	1	0	0	0	0	0
256	Potato chips,unsalted 10 chips (2.5 × 1.8 in)	.7 oz	110	1	0	1	2	0	2	2	4	0	0	0	1	1	0	0	0	0	0
257	Pretzels 1 oz	1.0 oz	110	1	1	1	1	0	0	0	0	0	5	0	0	0	0	0	0	0	0
258	Pretzels,soft,salty 1 oz	1.0 oz	90	1	1	1	1	0	0	0	0	0	4	0	0	0	0	0	0	0	0
259	Rusk or zweiback 2 pieces(3.5 in dia × .5)	.6 oz	80	1	1	1	1	0	0	0	0	0	0	0	0	0	0	0	0	0	0
260	Rye wafers 3 wafers (3 × 2 × 1/4 in)	.7 oz	70	1	1	1	2	0	0	0	0	0	2	0	0	1	1	0	0	1	1
261	Saltine crackers 6 crackers (1.8 in sq)	.6 oz	80	1	0	1	1	0	1	0	0	0	2	0	0	1	1	0	0	1	0
262	Soda crackers 6 crackers (1.8 in sq)	.6 oz	80	1	1	1	1	0	1	1	1	0	2	0	0	1	1	0	0	1	0
263	Snack crackers (ritz type) 5 crackers	.6 oz	90	1	0	1	1	N	1	1	1	0	2	0	0	1	1	0	1	1	0
264	Stoned wheat crackers 5 (1.5 in sq × 1/8 in)	.7 oz	80	1	1	1	2	0	1	1	0	0	1	0	0	1	1	0	0	1	0
265	Stoned wheat crackers,less salt 5 (1.5 in sq × 1/8 in)	.7 oz	80	1	1	1	2	0	1	1	0	0	0	0	0	0	0	0	0	0	0
266	Tortilla chips 1 oz, 3/4 cup	1.0 oz	140	1	1	1	3	0	2	3	0	1	2	0	0	0	0	0	1	1	1
267	Whole wheat biscuit crackers 10 crackers (1.5 in sq)	1.6 oz	210	2	1	2	2	0	2	1	1	0	2	0	0	2	2	0	0	1	1
268	Whole wheat thin crackers 20 crackers (1 in sq)	1.2 oz	180	2	1	2	2	0	2	2	0	0	2	0	0	2	2	0	0	1	1
Dressing and Stuffing																					
269	Bread stuffing,prepared dry 1/2 cup	2.5 oz	250	3	1	2	2	1	5	7	1	3	6	2	0	1	1	0	1	1	0

270 Bread stuffing w egg,moist 1/2 cup	3.5 oz	210	2	1	1	2	1	4	6	1	4	5	2	0	1	1	0	1	1	1
271 Croutons 1/4 cup	.4 oz	40	0	0	1	0	0	0	0	0	0	1	0	0	1	1	0	0	1	0
272 Oven stuffin mix,dry 1/4 cup	.6 oz	70	1	1	1	1	0	0	0	0	0	3	0	0	1	1	0	0	0	0
Macaroni, Noodles and Spaghetti																				
273 Macaroni,enr,ckd,firm,no salt 1/2 cup ckd	2.3 oz	100	1	1	1	1	0	0	0	0	0	0	0	0	2	1	0	0	1	0
274 Macaroni,enr,ckd firm,salted 1/2 cup ckd	2.3 oz	100	1	1	1	1	0	0	0	0	0	2	0	0	2	1	0	0	1	0
275 Macaroni,enr,ckd,tender,no salt 1/2 cup ckd	2.5 oz	80	1	1	1	1	0	0	0	0	0	0	0	0	1	1	0	0	1	0
276 Macaroni,enr,ckd tender,salted 1/2 cup ckd	2.5 oz	80	1	1	1	1	0	0	0	0	0	3	0	0	1	1	0	0	1	0
277 Noodles,chow mein 1/2 cup	.8 oz	110	1	1	1	1	0	2	1	0	0	2	0	0	0	0	0	0	0	0
278 Noodles,egg,enriched,no salt 1/2 cup ckd	2.8 oz	100	1	1	1	1	0	0	0	0	2	0	0	0	1	1	0	0	1	1
279 Noodles,egg,enr,ckd,salted 1/2 cup ckd	2.8 oz	100	1	1	1	1	0	0	0	0	2	3	0	0	1	1	0	0	1	1
280 Spaghetti,enr,ckd,no salt 1/2 cup ckd	2.5 oz	80	1	1	1	1	0	0	0	0	0	0	0	0	1	1	0	0	1	0
281 Spaghetti,enr,ckd,salted 1/2 cup ckd	2.5 oz	80	1	1	1	1	0	0	0	0	0	0	0	0	1	1	0	0	1	0
Muffins and Popovers																				
282 Blueberry muffin 2.3 in diam × 1.5 in	1.4 oz	110	1	1	1	1	1	1	1	1	2	3	0	0	1	1	0	1	1	0
283 Bran muffin 2.5 in diam × 1.5 in	1.4 oz	100	1	1	1	1	1	1	1	1	3	2	0	0	1	1	1	1	2	1
284 Cornmeal muffin 2.3 in diam × 1.5 in	1.4 oz	130	1	1	1	1	1	1	1	1	1	2	0	0	1	1	0	1	1	0
285 English muffin 1 average muffin	2.0 oz	140	1	1	2	2	1	0	0	0	0	3	0	0	3	3	0	2	2	1

continued

Breads, Pastas, and Grain Products

No.	Name/Portion Size		KCAL	CAL	PRO	CAR	FIB	SUG	FAT	SFA	PFA	CHL	SOD	A	C	THI	RIB	B6	CA	IRN	ZN
									NUTRI–UNITS												
286	Plain muffin 2.5 in diam × 1.5 in	1.4 oz	120	1	1	1	1	1	1	1	1	1	2	0	0	1	1	0	1	1	0
287	Popover 2.3 in diam × 4 in	1.4 oz	90	1	1	1	1	0	1	1	0	4	1	1	0	1	1	0	1	1	1
288	Whole wheat muffin 2.5 in diam × 1.5 in	1.4 oz	100	1	1	1	2	1	1	1	1	3	2	0	0	1	1	1	1	2	1
Rice and Grains																					
289	Barley 1/4 cup dry (1 c ckd)	2.0 oz	200	2	2	3	4	0	0	0	0	0	0	0	0	2	0	1	0	2	1
290	Brown rice,cooked,salted 1/2 cup	3.0 oz	100	1	1	2	2	0	0	0	0	0	2	0	0	1	0	1	0	0	1
291	Brown rice,cooked,no salt 1/2 cup	3.0 oz	100	1	1	2	2	0	0	0	0	0	0	0	0	1	0	1	0	0	1
292	Bulgar,cracked wheat, salt 1 cup	4.8 oz	250	2	3	3	2	1	1	1	1	0	6	0	0	1	1	3	1	2	N
293	Spanish rice,lo fat 1/2 cup	3.5 oz	90	1	1	1	1	0	1	0	0	0	3	3	5	1	0	1	0	1	1
294	Spanish rice,hi fat 1/2 cup	3.5 oz	230	2	0	1	1	0	5	4	3	0	4	0	0	1	0	1	0	1	0
295	White rice,enriched,ckd,salted 1/2 cup	3.2 oz	100	1	1	1	1	0	0	0	0	0	3	0	0	1	0	1	0	1	0
296	White rice,enriched,ckd,no salt 1/2 cup	3.2 oz	100	1	1	2	1	0	0	0	0	0	0	0	0	1	0	1	0	1	1
297	Wild rice,raw 1/2 cup	3.0 oz	300	3	4	4	2	N	0	0	0	0	0	0	0	5	6	N	0	4	2
Tortillas and Sopapillas																					
298	Tortilla,corn 1 6-inch	1.1 oz	110	1	1	2	4	0	0	0	0	0	1	0	0	1	0	1	0	1	1
299	Tortilla,white wheat flour 1 8-inch	1.3 oz	90	1	1	1	1	0	0	0	0	0	1	0	0	2	1	0	1	1	0

300 Sopapilla,vegetable fat 1 sopapilla	1.0 oz	90	1	0	1	1	0	1	1	1	0	1	0	0	1	1	0	0	1	0
301 Sopapilla,lard 1 sopapilla	1.0 oz	90	1	0	1	1	0	1	1	0	0	1	0	0	1	1	0	0	1	0
302 Sopapilla,veg fat,w honey 1 sop + 1/2 tbsp honey	1.3 oz	110	1	0	2	1	2	1	0	0	0	1	0	0	1	0	0	0	0	0
Spreads																				
303 Apple butter 1 tablespoon	.6 oz	30	0	0	1	0	2	0	0	0	0	0	0	0	0	0	0	0	0	0
304 Butter 2 teaspoons	.4 oz	70	1	0	0	0	0	2	5	0	1	1	1	0	0	0	0	0	0	0
305 Butter,unsalted 2 teaspoons	.4 oz	70	1	0	0	0	0	2	5	0	1	0	1	0	0	0	0	0	0	0
306 Marg:butter blend,60:40 2 teaspoons	.4 oz	70	1	0	0	0	0	2	2	2	0	1	1	0	0	0	0	0	0	0
307 Margarine,diet 2 teaspoons	.4 oz	40	0	0	0	0	0	1	1	1	0	1	1	0	0	0	0	0	0	0
308 Margarine,hard,p/s=1.5 2 teaspoons	.4 oz	70	1	0	0	0	0	2	1	2	0	1	1	0	0	0	0	0	0	0
309 Margarine,soft,p/s=2.0 2 teaspoons	.4 oz	70	1	0	0	0	0	2	1	3	0	1	1	0	0	0	0	0	0	0
310 Margarine,soft,p/s = 2.0 1 teaspoon	.2 oz	40	0	0	0	0	0	1	1	1	0	1	1	0	0	0	0	0	0	0
311 Margarine,safflower bar,p/s=2.5 2 teaspoons	.4 oz	70	1	0	0	0	0	2	1	3	0	1	1	0	0	0	0	0	0	0
312 Margarine,safflwr,soft,p/s=4.0 2 teaspoons	.4 oz	70	1	0	0	0	0	2	1	4	0	1	1	0	0	0	0	0	0	0
313 Margarine,soft,unsalted,p/s=1.7 2 teaspoons	.4 oz	70	1	0	0	0	0	2	1	2	0	0	1	0	0	0	0	0	0	0
314 Margarine,whipped,p/s=2.0 2 teaspoons	.2 oz	40	0	0	0	0	0	1	1	2	0	1	1	0	0	0	0	0	0	0
315 Honey 1 tablespoon	.7 oz	60	1	0	1	0	3	0	0	0	0	0	0	0	0	0	0	0	0	0

continued

Breads, Pastas, and Grain Products

										NUTRI–UNITS											
No.	Name/Portion Size		KCAL	CAL	PRO	CAR	FIB	SUG	FAT	SFA	PFA	CHL	SOD	A	C	THI	RIB	B6	CA	IRN	ZN
316	Jam,jelly and preserves 1 tablespoon	.7 oz	60	1	0	1	0	3	0	0	0	0	0	0	0	0	0	0	0	0	0
317	Jelly,lo cal 1 tablespoon	.7 oz	20	0	0	0	0	1	0	0	0	0	0	0	0	0	0	0	0	0	0
318	Marmalade 1 tablespoon	.7 oz	50	1	0	1	0	3	0	0	0	0	0	0	0	0	0	0	0	0	0
319	Mayonnaise 1 tablespoon	.5 oz	100	1	0	0	0	0	3	1	5	1	1	0	0	0	0	1	0	0	0
320	Mayonnaise,imitation,lo cal 1 tablespoon	.5 oz	30	0	0	0	0	0	1	0	1	0	1	0	0	0	0	0	0	0	0
321	Mayo type salad dressing 1 tablespoon	.5 oz	60	1	0	0	0	0	1	1	2	0	1	0	0	0	0	0	0	0	0
322	Mayo type sal drs,lo cal,lo sod 1 tablespoons	.5 oz	20	0	0	0	0	N	1	0	1	0	0	0	0	0	0	0	0	0	0
323	Mustard,brown 1 teaspoon	.2 oz	10	0	0	0	0	0	0	0	0	0	1	0	0	0	0	0	0	0	0
324	Mustard,yellow,prepared 1 teaspoon	.2 oz	0	0	0	0	0	0	0	0	0	0	1	0	0	0	0	0	0	0	0
325	Peanut butter,old fashioned 2 tablespoons	1.1 oz	180	2	3	0	2	0	5	4	2	0	1	0	0	0	0	1	0	1	1
326	P-nut butr,smal amt fat,sug,slt 2 tablespoons	1.1 oz	180	2	2	0	2	0	4	2	4	0	2	0	0	0	0	1	0	1	1
327	P-nut butr,mod amt fat,sug,salt 2 tablespoons	1.1 oz	180	2	2	0	2	0	5	3	4	0	2	0	0	0	0	1	0	1	1
328	P-nut butter,no salt 2 tablespoons	1.1 oz	180	2	2	0	2	0	4	2	4	0	0	0	0	0	0	1	0	1	1
329	Tahini,sesame butter 2 tablespoons	1.1 oz	180	2	2	0	4	N	5	2	6	0	0	0	0	5	2	0	3	3	2

Breakfast, All Items

Beverages

330 Buttermilk,cultured 1 8-oz glass	8.5 oz	100	1	2	1	0	2	1	1	0	1	3	0	1	1	4	1	6	0	1
331 Cafe almond or cafe mocha 1 8-oz cup	8.5 oz	80	1	0	1	0	2	0	0	0	0	0	0	0	0	0	0	0	0	0
332 Cafe capri or cafe viennese 1 8-oz cup	8.5 oz	60	1	0	1	0	2	0	0	0	0	0	0	0	0	0	0	0	0	0
333 Chocolate milk,2 percent fat 1 8-oz glass	8.8 oz	180	2	2	2	0	5	2	3	0	1	2	2	1	1	5	1	6	1	1
334 Chocolate milk,3.5 percent fat 1 8-oz glass	8.8 oz	210	2	2	2	0	5	3	5	0	2	1	1	1	1	5	1	6	1	1
335 Coffee,black,reg,inst or decaf 1 8-oz cup	8.5 oz	0	0	0	0	0	0	0	0	0	0	0	0	0	0	0	0	0	0	0
336 Egg nog,non alcoholic 1 8-oz glass	8.7 oz	340	3	3	2	0	6	6	9	0	10	1	3	2	1	6	1	6	1	2
337 Hot chocolate or cocoa 1 8-oz cup	8.8 oz	210	2	2	2	0	5	3	5	0	2	1	1	1	1	5	1	6	1	1
338 Instant breakfast, dry 1 serving	1.2 oz	120	1	2	1	N	4	0	0	0	0	1	4	18	2	1	0	2	5	N
339 Milk,skim 1 8-oz glass	8.6 oz	90	1	3	1	0	2	0	0	0	0	1	2	1	1	4	1	6	0	1
340 Milk,skim 1/2 cup	4.3 oz	40	0	1	0	0	1	0	0	0	0	1	1	0	1	2	0	3	0	1
341 Milk,1 percent fat,a+d fort 1 8-oz glass	8.7 oz	110	1	3	1	0	2	1	1	0	1	1	2	1	1	5	1	6	0	1
342 Milk,1 percent fat,a+d fort 1/2 cup	4.3 oz	50	1	1	0	0	1	0	1	0	0	1	1	0	1	3	1	3	0	1
343 Milk,2 percent fat,a+d fort 1 8-oz glass	8.7 oz	130	1	3	1	0	2	1	3	0	1	1	2	1	1	5	1	6	0	1
344 Milk,2 percent fat,a+d fort 1/2 cup	4.3 oz	60	1	1	0	0	1	1	1	0	1	1	1	0	1	3	1	3	0	1

continued

Breakfast, All Items

No.	Name/Portion Size		KCAL	CAL	PRO	CAR	FIB	SUG	FAT	SFA	PFA	CHL	SOD	A	C	THI	RIB	B6	CA	IRN	ZN
			NUTRI–UNITS																		
345	Milk,whole,3.5 percent fat 1 8-oz glass	8.6 oz	150	1	2	1	0	2	2	5	0	2	1	1	1	1	5	1	6	0	1
346	Milk,whole,3.5 percent fat 1/2 cup	4.3 oz	80	1	1	0	0	1	1	2	0	1	1	1	0	1	2	1	3	0	1
347	Ovaltine mix, dry 1 serving package	.7 oz	80	1	0	0	0	1	1	1	1	0	2	9	9	9	9	0	2	3	0
348	Orange juice 1 6-oz glass	6.6 oz	80	1	0	1	0	4	0	0	0	0	0	1	24	2	0	1	0	0	0
349	Tomato juice 1 6-oz glass	6.5 oz	40	0	1	1	0	1	0	0	0	0	4	6	10	1	1	1	0	2	0
350	Postum 1 8-oz cup	8.5 oz	20	0	0	0	0	0	0	0	0	0	0	0	0	1	0	0	0	1	0
351	Tea,instant or regular 1 8-oz cup	8.5 oz	10	0	0	0	0	0	0	0	0	0	0	0	0	0	0	0	0	0	0
Breads, Rolls and Pastries																					
352	Bagel 1 3-in diam	1.9 oz	170	2	2	2	2	0	0	0	0	1	2	0	0	3	2	0	0	2	0
353	Biscuit w sausage gravy 2.5-oz bisc,1/4 c gravy	4.9 oz	330	3	2	3	2	0	5	4	2	1	7	0	0	4	3	0	4	2	1
354	Cheese danish roll 3 3/4 in diam × 1 in	2.0 oz	240	2	1	2	1	2	4	3	1	2	2	1	0	0	0	0	1	1	1
355	Cinnamon roll (veg fat) 3 3/4 in diam × 2 in	4.0 oz	370	4	2	4	3	4	3	2	2	0	4	1	0	4	3	0	1	2	1
356	Corn fritter 2 in diam × 1/2 in	1.2 oz	130	1	1	1	1	N	2	2	1	2	2	1	0	1	1	1	0	1	0
357	Danish pastry 4 1/4 in diam × 1 in	2.3 oz	270	3	1	2	2	2	5	4	3	3	2	1	0	2	2	0	1	1	1
358	Doughnut,cake,plain 3 1/4 in diam × 1 in	1.5 oz	160	2	1	2	1	2	2	2	2	2	2	0	0	1	1	0	0	1	0
359	Doughnut,cake,cinnamon 3 1/4 in diam × 1 in	1.5 oz	170	2	0	2	1	2	3	2	2	1	2	0	0	1	1	0	0	0	0

360 Doughnut,cake w choc icing 3 1/4 in diam × 1 in	1.5 oz	200	2	1	1	1	2	4	3	2	0	1	0	0	1	1	0	0	1	0
361 Doughnut,cake w sugar icing 3 1/4 in diam × 1 in	1.5 oz	170	2	1	2	1	2	2	3	2	0	1	0	0	1	1	0	0	1	0
362 Doughnut,raised,plain 3 3/4 in diam × 1 1/4 in	1.5 oz	170	2	1	1	1	2	3	3	2	1	1	0	0	1	1	0	0	1	0
363 Doughnut,raised,glazed 3 3/4 in diam × 1 1/4 in	1.5 oz	170	2	1	1	1	2	3	2	2	1	1	0	0	1	1	0	0	1	0
364 English muffin 3 1/4 in diam × 1 in	2.0 oz	140	1	1	2	2	1	0	0	0	0	3	0	0	3	3	0	2	2	1
365 Croissant 1 medium, 2 oz	1.9 oz	220	2	1	2	1	1	4	4	4	1	3	0	0	4	2	0	0	1	1
366 French toast,plain 2 slices bread + egg mix	3.7 oz	260	3	3	2	1	1	4	3	2	13	4	2	0	2	2	1	1	2	1
367 French toast,butter + syrup 2 sl tst,2 tsp,2 tbsp	5.4 oz	430	4	3	4	1	6	6	7	2	15	5	3	0	2	2	1	2	2	1
368 French toast,soft marg. + syrup 2 sl tst,2 tsp,2 tbsp	5.4 oz	430	4	3	4	1	6	6	4	5	13	5	3	0	2	2	1	2	2	1
369 French toast w soft margarine 2 slices w 2 tsp marg	4.0 oz	330	3	3	2	1	1	6	4	5	13	5	3	0	2	2	1	1	2	1
370 Granola bar 1 oz bar	1.0 oz	130	1	1	1	3	1	1	1	2	1	1	0	0	1	0	1	0	1	1
371 Grits with 1/2 tbsp butter 1/2 cup	4.3 oz	210	2	1	2	3	0	3	5	0	2	6	2	0	2	1	0	0	1	0
372 Honey cinnamon bun 3 3/4 in diam × 1 in	1.9 oz	170	2	1	2	1	2	2	1	0	0	2	0	0	0	1	0	1	0	0
373 Pancake,buckwheat w egg 4 in diam × 3/8 in	1.2 oz	70	1	1	1	1	0	1	1	0	2	2	0	0	1	1	1	2	1	0
374 Pancake from mix,no egg 4 in diam × 3/8 in	1.2 oz	70	1	1	1	1	0	1	1	0	0	2	0	0	1	1	0	2	0	0
375 Pancake from mix,with egg 4 in diam × 3/8 in	1.2 oz	80	1	1	1	1	0	1	1	0	2	2	0	0	1	1	0	2	0	0
376 Pancake,homemade 4 in diam × 3/8 in	1.2 oz	80	1	1	1	1	0	1	1	0	1	1	0	0	1	1	0	1	1	0

continued

Breakfast, All Items

No.	Name/Portion Size		KCAL	CAL	PRO	CAR	FIB	SUG	FAT	SFA	PFA	CHL	SOD	A	C	THI	RIB	B6	CA	IRN	ZN
											NUTRI–UNITS										
377	Pancake,unenriched mix,no egg 4 in diam × 3/8 in	1.2 oz	70	1	1	1	1	0	1	1	0	0	2	0	0	0	1	0	2	0	0
378	Pancakes w hard marg. + syrup 3 4-in cks,1 tbsp,2 tbsp	6.2 oz	370	4	2	3	1	4	6	3	3	5	8	3	0	2	2	1	3	1	0
379	Poptart,strawberry 3 in × 4 1/2 in	1.8 oz	210	2	1	3	1	4	2	0	0	0	2	2	0	2	2	2	2	2	0
380	Super donut,fortified 2 oz	2.0 oz	250	3	2	2	2	2	4	0	0	0	3	4	8	4	2	0	2	5	0
381	Sweet roll 3 3/4 in diam × 1 in	1.9 oz	170	2	1	2	2	2	2	1	0	0	2	0	0	1	1	0	1	0	0
382	Toast,white,enriched 2 slices (18 per lb)	1.6 oz	140	1	1	2	1	1	0	0	0	0	3	0	0	2	1	0	1	2	0
383	Toast,whole wheat 2 slices (18 per lb)	1.6 oz	130	1	2	2	3	1	0	0	0	0	3	0	0	1	1	1	1	2	1
384	Toast,raisin bread 2 slices (18 per lb)	1.5 oz	130	1	1	2	2	2	0	0	0	0	2	0	0	2	1	0	1	2	0
385	Waffle,enriched 4 1/2 in square × 5/8 in	1.8 oz	140	1	1	1	1	1	1	1	1	4	2	1	0	2	2	0	1	1	1
386	Waffle,frozen 4 5/8 × 3 3/4 × 5/8 in	1.2 oz	90	1	1	1	1	0	1	0	0	3	2	0	0	1	1	0	1	1	0
387	Waffle from mix,no egg yolk 4 1/2 in square × 5/8 in	1.8 oz	150	2	1	1	1	1	2	1	0	0	3	0	0	1	1	0	1	1	0
388	Waffle w syrup + 1/2 tbsp but 5×3×5/8 in +1.5 oz syrup	2.3 oz	200	2	1	2	1	3	2	3	0	4	3	1	0	1	1	1	1	1	0
Cereals, Ready to Eat																					
389	All bran 1 oz (1/2 cup)	1.0 oz	70	1	1	1	8	1	0	0	0	0	3	5	5	5	5	5	0	5	5
390	Alpha bits 1 oz (1 cup)	1.0 oz	110	1	1	2	2	2	0	0	0	0	2	5	0	5	5	5	0	3	2
391	Apple jacks 1 oz (1 cup)	1.0 oz	110	1	0	2	1	3	0	0	0	0	1	5	5	5	5	5	0	5	5

392 Bran buds 1 oz (1/3 cup)	1.0 oz	70	1	1	1	8	1	0	0	0	0	2	5	5	5	5	5	0	5	5
393 Bran chex 1 oz (1/2 cup)	1.0 oz	90	1	1	2	5	1	0	0	0	0	3	0	5	5	2	5	0	5	2
394 Bran flakes,40 percent 1 oz (2/3 cup)	1.0 oz	90	1	1	2	5	1	0	0	0	0	2	5	0	5	5	5	0	5	5
395 Captain crunch 1 oz (3/4 cup)	1.0 oz	120	1	0	2	2	2	1	2	0	0	2	0	0	7	6	8	0	8	4
396 Captain crunch crunchberries 1 oz (3/4 cup)	1.0 oz	120	1	0	2	2	2	1	1	0	0	2	0	0	6	6	7	0	8	4
397 Captn crunch p-nut buttr cereal 1 oz (3/4 cup)	1.0 oz	120	1	1	1	2	2	1	1	1	0	2	0	0	6	7	8	0	8	4
398 Cheerios 1 oz (1 1/4 cup)	1.0 oz	110	1	1	1	2	0	1	0	1	0	3	5	5	5	5	5	1	5	1
399 Cocoa krispies 1 oz (1 cup)	1.0 oz	110	1	0	2	1	2	0	0	0	0	2	5	5	5	5	5	0	2	2
400 Cocoa pebbles,rice 1 oz (.8 cup)	1.0 oz	110	1	0	2	1	2	0	0	0	0	1	5	0	5	5	5	0	2	2
401 Cocoa pops 1 oz	1.0 oz	110	1	1	2	1	2	0	0	0	0	2	5	5	5	5	5	0	2	0
402 Cookie crisp 1 oz (1 cup)	1.0 oz	110	1	0	2	0	2	0	0	0	0	2	5	5	5	5	5	0	5	0
403 Corn bran 1 oz (1 cup)	1.0 oz	100	1	1	2	6	1	0	0	0	0	2	0	0	4	6	7	1	11	4
404 Corn chex 1 oz (1 cup)	1.0 oz	110	1	1	2	4	0	0	0	0	0	3	1	5	5	1	5	0	2	0
405 Corn flakes 1 oz (1 to 1.3 cup)	1.0 oz	110	1	1	2	3	0	0	0	0	0	4	5	5	5	5	5	0	2	0
406 Corn flakes,lo sod,unfortified 1 oz (1 to 1.3 cup)	1.0 oz	110	1	1	2	3	0	0	0	0	0	0	0	0	0	1	0	0	1	0
407 Corny snaps 1 oz (1 cup)	1.0 oz	120	1	1	2	2	3	0	0	0	0	2	5	5	5	5	5	0	2	0
408 Count chocula 1 oz (1 cup)	1.0 oz	110	1	1	2	1	2	0	0	0	0	2	5	5	5	5	5	0	2	0

continued

Breakfast, All Items

No.	Name/Portion Size		KCAL	CAL	PRO	CAR	FIB	SUG	FAT	SFA	PFA	CHL	SOD	A	C	THI	RIB	B6	CA	IRN	ZN
									NUTRI–UNITS												
409	Crisp rice,low sodium 1 oz (1 cup)	1.0 oz	110	1	0	2	1	0	0	0	0	0	0	0	0	0	1	0	0	1	1
410	CW Post family cereal 1 oz (1/4 cup)	1.0 oz	130	1	1	1	2	2	1	3	0	0	0	5	0	5	5	5	0	5	1
411	Crispy wheats n raisins 1 oz (2/3 cup)	1.0 oz	100	1	1	2	2	2	0	0	0	0	1	5	0	5	5	5	1	5	0
412	CW Post family cereal w raisins 1 oz (1/4 cup)	1.0 oz	120	1	1	1	1	2	1	3	0	0	0	5	0	5	5	5	0	5	1
413	Fortified oat flakes 1 oz (2/3 cup)	1.0 oz	100	1	2	1	3	1	0	0	0	0	3	5	0	5	5	5	1	9	1
414	Froot loops 1 oz (1 cup)	1.0 oz	110	1	1	2	1	3	0	0	0	0	1	5	5	5	5	5	0	5	5
415	Frosted miniwheats 1 oz (4 pieces)	1.0 oz	100	1	1	2	3	1	0	0	0	0	0	5	5	5	5	5	0	2	2
416	Frosted rice 1 oz (0.8 cup)	1.0 oz	110	1	0	2	1	2	0	0	0	0	2	5	5	5	5	5	0	2	0
417	Fruity pebbles 1 oz (7/8 cup)	1.0 oz	110	1	0	2	1	2	0	0	0	0	2	5	0	5	5	5	0	2	2
418	Golden grahams 1 oz (3/4 cup)	1.0 oz	110	1	0	2	2	2	0	1	0	0	3	5	5	5	5	5	0	5	0
419	Granola, homemade 1 oz (1/4 cup)	1.0 oz	140	1	1	1	3	1	2	1	4	0	0	0	0	2	1	1	0	1	1
420	Granola,nature valley 1 oz (1/4 cup)	1.0 oz	130	1	1	1	3	1	1	3	1	0	1	0	0	1	1	0	0	1	1
421	Grapenuts 1 oz (1/4 cup)	1.0 oz	100	1	1	2	3	0	0	0	0	0	2	5	0	5	5	5	0	1	1
422	Grapenut flakes 1 oz (7/8 cup)	1.0 oz	100	1	1	2	3	1	0	0	0	0	2	5	0	5	5	5	0	9	1
423	Heartland natural(oat+wht germ) 1 oz (1/4 cup)	1.0 oz	120	1	1	1	3	0	1	N	N	0	1	0	0	1	0	0	0	1	1

424 Heartland natural w raisins 1 oz (1/2 cup)	1.0 oz	120	1	1	1	3	1	1	N	N	0	1	0	0	1	0	1	0	1	1
425 Honeybran 1 oz (0.8 cup)	1.0 oz	100	1	1	2	8	1	0	0	0	0	2	5	5	5	5	5	0	5	1
426 Honeycomb 1 oz (1 1/3 cup)	1.0 oz	110	1	0	2	1	2	0	0	0	0	2	5	0	5	5	5	0	3	2
427 Honeynut cheerios 1 oz (7/8 cup)	1.0 oz	110	1	1	2	2	1	0	0	0	0	3	5	5	5	5	5	0	5	1
428 Honey nut cornflakes 1 oz (1 cup)	1.0 oz	110	1	1	2	3	1	0	0	0	0	2	5	5	5	5	5	0	2	0
429 King vitamin 1 oz (3/4 cup)	1.0 oz	110	1	0	2	3	1	0	1	0	0	2	13	15	16	17	16	0	19	0
430 Kix 1 oz (1 cup)	1.0 oz	110	1	1	2	3	0	0	0	0	0	3	5	5	5	5	5	1	9	0
431 Life 1 oz (2/3 cup)	1.0 oz	100	1	2	1	3	1	0	0	0	0	1	0	N	8	7	1	2	8	1
432 Lucky charm 1 oz	1.0 oz	110	1	1	2	2	2	0	0	0	0	2	5	5	5	5	5	1	5	1
433 Most 1 oz (1/2 cup)	1.0 oz	90	1	1	1	6	1	0	0	0	0	1	20	20	20	20	20	1	20	2
434 Mueslix 1 oz (1/2 cup)	1.0 oz	140	1	1	2	3	N	0	0	0	0	1	5	0	5	5	5	0	5	5
435 Nutri-grain barley 1 oz (2/3 cup)	1.0 oz	100	1	1	2	3	0	0	0	0	0	2	5	5	5	5	5	0	1	5
436 Nutri-grain corn 1 oz (2/3 cup)	1.0 oz	110	1	1	2	3	0	0	0	0	0	2	5	5	5	5	5	0	1	5
437 Nutri-grain rye 1 oz (2/3 cup)	1.0 oz	100	1	1	2	3	0	0	0	0	0	2	5	5	5	5	5	0	1	5
438 Nutri-grain wheat 1 oz (2/3 cup)	1.0 oz	100	1	1	2	3	0	0	0	0	0	2	5	5	5	5	5	0	1	5
439 Oat bran, dry 1/3 cup dry	1.0 oz	120	1	2	1	8	0	1	1	1	0	0	0	0	1	0	N	1	0	2
440 Pep wheat flakes 1 oz (1 cup)	1.0 oz	110	1	1	2	3	1	0	0	0	0	2	5	5	5	5	5	0	2	2

continued

Breakfast, All Items

No.	Name/Portion Size		KCAL	CAL	PRO	CAR	FIB	SUG	FAT	SFA	PFA	CHL	SOD	A	C	THI	RIB	B6	CA	IRN	ZN
										NUTRI–UNITS											
441	Post toasties 1 oz (1¼ cup)	1.0 oz	110	1	1	2	3	0	0	0	0	0	3	5	0	5	5	5	0	2	0
442	Product 19 1 oz (1 cup)	1.0 oz	110	1	1	2	3	1	0	0	0	0	3	20	20	20	20	20	0	20	1
443	Puffed rice 1 oz (2 cups)	1.0 oz	110	1	1	2	1	0	0	0	0	0	0	0	0	0	0	0	0	0	0
444	Puffed rice,fortified 1 oz (2 cups)	1.0 oz	110	1	1	2	1	0	0	0	0	0	0	0	0	10	6	0	0	10	0
445	Puffed wheat 1 oz (2 cups)	1.0 oz	100	1	1	2	4	0	0	0	0	0	0	0	0	1	1	0	0	1	1
446	Quisp 1 oz (1.2 cup)	1.0 oz	120	1	0	2	2	2	1	1	0	0	2	0	0	7	8	8	0	7	0
447	Raisin bran,iron fort. 1 oz (½ cup)	1.0 oz	90	1	1	1	6	2	0	0	0	0	2	4	0	4	4	4	0	14	4
448	Raisins rice n rye 1 oz (⅔ cup)	1.0 oz	90	1	0	2	2	3	0	0	0	0	2	4	0	4	4	4	0	4	4
449	Rice chex 1 oz (1⅛ cup)	1.0 oz	110	1	0	2	1	0	0	0	0	0	2	0	5	5	0	5	0	2	1
450	Rice krispies 1 oz (1 cup)	1.0 oz	110	1	1	2	1	0	0	0	0	0	3	5	5	5	5	5	0	2	1
451	Special K 1 oz (0.7 cup)	1.0 oz	110	1	2	1	2	0	0	0	0	0	3	5	5	5	5	5	0	5	5
452	Sugar smacks 1 oz (1 cup)	1.0 oz	100	1	1	2	1	3	0	0	0	0	1	5	5	5	5	5	0	2	0
453	Sugar corn pops 1 oz (1 cup)	1.0 oz	110	1	0	2	1	3	0	0	0	0	1	5	5	5	5	5	0	2	2
454	Sugar frosted flakes 1 oz (1.3 cup)	1.0 oz	110	1	0	2	1	2	0	0	0	0	2	5	5	5	5	5	0	2	0
455	Shredded wheat 1 biscuit 2 × 2.5 in	.8 oz	80	1	1	1	3	0	0	0	0	0	0	0	0	1	1	1	0	1	1

456 Super sugar crisp 1 oz (0.8 cup)	1.0 oz	110	1	1	2	1	3	0	0	0	0	0	5	0	5	5	5	0	2	2
457 Trix 1 oz (1 cup)	1.0 oz	110	1	0	2	2	2	0	0	0	0	2	5	5	5	5	5	0	5	0
458 Team 1 oz (2/3 cup)	1.0 oz	110	1	1	2	1	1	0	0	0	0	2	5	5	5	5	5	0	2	1
459 Tasteeos 1 oz (1 cup)	1.0 oz	110	1	1	2	3	0	0	0	0	0	2	5	5	5	5	5	0	5	1
460 Total 1 oz (7/8 cup)	1.0 oz	100	1	1	2	3	0	0	0	0	0	3	20	20	20	20	20	5	20	1
461 Waffelos 1 oz (1cup)	1.0 oz	110	1	0	2	2	3	0	0	0	0	1	5	5	5	5	5	0	5	0
462 Wheaties 1 oz (1 cup)	1.0 oz	100	1	1	2	3	0	0	0	0	0	3	5	5	5	5	5	1	5	1
463 Wheat chex 1 oz (2/3 cup)	1.0 oz	100	1	1	2	3	0	0	0	0	0	2	0	5	5	1	5	0	5	1
464 Wheat germ w brown sugar+honey 1 oz (1/4 cup)	1.0 oz	110	1	2	1	2	1	1	0	1	0	0	0	0	5	2	2	0	2	5
465 Wheat germ 1/4 cup (4 tablespoons)	1.0 oz	110	1	3	1	3	0	1	0	2	0	0	0	1	6	3	3	0	3	6
466 Wheat n raisin chex 1 oz (1/2 cup)	1.0 oz	100	1	1	2	2	2	0	0	0	0	2	0	0	4	4	4	0	4	1
Cooked Cereals																				
467 Bulgur,cnd 1 cup	4.8 oz	230	2	3	3	2	1	0	0	0	0	8	0	0	1	0	3	1	2	0
468 Corn grits,ckd w salt 1/2 cup	4.3 oz	70	1	1	1	3	N	0	0	0	0	3	0	0	2	1	0	0	1	0
469 Corn grits,ckd,no salt 1/2 cup	4.3 oz	70	1	1	1	3	N	0	0	0	0	0	0	0	2	1	0	0	1	0
470 Cornmeal,enr,ckd w salt 1/2 cup	4.2 oz	60	1	0	1	N	N	0	0	0	0	1	0	0	1	1	0	0	1	0
471 Cream of wheat,reg,ckd w salt 3/4 cup	6.6 oz	120	1	1	2	1	0	0	0	0	0	3	0	0	3	0	0	1	10	0

continued

Breakfast, All Items

No.	Name/Portion Size		KCAL	CAL	PRO	CAR	FIB	SUG	FAT	SFA	PFA	CHL	SOD	A	C	THI	RIB	B6	CA	IRN	ZN
			NUTRI–UNITS																		
472	Farina,enr,ckd w no salt 3/4 cup	6.5 oz	90	1	1	1	1	0	0	0	0	0	0	0	0	2	1	0	0	1	0
473	Farina,enr,ckd w salt 3/4 cup	6.5 oz	90	1	1	1	1	0	0	0	0	0	6	0	0	2	1	0	0	1	0
474	Farina,unenr,ckd w salt 3/4 cup	6.5 oz	90	1	1	1	1	0	0	0	0	0	6	0	0	0	0	0	0	0	0
475	Oat cereal,inst,fort,ckd,w salt 1 packet	6.2 oz	100	1	1	1	4	0	1	0	0	0	3	6	0	7	3	7	3	7	1
476	Oatmeal,ckd w salt 1 cup	8.5 oz	150	1	2	2	5	0	1	0	1	0	4	0	0	3	1	0	0	2	2
477	Oatmeal,ckd,no salt 1 cup	8.5 oz	150	1	2	2	5	0	1	0	1	0	0	0	0	3	1	0	0	2	2
478	Rice cereal,ckd w salt 1 cup	8.6 oz	130	1	1	2	1	0	0	0	0	0	4	0	0	0	0	1	0	1	2
479	Wheat cereal,instant,ckd w salt 1 cup	8.6 oz	140	1	2	2	1	N	0	0	0	0	6	0	0	0	1	0	0	2	2
Fruits																					
480	Banana $8^{3/4} \times 1^{3/8}$ inch	4.2 oz	110	1	0	2	4	4	0	0	0	0	0	0	4	1	1	7	0	0	0
481	Grapefruit 1/2 gpft (3 1/2 in diam)	3.4 oz	30	0	0	1	1	1	0	0	0	0	0	0	11	0	0	0	0	0	0
482	Orange 1 orange 2 5/8 in diam	4.6 oz	60	1	0	1	3	3	0	0	0	0	0	1	25	2	1	1	1	0	0
Meats or Eggs[a]																					
483	Bacon,crisp 2 slices (20/lb)	.5 oz	80	1	1	0	0	N	2	2	1	1	2	0	2	1	0	0	0	0	1
484	Canadian bacon,ckd 1 sl (3 3/8 in dia × 3/16)	.7 oz	40	0	2	0	0	0	1	1	0	1	3	0	2	2	0	1	0	0	0
485	Egg,fried,low fat 1 large	1.6 oz	80	1	2	0	0	0	2	2	1	14	1	1	0	0	1	1	1	1	1

486 Egg,hard cooked 1 large	1.8 oz	80	1	2	0	0	0	2	2	1	14	1	1	0	0	2	1	1	1	1
487 Egg,omelet 1 large egg	2.3 oz	100	1	2	0	0	0	2	3	1	13	2	1	0	1	2	1	1	1	1
488 Egg,omelet,with ham 1 large egg,1/2 tbsp ham	2.4 oz	160	2	2	0	0	0	4	6	1	16	2	4	0	1	2	1	1	2	1
489 Egg,poached 1 large	1.8 oz	80	1	2	0	0	0	2	2	1	14	1	1	0	0	1	1	1	1	1
490 Egg,spanish omelet 2 eggs,4 tbsp sauce	5.4 oz	330	3	4	1	0	1	8	8	1	25	3	8	4	1	3	5	2	2	2
491 Egg,scrambled 1 large	2.3 oz	100	1	2	0	0	0	2	3	1	13	2	1	0	1	2	1	1	1	1
492 Egg substitute 1/4 cup	2.1 oz	100	1	2	0	0	0	2	1	3	0	1	3	0	1	3	1	1	1	1
493 Egg substitute,low fat,low chol 3.3 tbsp	1.7 oz	80	1	2	0	0	0	2	1	3	0	1	3	0	1	2	1	1	1	1
494 Ham,fried,lean only 1 sl (4 × 2.3 × 1/4 in)	1.5 oz	110	1	4	0	0	N	2	2	1	3	0	0	0	7	2	2	0	0	1
495 Pork sausage,ckd 2 links (16/lb)	1.0 oz	100	1	2	0	0	0	3	3	1	1	3	0	0	3	1	1	0	0	1
Spreads and Condiments																				
496 Butter 2 teaspoons	.4 oz	70	1	0	0	0	0	2	5	0	1	1	1	0	0	0	0	0	0	0
497 Butter,unsalted 2 teaspoons	.4 oz	70	1	0	0	0	0	2	5	0	1	0	1	0	0	0	0	0	0	0
498 Cream,light coffee 1 tablespoon	.5 oz	30	0	0	0	0	0	1	2	0	1	0	0	0	0	0	0	0	0	0
499 Cream,non-dairy,liquid 1 tablespoon	.5 oz	20	0	0	0	0	0	0	0	0	0	0	0	0	0	0	0	0	0	0
500 Cream subst,polyrich,liquid 1 tablespoon	.5 oz	20	0	0	0	N	0	0	0	1	0	0	0	0	0	0	0	0	0	0

[a]Sodium values are for unsalted eggs except Spanish omelet.
Add 0.5 nutri-unit sodium for moderate or 1 nutri-unit for heavy salting.

continued

Cooking Ingredients and Sauces

No.	Name/Portion Size		KCAL	CAL	PRO	CAR	FIB	SUG	FAT	SFA	PFA	CHL	SOD	A	C	THI	RIB	B6	CA	IRN	ZN
501	Honey 1 tablespoon	.7 oz	60	1	0	1	0	3	0	0	0	0	0	0	0	0	0	0	0	0	0
502	Jam,jelly,and preserves 1 tablespoon	.7 oz	60	1	0	1	0	3	0	0	0	0	0	0	0	0	0	0	0	0	0
503	Jelly,lo cal 1 tablespoon	.7 oz	20	0	0	0	0	1	0	0	0	0	0	0	0	0	0	0	0	0	0
504	Marg:butter blend,60:40 2 teaspoons	.4 oz	70	1	0	0	0	0	2	2	2	0	1	1	0	0	0	0	0	0	0
505	Margarine,hard 2 teaspoons	.4 oz	70	1	0	0	0	0	2	1	2	0	1	1	0	0	0	0	0	0	0
506	Margarine,soft 2 teaspoons	.4 oz	70	1	0	0	0	0	2	1	3	0	1	1	0	0	0	0	0	0	0
507	Margarine,unsalted 2 teaspoons	.4 oz	70	1	0	0	0	0	2	1	2	0	0	1	0	0	0	0	0	0	0
508	Marmalade,citrus 1 tablespoon	.7 oz	50	1	0	1	0	3	0	0	0	0	0	0	0	0	0	0	0	0	0
509	Sugar 1 teaspoon	.1 oz	20	0	0	0	0	1	0	0	0	0	0	0	0	0	0	0	0	0	0
510	Syrup,cane and maple 2 tablespoons	1.4 oz	100	1	0	2	0	5	0	0	0	0	0	0	0	0	0	0	0	0	0

Cooking Ingredients and Sauces

Chocolate/Cocoa

No.	Name/Portion Size		KCAL	CAL	PRO	CAR	FIB	SUG	FAT	SFA	PFA	CHL	SOD	A	C	THI	RIB	B6	CA	IRN	ZN
511	Chocolate,bitter or baking 1 oz square	1.0 oz	140	1	1	1	1	N	4	7	0	0	0	0	0	0	1	0	0	2	0
512	Chocolate,semisweet 1 oz square	1.0 oz	140	1	0	1	N	3	3	5	0	0	0	0	0	0	0	0	0	1	0
513	Chocolate chips,semisweet 1 cup	6.0 oz	860	9	2	7	N	19	18	31	1	0	0	0	0	0	2	0	1	5	1
514	Cocoa powder,dry 1 oz (4 tablespoons)	1.0 oz	70	1	1	1	1	N	2	3	0	0	0	0	0	0	2	N	1	3	2

515 Milk chocolate 1 oz square	1.0 oz	150	1	1	1	N	3	3	5	0	0	0	0	0	0	1	0	1	0	0
Fats and Oils																				
516 Bacon drippings 1 tablespoon	.5 oz	100	1	0	0	0	0	3	3	1	1	0	0	0	0	0	N	0	0	0
517 Beef drippings 1 tablespoon	.5 oz	110	1	0	0	0	0	4	5	0	1	0	0	0	0	0	0	0	0	0
518 Butter 1/2 cup (1 stick)	4.0 oz	810	8	0	0	0	0	28	51	3	16	9	14	0	0	0	0	1	0	0
519 Butter 1 tablespoon	.5 oz	110	1	0	0	0	0	4	7	0	2	1	2	0	0	0	0	0	0	0
520 Butter,unsalted 1/2 cup (1 stick)	4.0 oz	810	8	0	0	0	0	28	51	3	16	0	14	0	0	0	0	1	0	0
521 Lard 1/2 cup	3.6 oz	920	9	0	0	0	0	31	36	10	6	0	0	0	0	0	0	0	0	0
522 Lard 1 tablespoon	.5 oz	120	1	0	0	0	0	4	5	1	1	0	0	0	0	0	0	0	0	0
523 Marg:butter blend,60:40 1 tablespoon	.5 oz	130	1	0	0	0	0	4	5	1	1	0	0	0	0	0	0	0	0	0
524 Margarine,hard,p/s=1.5 1/2 cup	4.0 oz	810	8	0	0	0	0	27	16	26	0	11	15	0	0	0	0	1	0	0
525 Margarine,hard,p/s=1.5 1 tablespoon	.5 oz	110	1	0	0	0	0	4	2	3	0	1	2	0	0	0	0	0	0	0
526 Margarine,bar,unsalted,p/s=1.5 1 tablespoon	.5 oz	110	1	0	0	0	0	4	2	3	0	0	2	0	0	0	0	0	0	0
527 Margarine,soft,p/s=2 1/2 cup	4.0 oz	810	8	0	0	0	0	27	14	32	0	12	15	0	0	0	0	1	0	0
528 Margarine,soft,p/s=2 1 tablespoon	.5 oz	110	1	0	0	0	0	4	2	4	0	2	2	0	0	0	0	0	0	0
529 Margarine,whipped,p/s=2 1 tablespoon	.3 oz	60	1	0	0	0	0	2	1	3	0	1	1	0	0	0	0	0	0	0
530 Oil, coconut 1 tablespoon	.5 oz	120	1	0	0	0	0	4	11	0	0	0	0	0	0	0	0	0	0	0

continued

Cooking Ingredients and Sauces

No.	Name/Portion Size		KCAL	CAL	PRO	CAR	FIB	SUG	FAT	SFA	PFA	CHL	SOD	A	C	THI	RIB	B6	CA	IRN	ZN
										NUTRI–UNITS											
531	Oil, corn 1 tablespoon	.5 oz	120	1	0	0	0	0	4	2	7	0	0	0	0	0	0	0	0	0	0
532	Oil, cottonseed 1 tablespoon	.5 oz	120	1	0	0	0	0	4	3	7	0	0	0	0	0	0	0	0	0	0
533	Oil, olive 1 tablespoon	.5 oz	120	1	0	0	0	0	4	2	1	0	0	0	0	0	0	0	0	0	0
534	Oil, palm 1 tablespoon	.5 oz	120	1	0	0	0	0	4	6	1	0	0	0	0	0	0	0	0	0	0
535	Oil, peanut 1 tablespoon	.5 oz	120	1	0	0	0	0	4	2	4	0	0	0	0	0	0	0	0	0	0
536	Oil, safflower 1 tablespoon	.5 oz	120	1	0	0	0	0	4	1	9	0	0	0	0	0	0	0	0	0	0
537	Oil, sesame 1 tablespoon	.5 oz	120	1	0	0	0	0	4	2	5	0	0	0	0	0	0	0	0	0	0
538	Oil, soybean 1 tablespoon	.5 oz	120	1	0	0	0	0	4	2	7	0	0	0	0	0	0	0	0	0	0
539	Turkey drippings 4 tablespoons	2.0 oz	40	0	1	0	0	0	1	1	1	0	0	0	0	0	0	0	0	0	0
540	Vegetable shortening 1/2 cup	3.5 oz	900	9	0	0	0	0	30	32	17	4	0	0	0	0	0	0	0	0	0
541	Vegetable shortening 1 tablespoon	.5 oz	120	1	0	0	0	0	4	4	2	0	0	0	0	0	0	0	0	0	0
Flours, Crumbs and Dry Cereals																					
˙542	Barley,dry 1/4 cup	1.8 oz	180	2	1	3	3	0	0	0	0	0	0	0	0	1	0	1	0	1	N
543	Breadcrumbs,dry,grated 1 cup	3.5 oz	390	4	4	5	4	2	1	1	1	0	7	0	0	5	4	0	2	5	1
544	Brewers yeast 1 tablespoon	.3 oz	20	0	1	0	0	0	0	0	0	0	0	0	0	17	4	2	0	2	1
545	Buckwheat flour,light 1 cup,sifted	3.7 oz	360	4	2	6	3	0	0	0	0	0	0	0	0	1	0	3	0	1	N

546 Corn flour 1 cup	4.1 oz	430	4	3	6	7	N	1	0	1	0	0	2	0	3	1	2	0	2	1
547 Cornmeal,whole grain 1 cup	4.4 oz	440	4	4	6	18	N	1	0	2	0	0	3	0	6	2	3	0	3	3
548 Cornmeal,degermed,enriched 1 cup	4.9 oz	510	5	3	8	13	N	1	0	0	0	0	2	0	8	4	3	0	5	1
549 Cornmeal,degermed,unenriched 1 cup	4.9 oz	510	5	3	8	13	N	1	0	0	0	0	2	0	3	1	3	0	2	2
550 Cornstarch 1/4 cup	1.1 oz	120	1	0	2	0	N	0	0	0	0	0	0	0	0	0	0	0	0	0
551 Cottonseed flour 4 oz	4.0 oz	400	4	17	3	N	N	2	2	3	0	0	0	0	18	11	11	6	16	N
552 Croutons 1/4 cup	.4 oz	40	0	0	1	1	0	0	0	0	0	1	0	0	1	1	0	0	1	0
553 Farina,enriched,uncooked 2 1/2 tablespoons	1.0 oz	100	1	1	1	1	0	0	0	0	0	1	0	0	2	1	0	1	9	1
554 Graham cracker crumbs,plain 1 cup,not packed	3.0 oz	330	3	2	4	9	5	2	2	2	0	6	0	0	1	6	0	1	3	1
555 Graham cracker crumbs,sugr coat 1 cup,not packed	3.0 oz	350	3	2	5	6	5	3	2	2	0	4	0	0	1	4	0	1	3	1
556 Masa harina,enriched 1 cup	4.1 oz	430	4	3	6	7	0	1	0	2	0	0	0	0	22	11	2	5	10	3
557 Oat bran,dry 1/3 cup	1.0 oz	120	1	2	1	8	0	1	1	1	0	0	0	0	1	0	N	1	0	2
558 Oatmeal,uncooked 1 cup,dry	2.8 oz	310	3	4	4	11	0	2	1	2	0	0	0	0	8	1	1	1	4	4
559 Rice cereal,uncooked 1/3 cup	2.0 oz	210	2	1	3	1	0	0	0	0	0	0	0	0	2	1	1	0	1	3
560 Rye flour,medium 1 cup	3.1 oz	310	3	3	5	4	N	0	0	0	0	0	0	0	4	1	1	0	3	4
561 Soy flour,low fat 1 cup,stirred	3.5 oz	360	4	13	3	14	1	2	1	3	0	0	0	0	11	4	60	5	10	N
562 Vanilla wafer crumbs 1 cup,crushed	2.8 oz	370	4	1	4	1	6	4	3	1	2	2	0	0	3	2	0	1	2	0

continued

Cooking Ingredients and Sauces

No.	Name/Portion Size		KCAL	CAL	PRO	CAR	FIB	SUG	FAT	SFA	PFA	CHL	SOD	A	C	THI	RIB	B6	CA	IRN	ZN
										NUTRI–UNITS											
563	Wheat bran + sugar and vit,dry 1/4 cup	1.1 oz	80	1	1	2	9	1	0	0	1	0	3	5	5	5	5	1	0	5	2
564	Wheat cereal,uncooked 1/4 cup,dry	1.0 oz	110	1	1	2	3	0	0	0	0	0	0	0	0	1	0	0	0	1	1
565	Wheat flour,all purpose,enr 1 cup,unsifted	4.4 oz	460	5	4	7	4	1	0	0	0	0	0	0	0	11	6	1	0	6	1
566	Wheat flour,cake or pastry 1 cup,unsifted	3.9 oz	400	4	3	6	2	1	0	0	0	0	0	0	0	0	0	0	0	1	0
567	Wheat germ,crude 4 tablespoons	1.4 oz	150	1	3	1	4	1	1	1	2	0	0	0	0	11	3	3	1	4	8
568	Whole wheat flour 1/2 cup	2.1 oz	200	2	2	3	6	0	0	0	1	0	0	0	0	4	1	2	0	2	2
Gravies and Sauces																					
569	Barbecue sauce 1/4 cup	2.1 oz	50	0	0	1	0	N	0	0	0	0	5	2	1	0	0	0	0	1	0
570	Brown gravy 1/4 cup	2.1 oz	21	0	0	0	0	N	0	0	0	0	3	0	0	0	0	0	0	0	0
571	Cheese sauce 1/4 cup	2.7 oz	80	1	1	0	0	N	1	2	0	1	4	0	0	0	2	0	3	0	0
572	Chili sauce,green 2 tablespoons	1.1 oz	10	0	0	0	0	0	0	0	0	0	0	1	7	0	0	0	0	0	0
573	Chili sauce,red 2 tablespoons	1.1 oz	10	0	0	0	1	0	0	0	0	0	0	12	3	0	0	0	0	0	N
574	Chili sauce,tomato 2 tablespoons	1.1 oz	30	0	0	1	1	1	0	0	0	0	4	2	2	0	0	0	0	0	0
575	Hollandaise sauce 1/4 cup	1.8 oz	180	2	1	0	0	0	6	6	2	19	3	4	0	0	0	0	0	1	1
576	Miso,fermented soy product 1/2 cup	4.9 oz	280	3	5	3	N	N	3	1	4	0	50	0	0	2	4	3	2	4	6
577	Mushroom sauce 2 tablespoons	1.1 oz	11	0	0	0	N	N	0	0	0	0	2	0	0	0	0	0	0	0	0

578 Natto,fermented soy product ½ cup	3.1 oz	190	2	5	1	N	N	3	1	5	0	0	0	4	2	2	1	4	8	4
579 Soy sauce 2 tablespoon	1.1 oz	20	0	0	0	N	N	0	0	0	0	17	0	0	0	0	1	0	1	0
580 Spagetti sauce ½ cup	4.4 oz	140	1	1	1	4	1	2	1	1	0	6	6	5	1	1	4	1	1	0
581 Spanish sauce ½ cup	4.3 oz	40	0	1	1	2	1	0	0	0	0	6	5	3	1	1	2	0	5	1
582 Steak sauce,lee and perrins 1 tablespoon	.5 oz	20	0	0	0	0	0	0	0	0	0	1	0	0	0	1	0	0	0	0
583 Sweet and sour sauce ¼ cup	2.1 oz	60	1	0	1	0	N	0	0	0	0	1	0	0	0	0	1	0	0	0
584 Taco sauce ¼ cup	2.0 oz	40	0	0	0	1	0	1	1	1	0	3	2	2	0	0	0	0	0	0
585 Tartar sauce 2 tablespoons	1.0 oz	150	1	0	0	0	0	5	3	7	1	2	0	0	0	0	0	0	0	0
586 Tartar sauce,low calorie 2 tablespoons	1.0 oz	60	1	0	0	0	0	2	1	3	1	2	0	0	0	0	0	0	0	0
587 Teriyaki sauce 2 tablespoons	1.1 oz	30	0	1	0	0	0	0	0	0	0	11	0	0	0	0	0	0	1	0
588 Tomato catsup 2 tablespoons	1.1 oz	30	0	0	1	1	1	0	0	0	0	3	2	1	0	0	0	0	0	0
589 Tomato sauce ¼ cup	2.2 oz	20	0	0	0	1	1	0	0	0	0	4	2	3	1	0	1	0	1	0
590 White sauce,thin ¼ cup	2.2 oz	80	1	1	0	0	0	2	3	0	1	2	1	0	0	1	0	2	0	0
591 White sauce,medium ¼ cup	2.2 oz	100	1	1	0	0	0	2	4	0	2	2	1	0	0	1	0	1	0	0
592 White sauce,thick ¼ cup	2.2 oz	120	1	1	0	0	0	3	5	0	2	2	1	0	1	1	0	1	0	0
593 Worchestershire sauce 1 teaspoon	.2 oz	0	0	0	0	0	0	0	0	0	0	0	0	0	0	0	0	0	0	0

continued

Cooking Ingredients and Sauces

No.	Name/Portion Size		KCAL	CAL	PRO	CAR	FIB	SUG	FAT	SFA	PFA	CHL	SOD	A	C	THI	RIB	B6	CA	IRN	ZN
			NUTRI–UNITS																		
Nuts, Peanut Butter and Raisins[b]																					
594	Coconut,dried,sweetned,shredded ½ cup	1.7 oz	260	3	1	2	11	5	6	15	0	0	0	0	0	0	0	0	0	1	0
595	Peanut butter ½ cup	4.2 oz	710	7	9	2	9	1	18	10	16	0	7	0	0	2	2	4	1	3	5
596	Raisins ½ cup	2.5 oz	220	2	1	4	5	10	0	0	0	0	0	0	1	1	1	2	1	2	0
597	Tahini,sesame butter 1 tablespoon	.5 oz	90	1	1	0	2	0	2	1	3	0	0	0	0	2	1	0	1	1	1
598	Walnuts,chopped ½ cup	2.3 oz	400	4	4	1	3	0	11	2	22	0	0	1	0	2	1	4	0	4	2
Sugars and Syrups																					
599	Corn syrup 1 cup	11.6 oz	950	10	0	17	0	37	0	0	0	0	2	0	0	0	0	0	3	15	0
600	Honey,strained 1 cup	11.9 oz	1020	10	0	19	0	52	0	0	0	0	0	0	1	0	2	1	0	2	0
601	Molasses,blackstrap 1 cup	11.3 oz	680	7	0	12	0	35	0	0	0	0	3	0	0	5	7	6	44	57	3
602	Molasses,light 1 cup	11.3 oz	810	8	0	15	0	42	0	0	0	0	0	0	0	3	2	6	11	15	1
603	Molasses,medium 2 tablespoons	1.4 oz	90	1	0	2	0	5	0	0	0	0	0	0	0	0	1	1	2	3	0
604	Molasses,medium 1 cup	11.3 oz	740	7	0	13	0	38	0	0	0	0	1	0	0	4	5	6	19	21	1
605	Sugar,brown 1 cup	7.9 oz	840	8	0	15	0	43	0	0	0	0	1	0	0	0	1	1	4	8	0
606	Sugar,confectioners,powdered 1 cup,stirred	4.5 oz	490	5	0	9	0	25	0	0	0	0	0	0	0	0	0	0	0	0	0
607	Sugar,granulated 1 cup	7.1 oz	770	8	0	14	0	40	0	0	0	0	0	0	0	0	0	0	0	0	0

608 Sugar substitute Equivalent of 1 c sugar	.6 oz	50	1	0	1	N	0	0	0	0	0	0	0	0	0	0	0	0	0	0
Vinegar and Leavening Agents																				
609 Baking powder 1 tablespoon	.3 oz	10	0	0	0	0	0	0	0	0	0	10	0	0	0	0	0	3	0	0
610 Baking soda 1 tablespoon	.3 oz	0	0	0	0	0	0	0	0	0	0	25	0	0	0	0	0	0	0	0
611 Bakers yeast dry or compressed 1/4 oz pkg or 1 cake	.2 oz	20	0	1	0	1	0	0	0	0	0	0	0	0	2	4	1	0	1	1
612 Salt 1 teaspoon	.2 oz	0	0	0	0	0	0	0	0	0	0	23	0	0	0	0	0	0	0	0
613 Vinegar,cider or distilled 1/4 cup	2.1 oz	10	0	0	0	0	0	0	0	0	0	0	0	0	0	0	0	0	0	0

Dairy Products and Eggs

Butter and Margarine																				
614 Butter 1 large pat,2 teaspoons	.4 oz	70	1	0	0	0	0	2	5	0	1	1	1	0	0	0	0	0	0	0
615 Butter,unsalted 1 large pat,2 teaspoons	.4 oz	70	1	0	0	0	0	2	5	0	1	0	1	0	0	0	0	0	0	0
616 Marg:butter blend,60:40 1 large pat,2 teaspoons	.4 oz	70	1	0	0	0	0	2	2	2	0	1	1	0	0	0	0	0	0	0
617 Margarine,bar,p/s = 1.5 1 large pat,2 teaspoons	.4 oz	70	1	0	0	0	0	2	1	2	0	1	1	0	0	0	0	0	0	0
618 Margarine,soft,p/s = 2.0 1 large pat,2 teaspoons	.4 oz	70	1	0	0	0	0	2	1	3	0	1	1	0	0	0	0	0	0	0
619 Margarine,soft,p/s = 2.5 1 large pat,2 teaspoons	.4 oz	70	1	0	0	0	0	2	1	3	0	1	1	0	0	0	0	0	0	0
620 Margarine,bar,p/s=1.5,unsalted 1 large pat,2 teaspoons	.4 oz	70	1	0	0	0	0	2	1	2	0	0	1	0	0	0	0	0	0	0
621 Margarine,safflower,bar,p/s=2.5 1 large pat,2 teaspoons	.4 oz	70	1	0	0	0	0	2	1	3	0	1	1	0	0	0	0	0	0	0

[b]See Appetizer and Snack section for additional nuts.

continued

Dairy Products and Eggs

No.	Name/Portion Size		KCAL	CAL	PRO	CAR	FIB	SUG	FAT	SFA	PFA	CHL	SOD	A	C	THI	RIB	B6	CA	IRN	ZN
										NUTRI–UNITS											
622	Margarine,saffl,soft,p/s=4.0 1 large pat,2 teaspoons	.4 oz	70	1	0	0	0	0	2	1	4	0	1	1	0	0	0	0	0	0	0
623	Margarine,diet 1 large pat,2 teaspoons	.4 oz	40	0	0	0	0	0	1	1	1	0	1	1	0	0	0	0	0	0	0
624	Margarine,whipped,p/s = 2.0 2 teaspoons	.2 oz	40	0	0	0	0	0	1	1	2	0	1	1	0	0	0	0	0	0	0
Cheese and Cheese Products																					
625	American,brick or cheddr cheese 1 oz (1 × 1 × 1.6 in pc)	1.0 oz	100	1	2	0	0	0	2	5	0	2	2	1	0	0	1	0	4	0	1
626	American,brick or cheddr cheese 1/4 cup,shredded	1.0 oz	100	1	2	0	0	0	2	5	0	2	2	1	0	0	1	0	4	0	1
627	Brie 1 oz (1/4 of 4.5 oz pkg)	1.0 oz	90	1	2	0	0	0	2	4	0	2	2	1	0	0	2	1	1	0	1
628	Blue or roquefort cheese 1 oz (1 × 1 × 1.6 in pc)	1.0 oz	100	1	2	0	0	0	2	5	0	1	4	1	0	0	1	0	3	0	1
629	Camembert cheese 1 oz (2 × 2 × 1 in pc)	1.0 oz	80	1	2	0	0	0	2	4	0	1	2	1	0	0	2	1	2	0	1
630	Cheddar cheese,low sodium 1 oz (1 × 1 × 1.6 in pc)	1.0 oz	110	1	2	0	0	0	3	5	0	2	0	1	0	0	1	0	4	0	1
631	Cheese,ched,swiss,lofat,less salt 1 oz (1 × 1 × 1.6 in pc)	1.0 oz	80	1	2	0	0	0	1	3	0	1	1	1	0	0	1	0	4	0	1
632	Cheese spread,pasteurized,proc 1 oz (2 tbsp)	1.0 oz	80	1	1	0	0	0	2	3	0	1	4	1	0	0	1	0	3	0	1
633	Cheese,past/proc,low sodium 1 oz(2 1/2 in sq × 1/4 in	1.0 oz	100	1	2	0	0	0	3	5	0	2	0	1	0	0	1	0	3	0	1
634	Cheese spread,pasteurized,proces 1 oz (2 tbsp)	1.0 oz	80	1	1	0	0	0	2	3	0	1	4	1	0	0	1	0	3	0	1
635	Cheese product,made w corn oil 1 oz (3 1/2 in sq × 1/8)	1.0 oz	100	1	2	0	0	0	2	0	2	0	4	1	0	0	1	0	3	0	1
636	Cottage cheese,creamed 1/2 cup	3.7 oz	110	1	4	0	0	1	1	3	0	1	4	1	0	0	2	1	1	0	1

637 Cottage cheese,2 percent fat $1/2$ cup	3.7 oz	90	1	4	0	0	1	1	1	0	1	4	0	0	0	2	1	1	0	1
638 Cottage cheese,dry curd,no salt $1/2$ cup	2.8 oz	70	1	4	0	0	0	0	0	0	0	0	0	0	0	1	1	1	0	1
639 Cream cheese 1 oz (2 tbsp)	1.0 oz	100	1	1	0	0	0	3	6	0	2	1	2	0	0	1	0	0	0	0
640 Gjetost (goat milk cheese) 1 oz	1.0 oz	130	1	1	1	0	2	2	5	0	2	2	1	0	1	5	1	2	0	0
641 Light natural cheese, lo fat 1 oz (1 × 1 × 1.6 in pc)	1.0 oz	80	1	2	0	0	0	1	3	0	1	1	1	0	0	1	0	4	0	1
642 Limburger cheese 1 oz ($1\frac{7}{8}$ in sq × $1/2$)	1.0 oz	90	1	2	0	0	0	2	4	0	2	2	1	0	0	2	0	3	0	1
643 Mozzarella,whole milk 1 oz (1 × 1 × 1.6 in pc)	1.0 oz	80	1	2	0	0	0	2	3	0	1	1	1	0	0	1	0	3	0	1
644 Mozzarella,lo moist,part skim 1 oz (1 × 1 × 1.6 in pc)	1.0 oz	80	1	2	0	0	0	1	3	0	1	1	1	0	0	1	0	4	0	1
645 Neufchatel 1 oz (2 tbsp)	1.0 oz	70	1	1	0	0	0	2	4	0	1	1	1	0	0	1	0	0	0	0
646 Parmesan $1/4$ cup grated	.7 oz	80	1	2	0	0	0	2	3	0	1	3	0	0	0	1	0	5	0	1
647 Pasteurized processed cheese 1 oz ($2\frac{1}{2}$ in sq × $1/4$)	1.0 oz	90	1	2	0	0	0	2	4	0	1	3	1	0	0	1	0	3	0	1
648 Ricotta $1/2$ cup	4.4 oz	220	2	4	0	0	1	5	9	0	4	1	2	0	0	3	1	5	1	2
649 Ricotta,part skim $1/2$ cup	4.4 oz	170	2	4	0	0	1	3	6	0	3	2	2	0	0	3	0	7	1	2
650 Swiss cheese 1 oz (2 × 2 × $1/2$ in)	1.0 oz	110	1	2	0	0	0	2	4	0	2	1	1	0	0	1	0	5	0	1
651 Skim American cheese 1 oz ($3\frac{1}{2}$ in sq × $1/8$)	1.0 oz	60	1	2	0	0	0	1	3	0	0	4	0	0	0	1	0	3	0	1
Cream Products																				
652 Cream,half + half $1/2$ cup	4.3 oz	160	2	1	0	0	1	4	8	0	3	0	2	0	1	2	0	3	0	1

continued

Dairy Products and Eggs

No.	Name/Portion Size		KCAL	CAL	PRO	CAR	FIB	SUG	FAT	SFA	PFA	CHL	SOD	A	C	THI	RIB	B6	CA	IRN	ZN
										NUTRI–UNITS											
653	Cream,half + half 1 tablespoon	.5 oz	20	0	0	0	0	0	1	1	0	0	0	0	0	0	0	0	0	0	0
654	Cream,light coffee 1 tablespoon	.5 oz	30	0	0	0	0	0	1	2	0	1	0	0	0	0	0	0	0	0	0
655	Cream subst,liq,m/w cocnt oil 1 tablespoon	.5 oz	20	0	0	0	0	0	0	1	0	0	0	0	0	0	0	0	0	0	0
656	Cream subst,liq,m/w hyd veg oil 1 tablespoon	.5 oz	20	0	0	0	0	0	0	0	0	0	0	0	0	0	0	0	0	0	0
657	Cream subst,powder,coc oil 1 teaspoon	.1 oz	10	0	0	0	0	0	0	1	0	0	0	0	0	0	0	0	0	0	0
658	Cream,light whipping 1 tbsp (2 tbsp whipped)	.5 oz	40	0	0	0	0	0	1	3	0	1	0	1	0	0	0	0	0	0	0
659	Cream,heavy whipping 1 tbsp (2 tbsp whipped)	.5 oz	50	1	0	0	0	0	2	3	0	1	0	1	0	0	0	0	0	0	0
660	Sour cream 1 tbsp	.4 oz	30	0	0	0	0	0	1	1	0	0	0	0	0	0	0	0	0	0	0
661	Sour cream,imitation 1 tbsp	.5 oz	30	0	0	0	0	0	1	2	0	0	0	0	0	0	0	0	0	0	0
Eggs[c]																					
662	Egg,fried,low fat 1 large	1.6 oz	80	1	2	0	0	0	2	2	1	14	1	1	0	0	1	1	1	1	1
663	Egg,hard cooked,no salt 1 large egg	1.8 oz	80	1	2	0	0	0	2	2	1	14	1	1	0	0	2	1	1	1	1
664	Egg,omelet,salted 1 large egg	2.3 oz	100	1	2	0	0	0	2	3	1	13	2	1	0	1	2	1	1	1	1
665	Egg,omelet,with ham,salted 1 large egg,1/2 tbsp ham	2.4 oz	160	2	2	0	0	0	4	6	1	16	2	4	0	1	2	1	1	2	1
666	Egg,poached,salted 1 large egg	1.8 oz	80	1	2	0	0	0	2	2	1	14	1	1	0	0	1	1	1	1	1
667	Egg,scrambled,salted 1 large egg	2.3 oz	100	1	2	0	0	0	2	3	1	13	2	1	0	1	2	1	1	1	1

668 Egg,spanish omelet,salted 2 eggs,4 tbsp sauce	5.4 oz	330	3	4	1	0	1	8	8	1	25	3	8	4	1	3	5	2	2	2
669 Egg substitute 1/4 cup (4 tbsp)	2.1 oz	100	1	2	0	0	0	2	1	3	0	1	3	0	1	3	1	1	1	1
670 Egg substitute,low fat,low chol 3.3 tbsp	1.7 oz	40	0	2	0	0	0	0	0	1	0	1	4	0	1	2	0	1	1	1
671 Egg white,no salt 1 large (2.2 tbsp)	1.2 oz	20	0	1	0	0	0	0	0	0	0	1	0	0	0	1	0	0	0	0
672 Egg yolk,no salt 1 large	.6 oz	60	1	1	0	0	0	2	2	1	14	0	1	0	1	1	1	1	1	1
Frozen Dairy Desserts																				
673 Ice cream,regular,10% fat 1/2 cup	2.5 oz	140	1	1	1	0	3	2	4	0	2	1	1	0	0	2	0	2	0	1
674 Ice cream,lite,7% fat 1/2 cup	3.0 oz	100	1	1	1	0	3	1	3	0	N	1	1	0	0	2	0	2	0	1
675 Ice cream,rich,16% fat 1/2 cup	2.6 oz	180	2	1	1	0	3	4	7	0	3	1	2	0	0	2	0	2	0	1
676 Ice cream,soft serve,13% fat 1/2 cup	3.1 oz	190	2	1	1	0	4	3	6	0	5	1	2	0	1	3	0	2	0	1
677 Ice milk,soft serve 1/2 cup	3.1 oz	110	1	1	1	0	4	1	1	0	0	1	0	0	1	3	1	3	0	1
678 Ice milk 1/2 cup	2.3 oz	90	1	1	1	0	3	1	2	0	1	1	0	0	1	2	0	2	0	0
679 Yogurt,frozen,4% fat 1/2 cup	3.1 oz	120	1	1	1	0	4	1	2	0	1	1	1	0	1	3	1	2	0	0
680 Yogurt,frozen,2% fat 1/2 cup	3.1 oz	90	1	1	1	0	3	0	1	0	0	1	0	0	0	2	0	3	0	1
Milk Products																				
681 Buttermilk,cultured 1 cup	8.6 oz	100	1	2	1	0	2	1	1	0	1	3	0	1	1	4	1	6	0	1

[c]Sodium values are for unsalted eggs except Spanish Omelet.
Add 0.5 sodium nutri-unit for moderate or 1 nutri-unit for heavy salting per serving.

continued

Dairy Products and Eggs

No.	Name/Portion Size		KCAL	CAL	PRO	CAR	FIB	SUG	FAT	SFA	PFA	CHL	SOD	A	C	THI	RIB	B6	CA	IRN	ZN
									NUTRI–UNITS												
682	Chocolate milk,2 percent fat 1 cup	8.8 oz	180	2	2	2	0	5	2	3	0	1	2	2	1	1	5	1	6	1	1
683	Chocolate milk,whole 1 cup	8.8 oz	210	2	2	2	0	5	3	5	0	2	1	1	1	1	5	1	6	1	1
684	Condensed milk,sweetened,canned 1/2 cup	5.4 oz	490	5	4	6	0	17	4	8	0	3	2	2	1	2	7	1	9	0	2
685	Dried milk,non fat,a+d fort. 1/3 cup (dry)	.8 oz	80	1	2	1	N	2	0	0	N	0	1	2	0	1	4	N	6	0	N
686	Evaporated milk,canned 1/2 cup	4.5 oz	170	2	3	1	0	3	3	5	0	3	1	1	1	1	5	1	7	0	1
687	Evaporated skim milk,cnd,unswt 1/2 cup	4.5 oz	100	1	3	1	0	3	0	0	0	0	1	2	1	1	5	1	7	0	2
688	Goat milk 1 cup	8.6 oz	170	2	3	1	0	2	3	6	0	2	1	2	1	2	4	1	7	0	1
689	Human milk 1 cup	8.6 oz	170	2	1	1	0	3	3	4	1	2	0	2	4	0	1	0	2	0	1
690	Skim milk 1 cup	8.7 oz	90	1	3	1	0	2	0	0	0	0	1	2	1	1	4	1	6	0	1
691	Part skim milk,1 percent fat 1 cup	8.7 oz	110	1	3	1	0	2	1	1	0	1	1	2	1	1	5	1	6	0	1
692	Part skim milk,2 percent fat 1 cup	8.7 oz	130	1	3	1	0	2	1	3	0	1	1	2	1	1	5	1	6	0	1
693	Whole milk 1 cup	8.7 oz	150	2	2	1	0	2	2	5	0	2	1	1	1	1	5	1	6	0	1
694	Whole milk, low sodium 1 cup	8.6 oz	150	1	2	1	0	2	3	5	0	2	0	1	1	1	3	1	5	0	1
Yogurt																					
695	Yogurt,lo fat,plain 8 oz container	8.0 oz	140	1	4	1	0	3	1	2	0	1	2	1	1	1	6	1	8	0	3
696	Yogurt,skim w nfdm,plain 8 oz container	8.0 oz	130	1	4	1	0	3	0	0	0	0	2	0	1	1	6	1	9	0	3

697 Yogurt,whole milk,plain 8 oz container	8.0 oz	140	1	2	1	0	2	2	4	0	2	1	1	0	1	4	1	5	0	2
698 Yogurt,frozen,4% fat 1/2 cup	3.1 oz	120	1	1	1	0	4	1	2	0	1	1	1	0	1	3	1	2	0	0
699 Yogurt,frozen,2% fat 1/2 cup	3.1 oz	90	1	1	1	0	3	0	1	0	0	1	0	0	0	2	0	3	0	1
700 Yogurt,fruit,part skim milk 8 oz container	8.0 oz	230	2	3	3	1	9	1	1	0	1	1	0	0	1	5	1	7	0	2
701 Yogurt,lo fat,van,coffee,lemon 8 oz container	8.0 oz	190	2	3	2	0	6	1	2	0	1	1	0	1	1	5	1	8	0	3

Desserts and Sweets

Cakes

702 Angelfood cake,from mix 1/12 of 10-in tube cake	1.4 oz	100	1	1	2	0	4	0	0	0	0	1	0	0	0	1	0	1	0	0
703 Applesauce cake w icing 2.75 in sq × 1.5 in piece	2.2 oz	230	2	1	3	2	4	2	2	1	2	1	0	0	1	1	1	1	0	0
704 Banana cake w icing 2.5 × 2 × 2 in piece	2.2 oz	210	2	0	2	1	4	3	2	2	2	1	1	1	0	0	1	0	0	0
705 Boston cream pie m/w butter 1/12 of 8-in 2-layer cake	2.4 oz	200	2	1	2	0	3	2	3	0	5	2	1	0	1	1	1	1	1	1
706 Boston cream pie m/w veg fat 1/12 of 8-in 2-layer cake	2.4 oz	210	2	1	2	0	3	2	2	1	4	1	1	0	1	1	1	1	1	1
707 Caramel cake m/w butter 1/16 of 9-in 2-layer cake	1.9 oz	200	2	1	2	0	3	3	4	0	4	2	1	0	1	1	0	1	1	0
708 Caramel cake m/w veg fat 1/16 of 9-in 2-layer cake	1.9 oz	210	2	1	2	0	3	3	2	2	3	2	0	0	1	1	0	1	1	0
709 Caramel cake,icing,m/w butter 1/16 of 9-in 2-layer cake	2.8 oz	290	3	1	3	0	6	3	5	0	5	3	2	0	1	1	0	1	2	0
710 Caramel cake,icing,m/w veg fat 1/16 of 9-in 2-layer cake	2.8 oz	300	3	1	3	0	6	4	3	2	3	2	1	0	1	1	0	1	2	0
711 Carrot cake w cream cheese icng 2.75 in sq × 1.5 in piece	2.3 oz	230	2	1	2	1	5	4	4	4	2	2	6	0	1	1	0	0	1	0

continued

Desserts and Sweets

No.	Name/Portion Size		KCAL	CAL	PRO	CAR	FIB	SUG	FAT	SFA	PFA	CHL	SOD	A	C	THI	RIB	B6	CA	IRN	ZN
			NUTRI–UNITS																		
712	Chocolate cake m/w butter 2 × 2 × 2 in piece	1.4 oz	140	1	1	1	0	2	2	3	0	2	2	1	0	1	1	0	1	1	0
713	Chocolate cake m/w veg fat 2 × 2 × 2 in piece	1.4 oz	140	1	1	1	0	2	2	2	1	2	1	0	0	1	1	0	1	1	0
714	Chocolate cake,icing,m/w butter 1/16 of 9-in 2-layer cake	2.6 oz	270	3	1	3	0	6	3	5	0	3	2	1	0	1	1	0	1	1	1
715	Chocolate cake,icng,m/w veg fat 1/16 of 9-in 2-layer cake	2.6 oz	280	3	1	3	0	6	3	4	1	2	2	1	0	1	1	0	1	1	1
716	Choc cake+icing,cream filling 1/16 of 9-in 2-layer cake	2.4 oz	260	3	1	2	0	5	5	5	1	2	1	1	0	1	1	0	1	1	1
717	Coffeecake,made w egg+milk 2.5× 2.75× 1.75 in piece	2.5 oz	230	2	1	3	1	5	2	2	1	3	3	0	0	2	2	0	1	1	1
718	Cottage pudding cake m/w butter 2 × 4 × 1.5 in piece	1.9 oz	180	2	1	2	0	3	2	3	0	3	2	1	0	2	1	0	1	1	1
719	Cottage puddng cake m/w veg fat 2 × 4 × 1.5 in piece	1.9 oz	190	2	1	2	0	3	2	2	1	2	2	0	0	2	1	0	1	1	1
720	Cottage pudd ck,choc sc,butter 2×4×1.5 in piece+sauce	2.6 oz	230	2	1	3	1	5	2	3	0	3	2	1	0	2	2	0	1	2	1
721	Cottage pudd ck,choc sc,veg fat 2×4×1.5 in piece+sauce	2.6 oz	240	2	1	3	1	5	2	2	1	2	2	0	0	2	2	0	1	2	1
722	Cott pudd ck,strawb sc,butter 2×4×1.5 in piece+sauce	2.5 oz	200	2	1	2	1	4	2	3	0	3	2	1	3	2	1	0	1	1	1
723	Cott pudd ck,strawb sc,veg fat 2×4×1.5 in piece+sauce	2.5 oz	200	2	1	2	1	4	2	2	1	2	2	0	3	2	1	0	1	1	1
724	Cranberry cake 2.75 in sq × 1.5 in piece	2.2 oz	200	2	1	2	1	3	3	4	0	6	1	2	0	1	1	0	1	1	0
725	Cupcake,plain,m/w butter 2.75 in diam cupcake	1.2 oz	120	1	0	1	0	2	1	2	0	2	1	1	0	1	1	0	0	1	0
726	Cupcake,plain,m/w veg fat 2.75 in diam cupcake	1.2 oz	120	1	0	1	0	2	1	1	1	1	1	0	0	1	1	0	0	1	0

727 Cupcake,choc icing,m/w butter 2.75 in diam cupcake	1.7 oz	170	2	1	2	0	4	2	3	0	2	1	1	0	1	1	0	1	1	0
728 Cupcake,choc icing,m/w veg fat 2.75 in diam cupcake	1.7 oz	170	2	1	2	0	4	2	2	1	2	1	0	0	1	1	0	1	1	0
729 Devilsfood cake w icing,frozen 1/16 of 9 in 2-layer cake	2.4 oz	260	3	1	3	0	6	4	6	1	2	3	1	0	1	1	0	1	1	1
730 Devilfood ck+icing,cream fillng 1/16 of 9-in 2-layer cake	2.4 oz	260	3	1	2	0	5	5	5	1	2	1	1	0	1	1	0	1	1	1
731 Dutch apple cake,w whip topping 2.5 × 2 × 2 in piece	2.3 oz	170	2	1	2	2	4	2	3	0	2	1	0	0	1	1	0	1	1	0
732 Fruitcake m/w butter 3.5 × 2.25 × .5 in piece	1.5 oz	160	2	1	2	1	4	2	2	1	1	1	1	0	1	1	0	1	1	0
733 Fruitcake m/w veg fat 3.5 × 2.25 × .5 in piece	1.5 oz	170	2	1	2	1	4	2	1	1	0	1	0	0	1	1	0	1	1	0
734 Gingerbread m/w butter 2.25 × 3 × 2 in piece	3.1 oz	260	3	1	3	1	5	3	4	0	4	3	1	0	2	1	0	1	3	1
735 Gingerbread m/w veg fat 2.25 × 3 × 2 in piece	3.1 oz	280	3	1	3	1	5	3	2	2	3	2	0	0	2	1	0	1	3	1
736 Honey spice cake w icing 1/16 of 9-in 2-layer cake	2.7 oz	270	3	1	3	1	6	2	2	1	3	2	0	0	1	1	0	1	1	0
737 Jelly roll w icing 1 slice	2.0 oz	170	2	1	2	0	3	1	1	1	0	1	0	0	2	2	0	1	1	0
738 Marble cake,boiled icing+butter 1/16 of 9-in 2-layer cake	2.3 oz	220	2	1	3	1	5	2	1	1	2	2	0	0	1	1	0	1	1	0
739 Peanut butter cake,w p-b icing 2 × 3.75 × 2 in piece	3.2 oz	340	3	2	3	2	6	5	4	3	5	3	1	0	1	1	0	1	2	1
740 Pineapple upsidedown cake 4 × 2.5 in piece	3.8 oz	310	3	1	3	1	6	4	3	3	2	2	1	1	1	1	1	2	1	1
741 Pound cake m/w butter 3.5 × 3 × .5 in slice	1.1 oz	130	1	1	1	0	1	2	4	0	4	1	1	0	0	0	0	0	0	0
742 Pound cake m/w veg fat 3.5 × 3 × .5 in slice	1.1 oz	140	1	1	1	0	1	3	2	2	3	0	0	0	1	1	0	0	1	0
743 Pound cake,cherry sc,whip toppn 3.5 × 3 × 1 in pc + sauce	3.2 oz	260	3	1	3	1	4	4	6	0	8	2	3	1	1	1	0	0	1	0

continued

Desserts and Sweets

No.	Name/Portion Size		KCAL	CAL	PRO	CAR	FIB	SUG	FAT	SFA	PFA	CHL	SOD	A	C	THI	RIB	B6	CA	IRN	ZN
										NUTRI–UNITS											
744	Pound cake,modified,m/w butter 3.5 × 3 × .5 in slice	1.0 oz	120	1	1	1	0	2	1	2	0	4	1	1	0	1	1	0	0	1	0
745	Pound cake,modified,m/w veg fat 3.5 × 3 × .5 in slice	1.0 oz	120	1	1	1	0	2	2	1	1	3	1	0	0	1	1	0	0	1	0
746	Spice cake w icing 2 × 2 × 2 in piece	1.8 oz	170	2	1	1	0	2	3	4	1	4	2	1	0	1	1	0	0	1	0
747	Sponge cake 1/12 of 10-in tube cake	2.3 oz	200	2	2	3	1	4	1	1	0	11	1	1	0	1	2	0	0	1	1
748	Strawbr shortck+1 tbsp whip top 3×4 in pc+0.4 cup berries	4.3 oz	290	3	1	3	2	6	3	6	0	4	2	2	8	2	1	0	1	1	0
749	Sweet potato cake 2.75 × 2 × 1.5 in piece	1.4 oz	120	1	0	1	1	2	1	1	2	1	1	2	1	1	1	0	0	0	0
750	White cake m/w butter 1/16 of 9-in 2-layer cake	1.9 oz	190	2	1	2	1	3	2	4	0	1	3	1	0	1	1	0	1	1	0
751	White cake m/w veg fat 1/16 of 9-in 2-layer cake	1.9 oz	200	2	1	2	1	3	3	2	2	0	2	0	0	1	1	0	1	1	0
752	White cake,icing,m/w butter 1/16 of 9-in 2-layer cake	2.8 oz	280	3	1	3	1	6	3	5	0	2	3	1	0	1	1	0	1	1	0
753	White cake,icing,m/w veg fat 1/16 of 9-in 2-layer cake	2.8 oz	290	3	1	3	1	6	3	3	2	0	2	0	0	1	1	0	1	1	0
754	Yellow cake m/w butter 1/16 of 9-in 2-layer cake	1.9 oz	190	2	1	2	1	3	2	3	0	3	2	1	0	1	1	0	1	1	0
755	Yellow cake m/w veg fat 1/16 of 9-in 2-layer cake	1.9 oz	200	2	1	2	1	3	2	2	1	2	1	0	0	1	1	0	1	1	0
756	Yellow cake,icing,m/w butter 1/16 of 9-in 2-layer cake	2.6 oz	260	3	1	3	1	6	3	4	0	3	2	1	0	1	1	0	1	1	0
757	Yellow cake,icing,m/w veg fat 1/16 of 9-in 2-layer cake	2.6 oz	270	3	1	3	1	6	3	3	1	2	2	0	0	1	1	0	1	1	0
758	Yellow cake w cherry topping 3 × 3 × 2 in piece+ sauce	2.3 oz	200	2	1	2	1	3	3	5	0	5	3	2	0	2	1	0	1	1	0

Cake Icings																				
759 Caramel icing 1 tbsp	.8 oz	80	1	0	1	0	3	0	1	0	0	0	0	0	0	0	0	0	0	0
760 Chocolate icing 1 tbsp	.6 oz	60	1	0	1	0	2	1	1	0	0	0	0	0	0	0	0	0	0	0
761 Coconut icing 1 tbsp	.4 oz	40	0	0	1	1	2	0	1	0	0	0	0	0	0	0	0	0	0	0
762 White icing,boiled 1 tbsp	.2 oz	20	0	0	0	0	1	0	0	0	0	0	0	0	0	0	0	0	0	0
763 White icing,uncooked 1 tbsp	.7 oz	80	1	0	1	0	3	0	1	0	0	0	0	0	0	0	0	0	0	0
Candy																				
764 Butterscotch candy 1 oz	1.0 oz	110	1	0	2	N	5	0	0	0	0	0	0	0	0	0	0	0	0	0
765 Candy bar,milk chocolate 1 oz	1.0 oz	150	1	1	1	N	3	3	5	0	0	0	0	0	0	1	0	1	0	0
766 Candy bar,milk choc w almonds 1 oz	1.0 oz	150	1	1	1	N	3	3	4	1	0	0	0	0	0	1	0	1	0	0
767 Candy bar,milk choc w peanuts 1 oz	1.0 oz	150	2	1	1	N	2	3	4	1	0	0	0	0	1	1	0	1	0	0
768 Candy bar,semisweet chocolate 1 oz	1.0 oz	140	1	0	1	N	3	3	5	0	0	0	0	0	0	0	0	0	1	0
769 Candy bar,sweet chocolate 1 oz	1.0 oz	150	1	0	1	N	3	3	5	0	0	0	0	0	0	0	0	1	0	0
770 Candy corn 20 7/8 × 1/2 × 1/4 pieces	1.0 oz	100	1	0	2	N	5	0	0	0	0	1	0	0	0	0	0	0	0	0
771 Candied fruit,all types 10 cherries or pieces	1.2 oz	120	1	0	2	N	6	0	0	0	0	0	0	1	0	0	0	0	0	0
772 Caramels,plain or chocolate 1 oz (3 medium pieces)	1.0 oz	110	1	0	2	N	4	1	1	0	0	1	0	0	0	1	0	1	0	0
773 Caramels,plain or choc,w nuts 1 oz (3 medium pieces)	1.0 oz	120	1	0	1	N	4	1	1	0	0	1	0	0	0	1	0	1	0	0

continued

Desserts and Sweets

No.	Name/Portion Size		KCAL	CAL	PRO	CAR	FIB	SUG	FAT	SFA	PFA	CHL	SOD	A	C	THI	RIB	B6	CA	IRN	ZN
			NUTRI–UNITS																		
774	Chewing gum,candy coated $3/4 \times 1/2 \times 1/4$ in piece	.1 oz	10	0	0	0	0	0	0	0	0	0	0	0	0	0	0	0	0	0	0
775	Chocolate coated almonds 1 oz (approx 6–8 nuts)	1.0 oz	160	2	1	1	N	2	4	2	1	0	0	0	0	0	2	0	1	1	0
776	Chocolate coated choclate fudge 1 oz	1.0 oz	120	1	0	1	N	4	1	1	0	0	1	0	0	0	0	0	1	0	0
777	Choc coated choc fudge w nuts 1 oz	1.0 oz	130	1	0	1	N	4	2	1	1	0	1	0	0	0	0	0	1	0	0
778	Chocolate coated coconut center 1 oz	1.0 oz	120	1	0	1	N	3	1	3	0	0	1	0	0	0	0	0	0	0	0
779	Chocolate coated fondant/ mints 2 mints ($1 3/8 \times 3/8$ in)	.8 oz	90	1	0	1	N	3	1	1	0	0	0	0	0	0	0	0	0	0	0
780	Choc coated fudge,carmel,peanuts 1 oz	1.0 oz	120	1	1	1	N	3	2	1	1	0	1	0	0	1	1	0	1	0	0
781	Choc coated fudge,p-nuts,carmel 1 oz	1.0 oz	130	1	1	1	N	3	2	2	1	0	0	0	0	1	0	0	1	0	0
782	Choc coat hrd candy/p-nut buttr 1 oz	1.0 oz	130	1	1	1	N	4	2	1	1	0	0	0	0	0	0	0	0	1	1
783	Choc coated nougat + caramel 1 oz	1.0 oz	120	1	0	1	N	4	1	1	0	0	0	0	0	0	1	0	1	0	0
784	Chocolate coated peanuts 1 oz (approx 8–16 nuts)	1.0 oz	160	2	1	1	N	2	3	3	2	0	0	0	0	1	1	1	1	0	1
785	Chocolate coated raisins 2 tbsp (50 sml, 18–28 lg)	1.0 oz	120	1	0	1	N	4	1	2	0	0	0	0	0	0	1	1	1	1	0
786	Chocolate coated vanilla cream 5 miniature	1.1 oz	130	1	0	1	0	4	2	1	0	0	1	0	0	0	0	0	1	0	0
787	Chocolate chips,semisweet $1/4$ cup	1.5 oz	210	2	1	2	0	5	5	8	0	0	0	0	0	0	0	0	0	1	0
788	Fondant 3 $1 1/2$ in dia $\times 1/2$ in pcs	1.0 oz	100	1	0	2	0	5	0	0	0	0	1	0	0	0	0	0	0	0	0

789 Fudge,chocolate 1 cubic inch	.7 oz	80	1	0	1	N	3	1	1	0	0	0	0	0	0	0	0	0	0	0
790 Fudge,chocolate,w nuts 1 cubic inch	.7 oz	90	1	0	1	N	3	1	1	1	0	0	0	0	0	0	0	0	0	0
791 Fudge,peanut butter 1 cubic inch	.7 oz	70	1	1	1	1	2	1	1	1	0	0	0	0	0	0	0	0	0	0
792 Fudge,vanilla 1 cubic inch	.7 oz	80	1	0	1	0	3	1	1	0	0	0	0	0	0	0	0	0	0	0
793 Fudge,vanilla,w nuts 1 cubic inch	.7 oz	90	1	0	1	N	3	1	1	1	0	0	0	0	0	0	0	0	0	0
794 Gum drops,starch,jelly pieces 3 lg(7/8 in dia) or 24 sm	1.1 oz	100	1	0	2	0	5	0	0	0	0	0	0	0	0	0	0	0	0	0
795 Hard candy,lifesavers 5 sq or 5 rings	.9 oz	100	1	0	2	0	5	0	0	0	0	0	0	0	0	0	0	0	1	0
796 Lollypop 1 pop,1 × 1.5 in	.9 oz	100	1	0	2	0	5	0	0	0	0	0	0	0	0	0	0	0	1	0
797 Jelly beans 10 beans (3/4 × 1/2 in)	1.0 oz	100	1	0	2	0	5	0	0	0	0	0	0	0	0	0	0	0	0	0
798 Marshmallows 1 cup,not pkd (.5 in dia)	1.6 oz	150	1	0	3	0	6	0	0	0	0	0	0	0	0	0	0	0	1	0
799 Peanut bar 1 oz	1.0 oz	140	1	2	1	N	2	3	2	2	0	0	0	0	2	0	0	0	1	1
800 Peanut brittle,no salt or soda 2 1/2 in sq × 3/8 in pc	.9 oz	110	1	0	1	N	4	1	1	1	0	0	0	0	1	0	0	0	1	1
801 Sugar coated almonds 8 nuts (1 × 5/8 in)	1.0 oz	130	1	1	1	N	4	2	0	1	0	0	0	0	0	1	0	1	1	1
802 Sugar coated chocolate discs 31 discs (1/2 in diam)	1.0 oz	130	1	0	1	N	4	2	3	0	0	0	0	0	0	1	0	1	0	0
Cookies																				
803 Animal crackers 7 crackers	.7 oz	90	1	0	1	1	1	1	0	0	0	1	0	0	1	1	0	0	0	0
804 Applesauce bars 2.5 in sq × .5 in bar	.7 oz	70	1	0	1	1	1	1	1	0	0	1	0	0	0	0	0	0	0	0

continued

Desserts and Sweets

No.	Name/Portion Size		KCAL	CAL	PRO	CAR	FIB	SUG	FAT	SFA	PFA	CHL	SOD	A	C	THI	RIB	B6	CA	IRN	ZN
				NUTRI–UNITS																	
805	Assorted cookies,pkg,commercial 2 2-in diameter cookies	.7 oz	100	1	0	1	0	1	1	1	0	1	1	0	0	0	0	0	0	0	0
806	Brownies w nuts,butter 1.7 in sq × .9 in brownie	.7 oz	90	1	0	1	0	2	2	2	1	1	1	0	0	1	0	0	0	0	0
807	Brownies w nuts,veg fat 1.7 in sq × .9 in brownie	.7 oz	100	1	0	1	0	2	2	1	1	1	1	0	0	1	0	0	0	0	0
808	Brownies w nuts,mix,w egg+water 2 × 2 × 0.7 in brownie	1.1 oz	130	1	0	1	1	2	2	1	1	1	0	0	0	1	0	0	0	1	1
809	Brownies w choc frosting 2.7 in sq × .9 in brownie	2.3 oz	260	3	1	2	1	5	4	4	2	3	1	1	0	1	1	0	1	1	0
810	Butter cookies,thin,rich 3 2-in dia × .2 in cookie	.5 oz	70	1	0	1	0	1	1	1	0	1	1	0	0	0	0	0	0	0	0
811	Chocolate chip,m/w butter 2 2.3-in diameter cookies	.7 oz	100	1	0	1	0	2	2	2	1	1	1	1	0	0	0	0	0	1	0
812	Chocolate chip,m/w veg fat 2 2.3-in diameter cookies	.7 oz	100	1	0	1	0	2	2	2	1	1	1	0	0	0	0	0	0	1	0
813	Chocolate cookies 2 2.3-in diameter cookies	.7 oz	90	1	0	1	0	2	1	1	0	1	0	0	0	1	1	0	0	1	0
814	Cinnamon crispies 1 crispie,large	1.3 oz	170	2	1	2	1	2	2	2	2	1	1	0	0	1	0	0	0	1	0
815	Coconut bars 2 (2.4 × 1.6 × .4 in)	.6 oz	90	1	0	1	1	1	1	2	1	1	0	0	0	0	0	0	0	1	0
816	Fig bars 2 (1.6-in sq × .4 in)	1.0 oz	100	1	0	1	1	2	0	0	0	1	1	0	0	1	1	0	0	1	0
817	Gingersnaps 3 2-in dia × .2 in cookie	.7 oz	90	1	0	1	0	2	1	0	0	1	1	0	0	1	1	0	0	1	0
818	Graham cracker,chocolate coated 2.5 × 2 & 0.2 in cracker	.5 oz	60	1	0	1	1	1	1	1	0	0	1	0	0	0	1	0	0	1	0
819	Granola bar 1 oz bar	1.0 oz	130	1	1	1	3	1	1	1	2	1	1	0	0	1	0	1	0	1	1

820 Ladyfingers 2 (3.2 × 1.4 × 1.1 in)	.8 oz	80	1	1	1	0	2	1	0	0	5	0	1	0	1	1	0	0	1	0
821 Macaroons 2.7 in dia × .2 in cookie	.7 oz	90	1	0	1	1	1	1	3	0	1	0	0	0	0	0	0	0	0	0
822 Marshmallow cookies 2 (1.7 in dia × .7 in)	.9 oz	110	1	0	1	0	2	1	2	0	1	1	0	0	0	0	0	0	0	0
823 Molasses cookies 3.6 in dia × .7 in cookie	.8 oz	100	1	0	1	0	2	1	1	0	1	1	0	0	1	1	0	0	1	0
824 Oatmeal cookies w raisins 2 (2.6 in dia × .2 in)	.9 oz	120	1	0	1	1	2	1	1	1	1	0	0	0	1	1	0	0	1	0
825 Peanut cookies 1.7 in dia × .5 in cookie	.4 oz	60	1	0	1	0	1	1	0	0	0	0	0	0	1	0	0	0	0	0
826 Peanut butter cookies 2.7 in dia × .5 in cookie	1.4 oz	190	2	1	1	1	3	3	3	2	2	1	1	0	1	0	0	0	1	1
827 Peanut butter raisin cookies 2.7 in dia × .5 in cookie	1.4 oz	170	2	1	1	1	3	3	2	2	2	1	0	0	1	1	0	0	1	0
828 Plain cookies 2.5 in dia × .2 in cookie	.4 oz	60	1	0	1	0	1	1	1	1	0	1	0	0	0	0	0	0	0	0
829 Pumpkin bars w frosting 2.6 × 2.7 × 1 in bar	1.7 oz	160	2	1	2	1	3	2	2	1	2	2	2	0	1	1	0	0	1	0
830 Raisin cookies 2 2.3-in diameter cookies	1.0 oz	110	1	0	2	1	2	0	0	0	1	0	0	0	1	1	0	0	1	0
831 Sandwich type cookies 2 (1.7 in dia × .4 in)	.7 oz	100	1	0	1	0	1	1	1	1	1	1	0	0	1	0	0	0	0	0
832 Shortbread cookies 3 (1.6 in sq × .2 in)	.8 oz1	120	1	1	1	0	2	2	1	1	1	0	0	0	1	1	0	0	1	0
833 Snickerdoodle cookies 2.7 in dia × .2 in cookie	.7 oz	80	1	0	1	0	1	1	2	0	1	1	1	0	1	0	0	0	0	0
834 Sugar cookies m/w butter 3 (2.5 in dia × .2 in)	.8 oz	100	1	0	1	0	2	1	2	0	1	1	1	0	1	1	0	0	1	0
835 Sugar cookies m/w veg fat 3 (2.5 in dia × .2 in)	.8 oz	110	1	0	1	0	2	1	1	1	1	1	0	0	1	1	0	0	1	0
836 Sugar wafers 5 (2.5 × .7 × .2 in)	.7 oz	100	1	0	1	0	2	1	1	1	1	0	0	0	1	0	0	0	0	0

continued

Desserts and Sweets

No.	Name/Portion Size		KCAL	CAL	PRO	CAR	FIB	SUG	FAT	SFA	PFA	CHL	SOD	A	C	THI	RIB	B6	CA	IRN	ZN
				NUTRI–UNITS																	
837	Vanilla wafers 5 (2.5 × .7 × .2 in)	.7 oz	90	1	0	1	0	2	1	1	0	1	1	0	0	1	1	0	0	1	0
Crisps, Cobblers, Shortcakes																					
838	Apple brown betty,m/w butter 1/2 cup	3.8 oz	160	2	1	2	3	5	1	1	0	1	2	0	0	1	1	0	0	1	0
839	Apple cobbler,m/w butter 1/2 cup	3.7 oz	260	3	1	3	3	5	2	3	0	5	2	2	0	2	1	0	1	2	0
840	Apple crisp,m/w veg fat 1/2 cup	4.1 oz	270	3	0	4	3	6	2	1	2	0	2	1	1	1	1	0	0	1	0
841	Cherry crisp,m/w veg fat 1/2 cup	3.7 oz	230	2	0	3	3	5	2	1	2	0	1	3	1	1	0	0	1	1	0
842	Peach cobbler,m/w veg fat 1/2 cup	3.4 oz	180	2	0	2	2	3	2	2	2	0	1	1	1	1	1	0	0	1	0
843	Peach cranberry crisp,m/w buttr 1/2 cup	3.5 oz	190	2	0	3	2	5	1	2	0	1	1	1	1	0	1	0	1	1	0
844	Strawberry shortcake w whp top 3×4 in ck/.4 cup berries	4.3 oz	290	3	1	3	2	6	3	6	0	4	2	2	8	2	1	0	1	1	0
Doughnuts, Pastries, Sweet Breads																					
845	Apple turnover 2 3/4 oz turnover	2.8 oz	230	2	0	2	2	3	4	3	2	0	0	0	0	1	1	0	0	1	0
846	Banana bread 3 × 5 × 1/2 in slice	2.0 oz	170	2	1	2	2	3	2	2	1	2	2	1	0	1	1	1	0	1	0
847	Cheese danish 2 oz danish	2.0 oz	240	2	1	2	1	2	4	3	1	2	2	1	0	0	0	0	1	1	1
848	Cinnamon crispie 2 oz crispie	2.0 oz	250	3	1	2	2	3	4	3	3	1	1	0	0	2	0	0	0	1	1
849	Cinnamon roll m/w veg fat 3 3/4 in diam × 2 in roll	4.0 oz	370	4	2	4	3	4	3	2	2	0	4	1	0	4	3	0	1	2	1
850	Danish pastry 1/8 of 12 oz package	1.5 oz	180	2	1	1	1	1	3	3	2	2	2	1	0	2	1	0	0	1	0

851 Doughnut, cake type 3¼ in diam × i in	1.5 oz	160	2	1	2	1	2	2	2	2	2	2	0	0	1	1	0	0	1	0
852 Doughnut,cake,cinnamon 3¼ in diam × 1 in	1.5 oz	170	2	0	2	1	2	3	2	2	1	2	0	0	1	1	0	0	0	0
853 Doughnut,cake w choc icing 3¼ in diam × 1 in	1.5 oz	200	2	1	1	1	2	4	3	3	0	1	0	0	1	1	0	0	1	0
854 Doughnut,cake w sugar icing 3¼ in diam × 1 in	1.5 oz	170	2	1	2	1	2	2	2	2	0	0	0	0	1	1	0	0	1	0
855 Doughnut, yeast,plain 3¾ in diam × 1¼ in	1.5 oz	170	2	1	1	1	2	3	3	2	1	1	0	0	1	1	0	0	1	0
856 Doughnut,yeast,glazed 3¾ in diam × 1¼ in	1.5 oz	170	2	1	1	1	2	3	2	2	1	1	0	0	1	1	0	0	1	0
857 Eclair,custard fill,choc icing 5 × 2 × 1¾ in eclair	3.5 oz	240	2	2	2	1	2	4	4	2	9	1	1	0	1	2	0	2	1	1
858 Long john 2 oz long john	2.0 oz	130	1	1	1	1	2	2	2	1	5	0	1	0	0	1	0	1	0	0
859 Sopapilla w honey 1 sopapilla+ 1 tbsp honey	1.3 oz	110	1	0	2	1	2	1	0	0	0	1	0	0	1	0	0	0	0	0
860 Strawberry poptart 3 × 4½ in tart	1.8 oz	210	2	1	3	1	4	2	0	0	0	2	2	0	2	2	2	2	2	0
861 Super donut 2 oz donut	2.0 oz	250	3	2	2	2	2	4	0	0	0	0	4	8	4	2	0	2	5	0
Frozen Desserts																				
862 Banana split w soft serve 1 banana split	13.5 oz	540	5	3	6	3	18	5	10	0	5	1	3	6	8	7	7	7	2	3
863 Cone,choc dipped,soft serve,med 1 cone	5.5 oz	300	3	2	3	0	8	4	6	0	2	2	1	0	1	4	1	4	0	1
864 Cone,soft serve,small 1 cone	2.5 oz	110	1	1	1	0	3	1	2	0	1	1	0	0	0	2	0	2	0	0
865 Cone,soft serve,medium 1 cone	5.0 oz	230	2	2	2	0	5	2	3	0	1	2	1	0	1	3	1	4	0	1
866 Cone,soft serve,large 1 cone	7.5 oz	340	3	3	4	0	8	3	5	0	2	2	2	0	2	5	1	6	0	1

continued

Desserts and Sweets

No.	Name/Portion Size		KCAL	CAL	PRO	CAR	FIB	SUG	FAT	SFA	PFA	CHL	SOD	A	C	THI	RIB	B6	CA	IRN	ZN
										NUTRI–UNITS											
867	Dreamsicle 2 oz bar	2.0 oz	90	1	0	1	0	3	1	1	0	0	0	0	0	0	0	0	1	0	0
868	Fruitsicle 4 oz bar	4.1 oz	60	1	0	1	0	3	0	0	0	0	0	0	1	0	0	0	0	0	0
869	Hot fudge brownie w soft serve 1 serving	9.4 oz	560	6	3	6	2	13	6	11	0	2	2	2	0	6	5	1	6	1	2
870	Ice cream bar 2 oz bar	2.0 oz	150	2	1	1	0	3	3	5	0	0	0	1	0	0	1	0	1	0	0
871	Ice cream cone (no ice cream) 1 cone	.4 oz	50	0	0	1	0	0	0	0	0	0	0	0	0	0	0	0	0	0	0
872	Ice cream,10 percent fat 1/2 cup	2.3 oz	130	1	1	1	0	3	2	4	0	2	1	1	0	0	2	0	2	0	1
873	Ice cream,light,7 percent fat 1/2 cup	3.0 oz	100	1	1	1	0	3	1	2	0	1	1	1	0	0	2	0	2	0	1
874	Ice cream,rich,16 percent fat 1/2 cup	2.6 oz	180	2	1	1	0	3	4	7	0	3	1	2	0	0	2	0	2	0	1
875	Ice cream,soft serv,13 pcnt fat 1/2 cup	3.1 oz	190	2	1	1	0	4	3	6	0	5	1	2	0	1	3	0	2	0	1
876	Ice milk, soft serve,3 pcnt fat 1/2 cup	3.1 oz	110	1	1	1	0	4	1	1	0	0	1	0	0	1	3	1	3	0	1
877	Ice milk,5 percent fat 1/2 cup	2.3 oz	90	1	1	1	0	3	1	2	0	1	1	0	0	1	2	0	2	0	0
878	Ice,water,lime 1/2 cup	3.0 oz	110	1	0	2	0	5	0	0	0	0	0	0	0	0	0	0	0	0	0
879	Parfait,soft serve 1 parfait	10.0 oz	460	5	3	6	0	16	3	6	0	2	3	2	0	2	5	5	6	2	2
880	Sandwich,soft serve 1 sandwich	2.1 oz	140	1	1	2	0	4	1	2	0	1	1	0	0	0	2	0	1	0	0
881	Sherbet,orange 1/2 cup	3.4 oz	130	1	0	2	0	6	1	1	0	0	0	0	1	0	1	0	1	0	1

882 Sundae,chocolate,soft serve med 1 sundae	6.5 oz	300	3	2	4	0	10	2	3	0	1	2	1	0	1	3	1	4	1	1
883 Sundae,deluxe,soft serve 1 sundae	9.5 oz	570	6	3	6	0	16	6	11	0	2	2	1	0	3	3	5	4	0	2
884 Yogurt,frozen,4% fat 1/2 cup	3.1 oz	120	1	1	1	0	4	1	2	0	1	1	1	0	1	3	1	2	0	0
885 Yogurt,frozen,2% fat 1/2 cup	3.1 oz	90	1	1	1	0	3	0	1	0	0	1	0	0	0	2	0	3	0	1
Refrigerated Desserts																				
886 Apple tapioca dessert 1/2 cup	4.4 oz	150	1	0	3	N	N	0	0	0	0	1	0	0	0	0	0	0	0	0
887 Banana pudding w whip topping 1/2 cup incl 2.5 tbsp ban	4.6 oz	240	2	1	3	0	4	2	4	0	1	1	1	0	0	1	N	2	0	0
888 Bread pudding w raisins 3/4 cup	6.3 oz	340	3	3	4	4	5	3	5	1	8	4	2	1	2	4	2	4	2	2
889 Charlotte russe,whip crm fillng 4 lady fingrs+1/3 c filln	4.0 oz	330	3	2	3	N	7	5	7	1	15	0	3	0	2	2	1	1	1	0
890 Cheesecake,plain 1/8 of 8 in diam cake	3.0 oz	250	3	2	2	N	4	4	5	1	7	2	1	0	1	2	N	2	1	0
891 Cheesecake w cherry topping, fz 1/8 of 8 in diam cake	3.0 oz	220	2	1	2	1	3	3	5	2	7	1	1	3	0	1	1	1	1	0
892 Cream puff w custard filling 3 1/2 in dia × 2 in puff	4.6 oz	300	3	3	2	1	2	5	5	3	12	1	2	0	1	3	0	2	1	1
893 Custard,baked 1/2 cup	4.7 oz	150	2	2	1	0	3	2	3	0	9	1	2	0	1	3	1	3	1	1
894 Eclair w custd fillng,choc icng 5 × 2 × 1 3/4 in eclair	3.5 oz	240	2	2	2	1	2	4	4	2	9	1	1	0	1	2	0	2	1	1
895 Gelatin dessert,plain 1/2 cup	3.9 oz	70	1	1	1	0	3	0	0	0	0	1	0	0	0	0	0	0	0	0
896 Gelatin dessert,low-cal 1/2 cup	3.9 oz	10	0	1	0	0	0	0	0	0	0	0	0	0	0	0	0	0	0	0
897 Gelatin dessert w mixed fruit 1/2 cup	3.9 oz	70	1	0	1	0	3	0	0	0	0	0	0	1	0	0	0	0	0	0

continued

Desserts and Sweets

No.	Name/Portion Size		KCAL	CAL	PRO	CAR	FIB	SUG	FAT	SFA	PFA	CHL	SOD	A	C	THI	RIB	B6	CA	IRN	ZN
									NUTRI–UNITS												
898	Gelatin dessert w bananas 1/2 cup incl 1.5 tbsp ban	3.9 oz	90	1	0	2	0	4	0	0	0	0	0	0	3	0	0	0	0	0	0
899	Gelatin dessert,lime,w pears 1/2 cup	3.9 oz	80	1	0	1	0	4	0	0	0	0	0	0	0	0	0	0	0	0	0
900	Gelatin dessert,orange,w oranges 1/3 cup + 1/6 cup oranges	3.5 oz	60	1	0	1	0	3	0	0	0	0	0	0	2	0	0	0	0	0	0
901	Gelatin dessert w whip topping 1/2 cup w whip topping	4.1 oz	120	1	0	1	0	4	2	5	0	0	1	0	0	0	0	1	0	0	0
902	Lemon refrigerator dessert 1/2 cup	3.9 oz	230	2	3	2	0	4	3	4	0	7	2	2	1	0	2	0	2	1	1
903	Prune whip 1/2 cup	2.3 oz	100	1	1	2	0	4	0	0	0	0	1	1	0	0	1	0	0	1	N
904	Pudding,chocolate,home recipe 1/2 cup	4.8 oz	200	2	1	2	0	5	2	3	0	1	1	1	0	0	2	0	3	1	1
905	Pudding,choc,mix,ckd w milk 1/2 cup	4.6 oz	160	2	1	2	0	5	1	2	0	1	2	1	0	0	2	0	3	0	1
906	Pudding,choc/van/butrsct,canned 1 can	5.0 oz	180	2	1	2	0	5	1	3	0	1	3	0	0	0	2	0	2	1	1
907	Pudding,custard,mix,ckd w milk 1/2 cup	4.6 oz	170	2	1	2	0	5	1	2	0	1	1	1	0	0	2	1	3	0	2
908	Pudding,lemon,canned 1/2 cup	4.0 oz	120	1	0	2	0	4	0	0	0	0	1	0	0	0	0	0	0	0	0
909	Pudding,lo cal,w nonfat milk 1/2 cup	4.6 oz	70	1	2	1	0	0	0	0	0	0	0	0	0	0	0	1	0	0	0
910	Pudding,pistach,mix,ckd w milk 1/2 cup	4.6 oz	170	2	1	2	0	4	2	3	0	0	2	1	0	1	2	1	0	0	0
911	Pudding,vanilla,home recipe 1/2 cup	4.4 oz	140	1	1	1	0	3	1	2	0	1	1	1	0	0	2	0	3	0	1
912	Rennin dessert,home recipe 1/2 cup	4.5 oz	110	1	1	1	0	3	1	2	0	1	1	1	0	1	2	0	3	0	1

913 Rennin dessert,choc,mix,w milk ½ cup	4.5 oz	130	1	1	1	0	3	1	2	0	1	1	1	0	1	2	0	3	0	1
914 Rennin desrt,othr flav,mix,milk ½ cup	4.4 oz	120	1	1	1	N	3	1	2	0	1	1	1	0	0	2	0	3	0	0
915 Rice pudding w raisins ½ cup	4.6 oz	190	2	1	2	1	4	1	2	0	1	1	1	0	1	2	1	3	1	1
916 Tapioca cream pudding ½ cup	2.9 oz	110	1	1	1	N	3	1	2	0	5	1	1	0	0	2	0	2	0	0
917 Yogurt,plain,part skim milk 1 8-oz container	8.0 oz	140	1	4	1	0	3	1	2	0	1	2	1	1	1	6	1	8	0	3
918 Yogurt,part skim,fruit flavors 1 8-oz container	8.0 oz	230	2	3	3	0	8	1	2	0	1	1	0	0	1	4	1	6	0	2
919 Yogurt,plain,skim milk w nfdm 1 8-oz container	8.0 oz	130	1	4	1	0	3	0	0	0	0	2	0	1	1	6	1	9	0	3
920 Yogurt,plain,whole milk 1 8-oz container	8.0 oz	140	1	2	1	0	2	2	4	0	2	1	1	0	1	4	1	5	0	2
Pies[d]																				
921 Apple pie m/w lard 1/6 of 9 in diam pie	5.5 oz	400	4	1	4	3	7	5	6	2	1	5	0	1	2	1	3	0	2	0
922 Apple pie m/w veg fat 1/6 of 9 in diam pie	5.5 oz	400	4	1	4	3	7	5	4	3	0	5	0	1	2	1	3	0	2	0
923 Apple pie,frozen,baked 1/6 of 8 in diam pie	3.2 oz	230	2	1	3	2	6	3	2	2	0	2	0	0	1	1	0	0	1	0
924 Apple pie,deep fried,individ 1 pie	3.2 oz	270	3	1	2	2	4	5	5	1	1	4	0	1	0	0	0	0	1	0
925 Banana custard pie m/w lard 1/6 of 9 in diam pie	5.4 oz	340	3	2	3	2	4	4	5	1	6	4	2	1	2	3	1	2	2	1
926 Banana custard pie m/w veg fat 1/6 of 9 in diam pie	5.4 oz	340	3	2	3	2	4	4	4	2	6	4	2	1	2	3	1	2	2	1
927 Blackberry pie m/w lard 1/6 of 9 in diam pie	5.5 oz	380	4	1	4	4	7	5	6	2	1	6	1	2	2	2	0	1	2	0

[d]For 1/8 of 9-inch pie, multiply nutri-units by 0.75.
For pies with saltless crusts, subtract 2 nutri-units sodium per serving.

continued

Desserts and Sweets

No.	Name/Portion Size		KCAL	CAL	PRO	CAR	FIB	SUG	FAT	SFA	PFA	CHL	SOD	A	C	THI	RIB	B6	CA	IRN	ZN
									NUTRI–UNITS												
928	Blackberry pie m/w veg fat 1/6 of 9 in diam pie	5.5 oz	380	4	1	4	4	7	5	4	3	0	6	1	2	2	2	0	1	2	0
929	Blueberry pie m/w lard 1/6 of 9 in diam pie	5.5 oz	380	4	1	4	4	7	5	6	2	1	6	0	2	2	2	0	0	2	0
930	Blueberry pie m/w veg fat 1/6 of 9 in diam pie	5.5 oz	380	4	1	4	4	7	5	4	3	0	6	0	2	2	2	0	0	2	0
931	Butterscotch pie m/w lard 1/6 of 9 in diam pie	5.4 oz	410	4	2	4	1	6	5	6	1	6	5	2	0	1	3	1	2	2	1
932	Butterscotch pie m/w veg fat 1/6 of 9 in diam pie	5.4 oz	410	4	2	4	1	6	5	5	2	5	5	2	0	1	3	1	2	2	1
933	Cherry pie m/w lard 1/6 of 9 in diam pie	5.5 oz	410	4	1	4	3	8	5	6	2	1	5	3	0	3	2	0	0	2	0
934	Cherry pie m/w veg fat 1/6 of 9 in diam pie	5.5 oz	410	4	1	4	3	8	5	4	3	0	5	3	0	3	2	0	0	2	0
935	Cherry pie,frozen,baked 1/6 of 8 in diam pie	3.4 oz	280	3	1	3	2	6	3	3	2	0	2	1	1	2	1	0	0	1	0
936	Cherry pie,deep fried,individ 1 pie	3.2 oz	270	3	1	2	2	4	4	5	1	1	5	1	0	0	0	0	0	1	0
937	Chocolate chiffon pie w lard 1/6 of 9 in diam pie	3.8 oz	350	4	2	3	1	6	5	6	1	10	4	1	0	1	2	0	1	2	1
938	Chocolate chiffon pie w veg fat 1/6 of 9 in diam pie	3.8 oz	350	4	2	3	1	6	5	5	2	10	4	1	0	1	2	0	1	2	1
939	Chocolate meringue pie w lard 1/6 of 9 in diam pie	5.4 oz	380	4	2	4	1	8	5	7	1	6	4	1	0	1	3	1	2	2	1
940	Chocolate meringue pie/veg fat 1/6 of 9 in diam pie	5.4 oz	380	4	2	4	1	8	5	6	2	6	4	1	0	1	3	1	2	2	1
941	Coconut custard pie m/w lard 1/6 of 9 in diam pie	5.4 oz	360	4	3	3	3	4	6	8	1	11	4	1	0	2	4	1	3	2	1
942	Coconut custard pie m/w veg fat 1/6 of 9 in diam pie	5.4 oz	360	4	3	3	3	4	6	7	2	10	4	1	0	2	4	1	3	2	1

943 Coconut custard pie,frozen 1/6 of 8 in diam pie	3.5 oz	250	2	2	2	2	3	4	4	1	7	3	1	0	2	3	1	2	1	1
944 Custard pie m/w lard 1/6 of 9 in diam pie	5.4 oz	330	3	3	2	1	4	5	6	1	11	4	1	0	2	4	1	3	2	1
945 Custard pie m/w veg fat 1/6 of 9 in diam pie	5.4 oz	330	3	3	2	1	4	5	5	2	11	4	1	0	2	4	1	3	2	1
946 Lemon chiffon m/w lard 1/6 of 9 in diam pie	3.8 oz	340	3	2	3	1	7	4	4	1	13	4	1	1	1	2	1	0	2	0
947 Lemon chiffon pie m/w veg fat 1/6 of 9 in diam pie	3.8 oz	340	3	2	3	1	7	4	3	2	12	4	1	1	1	2	1	0	2	0
948 Lemon meringue pie m/w lard 1/6 of 9 in diam pie	4.9 oz	360	4	2	4	1	8	4	5	1	9	4	1	1	1	2	0	0	2	0
949 Lemon meringue pie m/w veg fat 1/6 of 9 in diam pie	4.9 oz	360	4	2	4	1	8	4	4	2	9	4	1	1	1	2	0	0	2	0
950 Mince pie m/w lard 1/6 of 9 in diam pie	5.5 oz	430	4	1	5	4	8	5	6	2	1	7	0	1	2	2	1	1	3	N
951 Mince pie m/w veg fat 1/6 of 9 in diam pie	5.5 oz	430	4	1	5	4	8	5	4	3	0	7	0	1	2	2	1	1	3	N
952 Peach pie m/w lard 1/6 of 9 in diam pie	5.5 oz	400	4	1	4	2	6	5	6	2	1	6	5	2	2	2	0	0	2	0
953 Peach pie m/w veg fat 1/6 of 9 in diam pie	5.5 oz	400	4	1	4	2	6	5	4	3	0	6	5	2	2	2	0	0	2	0
954 Pecan pie m/w lard 1/6 of 9 in diam pie	4.8 oz	570	6	2	5	2	8	9	5	5	6	5	1	0	4	2	1	1	5	1
955 Pecan pie m/w veg fat 1/6 of 9 in diam pie	4.8 oz	570	6	2	5	2	8	9	4	6	6	5	1	0	4	2	1	1	5	1
956 Pineapple pie m/w lard 1/6 of 9 in diam pie	5.5 oz	400	4	1	4	1	6	5	6	2	1	6	0	1	3	2	1	0	2	0
957 Pineapple pie m/w veg fat 1/6 of 9 in diam pie	5.5 oz	400	4	1	4	1	6	5	4	3	0	6	0	1	3	2	1	0	2	0
958 Pineapple chiffon pie m/w lard 1/6 of 9 in diam pie	3.8 oz	310	3	2	3	1	6	4	4	1	11	4	2	0	2	2	1	1	2	0
959 Pineapple chiffon m/w veg fat 1/6 of 9 in diam pie	3.8 oz	310	3	2	3	1	6	4	3	2	11	4	2	0	2	2	1	1	2	0

[d]For 1/8 of 9-inch pie, multiply nutri-units by 0.75.
For pies with saltless crusts, subtract 2 nutri-units sodium per serving.

continued

Desserts and Sweets

No.	Name/Portion Size		KCAL	CAL	PRO	CAR	FIB	SUG	FAT	SFA	PFA	CHL	SOD	A	C	THI	RIB	B6	CA	IRN	ZN
										NUTRI–UNITS											
960	Pineapple custard pie m/w lard 1/6 of 9 in diam pie	5.4 oz	330	3	2	3	1	6	4	5	1	6	4	1	1	2	2	1	2	1	1
961	Pineapp custard pie m/w veg fat 1/6 of 9 in diam pie	5.4 oz	330	3	2	3	1	6	4	4	2	6	4	1	1	2	2	1	2	1	1
962	Pumpkin pie m/w lard 1/6 of 9 in diam pie	5.4 oz	320	3	2	3	2	6	5	7	1	7	5	15	0	2	3	1	2	2	0
963	Pumpkin pie m/w veg fat 1/6 of 9 in diam pie	5.4 oz	320	3	2	3	2	6	5	5	2	6	5	15	0	2	3	1	2	2	0
964	Raisin pie m/w lard 1/6 of 9 in diam pie	5.5 oz	420	4	1	5	5	9	5	6	2	1	4	0	1	2	2	N	1	3	0
965	Raisin pie m/w veg fat 1/6 of 9 in diam pie	5.5 oz	420	4	1	5	5	9	5	4	3	0	4	0	1	2	2	N	1	3	0
966	Rhubarb pie m/w lard 1/6 of 9 in diam pie	5.5 oz	400	4	1	4	3	8	5	6	2	1	6	0	2	2	2	1	2	2	0
967	Rhubarb pie m/w veg fat 1/6 of 9 in diam pie	5.5 oz	400	4	1	4	3	8	5	4	3	0	6	0	2	2	2	1	2	2	0
968	Strawberry pie m/w lard 1/6 of 9 in diam pie	4.4 oz	250	2	1	3	3	5	3	3	1	1	4	0	10	1	1	1	0	2	0
969	Strawberry pie m/w veg fat 1/6 of 9 in diam pie	4.4 oz	250	2	1	3	3	5	3	2	2	0	4	0	10	1	1	1	0	2	0
970	Sweetpotato pie m/w lard 1/6 of 9 in diam pie	5.4 oz	320	3	2	3	3	6	5	7	1	6	5	15	2	2	3	0	2	2	0
971	Sweetpotato pie m/w veg fat 1/6 of 9 in diam pie	5.4 oz	320	3	2	3	3	6	5	6	2	5	5	15	2	2	3	0	2	2	0
Piecrust[e]																					
972	Graham cracker piecrust 1/6 of 8–9 in pie shell	1.1 oz	160	2	0	1	1	2	3	3	3	0	2	1	0	0	0	0	0	0	0
973	Piecrust m/w lard 1/6 of 8–9 in pie shell	1.1 oz	150	1	1	1	1	0	3	3	1	1	2	0	0	1	1	0	0	1	0
974	Piecrust m/w veg fat 1/6 of 8–9 in pie shell	1.1 oz	150	1	1	1	1	0	3	2	2	0	2	0	0	1	1	0	0	1	0

975 Piecrust,m/w veg fat,no salt 1/6 of 8–9 in pie shell	1.1 oz	150	1	1	1	1	0	3	2	2	0	0	0	0	1	1	0	0	1	0
976 Piecrust from mix,unenriched 1/6 of 8–9 in pie shell	1.0 oz	130	1	1	1	1	0	2	2	2	0	2	0	0	1	1	0	0	1	0
Toppings and Sauces																				
977 Butterscotch topping 3 tablespoons	1.8 oz	160	2	0	3	0	8	0	0	0	0	1	0	0	0	0	0	0	0	0
978 Cherry topping 3 tablespoons	1.8 oz	150	1	0	3	4	7	0	0	0	0	0	0	0	0	0	0	0	0	0
979 Chocolate pudding sauce 1/4 cup	2.3 oz	80	1	1	1	0	2	1	1	0	1	1	0	0	0	1	0	1	0	0
980 Chocolate syrup,thin 2 tablespoons	1.4 oz	100	1	0	2	0	5	0	0	0	0	0	0	0	0	0	0	0	1	0
981 Chocolate syrup,fudge 2 tablespoons	1.4 oz	130	1	1	2	0	4	2	3	0	0	0	0	0	0	1	0	1	1	1
982 Cranberry sauce 1/4 cup	2.4 oz	100	1	0	2	1	4	0	0	0	0	0	0	0	0	0	0	0	0	0
983 Custard sauce 1/4 cup	2.5 oz	90	1	1	1	0	1	1	2	1	6	1	1	0	1	3	0	1	0	0
984 Cream,light whipping 2 tbsp (1/4 cup whipped)	1.1 oz	90	1	0	0	0	0	3	5	0	2	0	1	0	0	0	0	0	0	0
985 Cream,heavy whipping 2 tbsp (1/4 cup whipped)	1.1 oz	100	1	0	0	0	0	3	6	0	3	0	2	0	0	0	0	0	0	0
986 Cream subst dessert topping,frz 1/4 cup	.6 oz	50	1	0	0	N	N	1	3	0	0	0	1	0	0	0	0	0	0	0
987 Hard sauce made w butter 2 tablespoons	.7 oz	100	1	0	1	0	2	2	3	0	1	1	1	0	0	0	0	0	0	0
988 Lemon sauce 1/4 cup	1.9 oz	130	1	0	2	0	5	1	1	0	0	1	0	1	0	0	0	0	0	0
989 Raisin sauce 1/4 cup	1.7 oz	130	1	0	2	2	5	1	1	0	0	0	1	2	0	0	0	0	0	0

[e]For 1/8 of 9-inch pie multiply nutri-units by 0.75.
For pies with saltless crusts, subtract 2 nutri-units sodium per serving.

continued

Eating Out, Fast Foods

No.	Name/Portion Size		KCAL	CAL	PRO	CAR	FIB	SUG	FAT	SFA	PFA	CHL	SOD	A	C	THI	RIB	B6	CA	IRN	ZN
990	Strawberry topping 3 tablespoons	1.8 oz	140	1	0	2	1	7	0	0	0	0	0	0	0	0	0	0	0	0	0
991	Strawberries,frozen,sweetened 1/4 cup	2.2 oz	60	1	0	1	1	3	0	0	0	0	0	0	9	0	0	N	0	0	0
992	Sour cream 2 tablespoons	.9 oz	50	1	0	0	0	0	2	3	0	1	0	1	0	0	0	0	1	0	0
993	Sour cream,imitation 2 tablespoons	1.0 oz	60	1	0	0	0	0	2	4	0	0	0	0	0	0	0	0	0	0	0

NUTRI–UNITS: columns CAL through ZN.

Eating Out, Fast Foods[f]

Beverages

No.	Name/Portion Size		KCAL	CAL	PRO	CAR	FIB	SUG	FAT	SFA	PFA	CHL	SOD	A	C	THI	RIB	B6	CA	IRN	ZN
994	Burger King shake,vanilla 1 medium,	14.0 oz	330	3	3	4	0	13	3	5	0	3	2	0	0	0	0	2	8	0	2
995	Dairy Queen float 1 serving,	14.0 oz	330	3	2	4	0	12	2	4	0	1	4	0	0	3	2	0	4	0	0
996	Dairy Queen freeze 1 serving,	14.0 oz	520	5	3	6	0	17	4	7	0	3	4	1	0	2	4	2	6	0	0
997	Dairy Queen choclate malt,small 1 small,	8.5 oz	340	3	3	4	0	8	4	7	0	2	2	2	1	1	4	1	6	2	2
998	Dairy Queen choclate malt,med 1 medium,	14.7 oz	600	6	5	6	0	13	6	11	0	3	4	3	1	1	6	2	10	4	4
999	Dairy Queen choclate malt,large 1 large,	20.7 oz	840	8	7	9	0	19	9	16	0	4	5	3	2	2	9	3	12	6	5
1000	Dairy Queen misty float 1 serving,	14.3 oz	440	4	2	6	0	17	2	4	0	1	4	0	0	2	2	0	4	0	0
1001	Dairy Queen misty freeze 1 serving,	14.5 oz	500	5	3	6	0	17	4	6	0	3	4	1	0	2	4	2	6	0	0
1002	Jack in Box chocolate shake 1 serving,	11.2 oz	370	4	3	4	0	11	3	6	0	2	3	2	1	2	7	2	7	1	2
1003	Jack in Box strawberry shake 1 serving,	11.6 oz	380	4	3	4	0	11	3	6	0	2	3	2	1	2	7	2	7	0	1

1004 Jack in Box vanilla shake 1 serving,	11.1 oz	340	3	3	4	0	11	3	6	0	2	3	2	1	2	6	3	7	3	1
1005 McDonalds chocolate shake 1 serving,	10.2 oz	360	4	3	4	0	10	3	5	0	2	3	1	1	2	5	1	7	1	2
1006 McDonalds strawberry shake 1 serving,	10.3 oz	350	3	3	4	0	10	3	5	0	2	3	1	1	2	5	1	7	0	2
1007 McDonalds vanilla shake 1 serving,	10.2 oz	320	3	3	4	0	10	3	5	0	2	3	1	1	2	8	1	7	0	1
1008 Wendy's frosty 1 serving,	8.8 oz	390	4	3	4	0	11	5	9	0	3	2	1	0	3	7	1	5	1	1
Breakfast																				
1009 Jack in Box breakfast jack 1 serving,	4.3 oz	380	4	6	2	1	0	4	4	3	12	10	2	1	5	6	1	4	3	2
1010 Jack in Box scrambled eggs 1 serving,	9.4 oz	390	4	8	0	0	2	9	11	3	69	8	5	0	9	7	3	5	6	4
1011 J in b omelette,double cheese 1 serving,	5.9 oz	420	4	6	2	0	1	8	7	1	25	9	3	1	4	8	1	6	4	3
1012 J in b omelette,ham and cheese 1 serving,	6.1 oz	430	4	6	2	0	1	7	6	2	24	10	3	1	5	8	2	5	4	3
1013 J in b omelette,ranchero 1 serving,	6.9 oz	410	4	6	2	0	1	7	9	2	23	11	3	1	4	9	2	6	4	3
1014 Jack in Box pancakes 1 serving,	8.2 oz	630	6	5	6	1	2	8	4	4	6	17	2	0	8	5	2	2	3	3
1015 McDonalds biscuit w spread 1 serving,	3.0 oz	330	3	2	3	N	N	5	5	4	1	8	1	0	3	2	N	1	1	1
1016 McDonalds biscuit+bacon,egg,chee 1 serving,	5.1 oz	480	5	5	2	N	N	9	12	4	17	13	3	1	4	5	N	4	3	N
1017 McDonalds biscuit+sausage 1 serving,	4.3 oz	470	5	4	2	N	N	9	11	4	3	12	0	0	7	3	N	2	2	N
1018 McDonalds biscuit+sausage,egg 1 serving,	6.2 oz	590	6	6	3	N	N	12	11	4	19	13	2	1	7	6	N	2	4	N

continued

[f] Some nutrients are estimated based on similar items.

Eating Out, Fast Foods

No.	Name/Portion Size		KCAL	CAL	PRO	CAR	FIB	SUG	FAT	SFA	PFA	CHL	SOD	A	C	THI	RIB	B6	CA	IRN	ZN
			NUTRI–UNITS																		
1019	McDonalds egg mcmuffin 1 serving,	4.7 oz	310	3	6	2	1	0	4	6	1	15	8	1	1	5	7	2	4	3	2
1020	McDonalds hashbrowns 1 piece,	1.9 oz	130	1	1	1	1	0	2	1	1	0	3	0	1	1	0	1	0	0	0
1021	McDonalds sausage mcmuffin 1 serving,	4.1 oz	430	4	5	2	N	N	8	10	2	4	9	2	0	9	3	N	3	2	N
1022	McDonalds sausage mcmuffin+egg 1 serving,	5.8 oz	520	5	7	2	N	N	10	12	2	19	10	3	1	11	6	N	4	4	N
1023	McD scrambled eggs 1 serving,	2.7 oz	140	1	3	0	0	0	3	4	0	18	2	2	0	1	4	1	1	2	2
1024	McD english muffin,buttered 1 serving,	2.2 oz	190	2	2	2	1	0	2	3	0	1	3	0	0	3	2	0	2	2	1
1025	McD hot cakes,butter and syrup 1 serving,	7.3 oz	480	5	2	6	1	8	3	4	0	2	10	1	1	3	4	1	3	3	1
1026	McD pork sausage 1 serving,	1.7 oz	180	2	3	0	0	0	5	6	1	3	6	0	0	3	1	2	0	1	2
Desserts																					
1027	Arby's apple turnover 1 turnover,	3.0 oz	290	3	1	2	1	3	6	6	1	2	2	0	1	0	0	0	0	0	0
1028	Arby's blueberry turnover 1 turnover,	3.0 oz	320	3	1	2	1	3	6	6	1	2	2	0	1	0	0	0	0	0	0
1029	Arby's cherry turnover 1 turnover,	3.0 oz	300	3	1	2	1	3	6	6	1	2	2	0	1	0	0	0	0	0	0
1030	Dairy Queen banana split 1 serving,	13.5 oz	540	5	3	6	2	18	5	10	0	5	1	3	6	8	7	7	7	2	3
1031	Dairy Queen buster bar 1 serving,	5.3 oz	390	4	3	3	0	7	7	12	1	6	1	1	0	1	4	1	4	1	2
1032	Dairy Queen cone,small 1 serving,	2.5 oz	110	1	1	1	0	3	1	2	0	1	1	0	0	0	2	0	2	0	0
1033	Dairy Queen cone,medium 1 serving,	5.0 oz	230	2	2	2	0	5	2	3	0	1	2	1	0	1	3	1	4	0	1

1034	Dairy Queen cone,large 1 serving,	7.5 oz	340	3	3	4	0	8	3	5	0	2	2	2	0	2	3	1	6	0	1
1035	DQ choc dipped cone,small 1 cone,	2.8 oz	150	1	1	1	0	4	2	3	0	1	1	0	0	0	2	0	2	0	0
1036	DQ choc dipped cone,medium 1 cone,	5.5 oz	300	3	2	3	0	8	4	6	0	2	2	1	0	1	4	1	4	0	1
1037	DQ choc dipped cone,large 1 cone,	8.3 oz	450	4	3	4	0	12	6	8	0	2	3	2	0	2	6	1	6	0	1
1038	DQ chocolate sundae,small 1 serving,	3.7 oz	170	2	1	2	0	6	1	2	0	1	1	0	0	0	2	0	2	1	1
1039	DQ chocolate sundae,medium 1 serving,	6.5 oz	300	3	2	4	0	10	2	3	0	1	2	1	0	1	3	1	4	1	1
1040	DQ chocolate sundae,large 1 serving,	8.7 oz	400	4	3	5	0	14	3	4	0	2	2	2	0	1	5	1	6	2	2
1041	Dairy Queen dilly bar 1 serving,	3.0 oz	240	2	1	2	N	4	4	8	0	1	1	0	0	1	2	0	2	0	0
1042	Dairy Queen fiesta sundae 1 serving,	9.5 oz	570	6	3	6	0	16	6	11	0	2	2	1	0	3	3	5	4	0	2
1043	Dairy Queen frozen dessert 1 serving,	4.0 oz	180	2	2	2	0	5	2	3	0	1	1	0	0	1	2	N	3	1	2
1044	Dairy Queen parfait 1 serving,	10.0 oz	460	5	3	6	0	16	3	6	0	2	3	2	0	2	5	5	6	2	2
1045	Dairy Queen sandwich 1 serving,	2.1 oz	140	1	1	2	0	4	1	2	0	1	1	0	0	0	2	0	1	0	0
1046	McDonalds apple pie 1 serving,	3.2 oz	270	3	1	2	2	4	5	5	1	1	4	0	1	0	0	0	0	1	0
1047	McDonalds cherry pie 1 serving,	3.2 oz	270	3	1	2	2	4	4	5	1	1	5	1	0	0	0	0	0	1	0
1048	McDonalds cookies 1 box,	2.2 oz	290	3	1	3	1	3	3	2	1	1	3	0	0	4	3	0	0	2	0
1049	McDonalds sundae,caramel 1 serving,	5.8 oz	330	3	2	3	0	9	3	6	0	2	2	1	1	1	4	0	4	0	1
1050	McDonalds sundae,hot fudge 1 serving,	5.8 oz	310	3	2	3	0	9	3	6	1	1	2	1	1	1	4	1	4	1	1

[f]Some nutrients are estimated based on similar items.

continued

Eating Out, Fast Foods

No.	Name/Portion Size		KCAL	CAL	PRO	CAR	FIB	SUG	FAT	SFA	PFA	CHL	SOD	A	C	THI	RIB	B6	CA	IRN	ZN
											NUTRI–UNITS										
1051	McDonalds sundae,strawberry 1 serving,	5.8 oz	290	3	2	3	3	9	3	5	1	1	1	1	1	1	3	0	3	0	1
French Fries, Etc.																					
1052	Arby's potato cakes 1 serving, 2 cakes	5.8 oz	300	3	1	3	3	0	4	3	3	0	0	0	10	2	1	1	0	0	1
1053	Burger King french fr,no salt 1 serving, small,	3.7 oz	210	2	1	2	3	0	3	4	1	1	0	0	5	0	0	2	0	1	0
1054	Dairy Queen french fr,salted 1 serving,	2.5 oz	200	2	1	2	2	0	3	3	1	1	1	0	1	1	0	2	0	0	0
1055	Dairy Queen french fr,salted 1 serving,	4.0 oz	320	3	1	3	3	0	5	5	1	2	2	0	2	1	0	3	0	1	0
1056	McDonalds french fries,salted 1 serving,	2.4 oz	210	2	1	2	2	0	3	5	0	1	1	0	4	2	0	2	0	1	0
1057	Wendys french fries,salted 1 serving,	4.2 oz	330	3	2	3	2	0	5	3	3	0	1	0	2	2	1	4	0	1	1
1058	Hush puppies 1 serving, 3 pieces	1.6 oz	150	2	1	1	1	0	2	1	4	0	2	0	0	1	1	0	0	1	0
1059	Dairy Queen onion rings 1 serving,	3.0 oz	300	3	2	2	1	0	5	13	2	0	2	0	1	1	0	1	0	0	0
1060	Jack in Box onion rings 1 serving,	3.0 oz	350	4	2	2	1	0	7	11	2	2	3	N	0	3	1	1	1	2	1
Fried Chicken and Fish																					
1061	Kentucky Fried,orig,3 pieces 3 pieces,	7.6 oz	360	4	21	0	0	0	2	2	1	12	2	0	0	2	3	13	1	2	3
1062	KFC extra crispy dinner 2 pc,pot,gravy,slaw,roll	15.4 oz	950	9	16	4	2	0	16	12	12	17	19	3	9	5	6	10	3	4	8
1063	Kentucky Fried,drumstick,orig 1 serving,	1.9 oz	140	1	4	0	0	0	2	2	1	5	1	0	0	0	1	2	0	1	2
1064	Kentucky Fried,keel,orig 1 serving,	3.4 oz	280	3	8	0	0	0	4	3	2	6	3	0	0	1	1	3	1	1	3

1065 Kentucky Fried,rib,orig 1 serving,	2.9 oz	240	2	6	1	0	0	4	4	2	6	2	0	0	1	2	3	1	1	1
1066 Kentucky Fried,thigh,orig 1 serving,	3.4 oz	270	3	6	1	0	0	6	4	4	10	3	0	0	1	3	3	1	1	4
1067 Kentucky Fried,wing,orig 1 serving,	1.6 oz	150	2	3	0	0	0	3	2	2	5	1	0	0	0	1	1	0	1	2
1068 Kentucky Fr Chick,orig dinner 2 pc,pot,gravy,slaw,roll	15.0 oz	830	8	16	4	2	0	14	11	11	19	23	3	9	5	6	10	3	5	7
1069 McDonalds chicken mcnuggets 1 serving, 6 pc	3.9 oz	270	3	6	1	0	0	5	4	4	5	5	0	2	1	2	4	0	1	2
1070 McDonalds chicken mcnuggets 1 serving, 9 pc	5.9 oz	400	4	9	1	1	0	7	6	5	8	8	1	3	2	3	6	1	1	2
1071 McDonalds chicken mcnuggets 1 serving, 20 pc	13.1 oz	900	9	19	3	1	0	17	14	12	17	17	1	7	5	7	14	1	2	5
1072 Barbeque sauce 1 serving,	1.3 oz	30	0	0	0	N	N	0	0	0	0	3	1	1	0	0	0	0	0	0
1073 Mustard sauce 1 serving, 1 tablespoon	.6 oz	40	0	0	0	0	0	1	0	1	0	2	0	0	0	0	N	0	0	0
1074 Sweet and sour sauce 1 serving,	1.1 oz	50	1	0	1	N	0	0	0	0	0	2	0	0	0	0	0	0	0	0
1075 Fish,batter fried 2 pieces,	4.8 oz	370	4	4	2	0	0	7	9	5	2	2	0	0	1	1	3	0	1	1
Mexican Foods																				
1076 Jack in Box taco,regular 1 serving,	2.9 oz	190	2	2	1	0	0	3	4	0	1	5	1	0	1	2	1	2	1	2
1077 Jack in Box taco,super 1 serving,	5.1 oz	290	3	4	1	1	0	5	7	0	2	10	2	1	1	1	2	4	2	3
1078 Taco Bell bean burrito 1 serving,	6.7 oz	360	4	4	4	7	0	3	5	1	1	9	1	1	9	5	6	2	2	3
1079 Taco Bell beef burrito 1 serving,	6.7 oz	400	4	7	3	6	0	5	8	0	4	10	2	0	5	5	7	2	2	4
1080 Taco Bell beefy tostada 1 serving,	6.5 oz	320	3	5	1	4	0	3	9	0	3	8	4	2	3	3	3	4	2	6

[f]Some nutrients are estimated based on similar items.

continued

Eating Out, Fast Foods

No.	Name/Portion Size		KCAL	CAL	PRO	CAR	FIB	SUG	FAT	SFA	PFA	CHL	SOD	A	C	THI	RIB	B6	CA	IRN	ZN
1081	Taco Bell burrito supreme 1 serving,	8.7 oz	420	4	5	3	8	0	6	8	1	2	10	4	3	6	5	4	3	3	3
1082	Taco Bell combination burrito 1 serving,	6.7 oz	380	4	5	3	6	0	4	6	1	2	10	2	1	7	5	4	2	2	2
1083	Taco Bell enchirito 1 serving,	7.5 oz	380	4	6	2	5	0	6	9	2	3	13	4	1	5	5	5	5	2	4
1084	Taco Bell pintos and cheese 1 serving,	4.5 oz	190	2	3	1	8	0	3	4	0	1	7	2	0	6	3	2	3	2	2
1085	Taco Bell taco 1 serving,	2.8 oz	180	2	3	1	1	0	3	6	0	2	3	1	0	1	2	3	2	1	1
1086	Taco Bell tostada 1 serving,	5.5 oz	240	2	3	2	1	0	3	5	1	1	7	2	1	5	3	4	3	2	1
Pizza																					
1087	Pizza Hut pizza,thin,cheese 1/4 of 13 in pizza	4.6 oz	340	3	6	3	2	1	3	4	1	1	9	2	0	6	6	2	10	4	3
1088	Pizza H,thin,superstyle,cheese 1/4 of 13 in pizza	5.3 oz	410	4	8	3	2	1	4	5	1	2	11	3	0	7	7	2	16	4	3
1089	Pizza H,thin,pepperoni 1/4 of 13 in pizza	4.6 oz	370	4	6	3	2	1	4	5	1	2	10	3	0	6	5	2	8	4	2
1090	Pizza H,thin,suprstyle,peppróni 1/4 of 13 in pizza	5.3 oz	430	4	7	3	2	1	6	6	1	2	12	3	0	8	5	2	11	4	2
1091	Pizza H,thin,pork w mushroom 1/4 of 13 in pizza	4.6 oz	380	4	6	3	2	1	4	4	1	2	12	3	0	7	6	2	2	5	2
1092	Pizza H,thin,super,pork w mushr 1/4 of 13 in pizza	5.3 oz	450	4	8	3	2	1	6	6	1	3	14	3	0	8	7	2	3	7	2
1093	Pizza H,thin,supreme 1/4 of 13 in pizza	5.3 oz	400	4	6	3	2	1	5	5	1	1	12	3	0	9	6	2	8	5	2
1094	Pizza H,thin,super,supreme 1/4 of 13 in pizza	6.3 oz	520	5	9	3	2	1	8	6	2	3	15	4	0	14	8	2	11	6	3
1095	Pizza H,thick,cheese 1/4 of 13 in pizza	5.3 oz	390	4	7	4	2	1	3	4	1	1	8	3	0	10	14	2	12	5	3

1096 Pizza H,thick,superstyle,cheese ¼ of 13 in pizza	6.0 oz	450	4	10	4	2	1	4	5	1	1	10	4	0	11	8	2	19	5	3
1097 Pizza H,thick,pepperoni ¼ of 13 in pizza	5.3 oz	450	4	8	4	2	1	5	6	1	1	9	6	0	11	8	2	10	5	3
1098 Pizza H,thick,suprstyl,pepproni ¼ of 13 in pizza	6.0 oz	490	5	8	4	2	1	6	7	2	2	12	4	0	11	8	2	10	4	3
1099 Pizza H,thick,pork w mushroom ¼ of 13 in pizza	5.3 oz	430	4	8	4	2	1	4	5	1	1	10	4	0	12	8	2	8	6	3
1100 Pizza H,thick,super,pork w mush ¼ of 13 in pizza	6.0 oz	500	5	9	4	2	1	5	6	2	1	12	4	0	12	8	2	11	7	3
1101 Pizza H,thick,supreme ¼ of 13 in pizza	6.0 oz	480	5	9	4	0	1	5	6	2	2	10	4	0	12	9	2	11	6	3
1102 Pizza H,super,supreme ¼ of 13 in pizza	7.1 oz	590	6	10	4	2	1	8	8	2	3	14	4	0	16	11	3	11	7	3
Salads (see dressings in salad section)																				
1103 McDonalds chef salad 1 serving,	9.6 oz	220	2	6	0	N	N	4	5	1	6	7	5	3	7	4	N	4	7	N
1104 McDonalds chicken salad oriental 1 serving,	9.9 oz	150	1	7	0	N	N	1	1	1	6	3	5	7	2	2	N	1	2	N
1105 McDonalds garden salad 1 serving,	7.2 oz	90	1	2	0	N	N	2	2	0	7	1	3	3	1	2	N	2	1	N
1106 McDonalds side salad 1 serving,	4.0 oz	50	0	1	0	N	N	1	1	0	3	0	2	2	1	1	N	1	0	N
1107 McDonalds shrimp salad 1 serving,	9.3 oz	100	1	4	0	N	N	1	1	0	13	6	3	3	2	2	N	1	1	N
Sandwiches																				
1108 Arbys chicken breast sandwich 1 serving,	7.2 oz	550	6	8	4	1	0	8	6	4	4	12	1	0	6	6	2	3	5	1
1109 Arbys roast beef sandwich 1 serving,	5.3 oz	350	3	7	2	1	0	5	5	1	3	9	0	0	6	6	2	2	3	1
1110 Arbys junior roast bf sandwich 1 serving,	3.2 oz	220	2	4	1	1	0	3	3	0	2	5	0	0	2	2	1	1	1	0
1111 Arbys beef and cheddar sandwich 1 serving,	6.3 oz	480	5	9	3	1	0	6	7	0	5	17	0	0	15	8	3	7	2	5

[f] Some nutrients are estimated based on similar items.

continued

Eating Out, Fast Foods

No.	Name/Portion Size	KCAL	CAL	PRO	CAR	FIB	SUG	FAT	SFA	PFA	CHL	SOD	A	C	THI	RIB	B6	CA	IRN	ZN
		NUTRI–UNITS																		
1112	Arbys super roast beef sandwich 1 serving, 10.3 oz	620	6	9	4	2	0	8	10	2	6	14	0	0	19	14	3	5	10	2
1113	Arbys ham+cheese sandwich 1 serving, 8.7 oz	480	5	9	3	2	0	6	7	3	5	17	0	0	21	12	5	10	3	3
1114	Arbys sub (no dressing) 1 serving, 10.1 oz	480	5	11	5	3	0	9	10	5	4	14	4	2	11	11	3	9	8	3
1115	Arbys sauce 1 serving, 1.1 oz	30	0	0	0	0	0	1	0	1	0	2	0	1	0	0	1	0	0	0
1116	Arbys horsey sauce 1 serving, 1.1 oz	50	1	0	0	0	0	1	1	0	0	3	0	0	0	1	0	0	0	0
1117	Burger King,cheeseburger 1 serving, 4.2 oz	310	3	5	2	1	0	4	5	1	4	6	1	0	3	0	2	3	2	3
1118	Burger King,hamburger 1 serving, 3.7 oz	250	3	4	2	1	0	3	4	1	3	4	0	0	3	0	1	1	2	4
1119	Burger King,whopper 1 serving, 10.0 oz	610	6	9	4	3	0	9	13	0	8	9	3	4	10	0	4	1	7	10
1120	Jack in Box hamburger 1 serving, 3.4 oz	260	3	4	2	1	0	3	3	1	2	6	0	0	4	2	1	2	3	2
1121	Jack in Box cheeseburger 1 serving, 3.4 oz	280	3	4	2	2	0	4	6	0	2	8	1	0	3	2	1	3	3	3
1122	Jack in Box jumbo jack burger 1 serving, 3.8 oz	240	2	4	1	1	0	4	4	1	2	5	0	1	3	2	1	1	2	2
1123	J in b jumbo burger w cheese 1 serving, 8.7 oz	570	6	9	3	4	0	10	14	0	7	15	3	1	6	4	3	5	5	6
1124	J in b moby jack sandwich 1 serving, 5.0 oz	460	5	5	3	2	0	8	7	6	4	8	0	0	4	2	11	3	2	1
1125	McDonalds big mac 1 serving, 6.6 oz	520	5	7	3	2	0	9	14	0	5	10	1	1	5	4	2	4	4	5
1126	McDonalds cheeseburger 1 serving, 4.0 oz	310	3	5	2	1	0	4	5	1	3	8	1	1	3	3	1	3	3	3

1127 McDonalds filet of fish 1 serving,	4.6 oz	400	4	5	2	2	0	7	6	6	3	7	1	1	3	3	1	2	2	1
1128 McDonalds hamburger 1 serving,	3.5 oz	260	3	4	2	1	0	3	4	0	2	5	0	1	3	3	1	1	3	3
1129 McDonalds quarter pounder 1 serving,	5.8 oz	420	4	7	2	2	0	5	9	0	5	7	1	1	4	5	3	2	5	7
1130 McD quarter pounder w cheese 1 serving,	6.8 oz	520	5	10	2	3	0	9	11	0	6	12	3	1	4	4	2	5	5	8
1131 Bellbeefer 1 serving,	4.3 oz	220	2	5	2	1	0	2	3	0	4	2	12	3	2	2	2	1	3	5
1132 Bellbeefer w cheese 1 serving,	4.8 oz	280	3	6	2	2	0	4	5	0	4	3	13	3	2	3	2	3	3	4
1133 Wendy's single burger 1 serving,	7.1 oz	470	5	8	2	2	0	8	11	0	5	8	0	0	3	4	3	2	6	6
1134 Wendy's single burger w cheese 1 serving,	8.5 oz	580	6	10	2	3	0	10	14	2	6	11	1	0	5	5	2	5	6	7
1135 Wendy's double burger 1 serving,	10.1 oz	670	7	14	2	3	0	12	17	0	7	10	1	1	6	7	5	3	9	12
1136 Wendy's double burger w cheese 1 serving,	11.5 oz	800	8	15	3	4	0	14	19	3	10	14	2	1	6	9	3	4	12	13
1137 Wendy's triple burger 1 serving,	12.7 oz	840	8	20	2	4	0	15	21	0	14	12	1	1	6	8	6	2	12	18
1138 Wendy's triple burger w cheese 1 serving,	14.1 oz	1040	10	22	2	5	0	20	29	4	15	18	2	1	11	10	4	7	12	19

Soups

1139 Wendy's chili w beans 1 serving,	8.8 oz	230	2	6	1	6	0	2	2	0	2	11	5	1	3	3	2	2	5	5
1140 Clam chowder(potato base) 1 serving,	8.8 oz	220	2	3	1	1	3	4	7	0	3	12	1	0	1	4	1	5	1	3

Fruits and Fruit Juices

Fruits

1141 Apples,raw,w skin $2^3/_4$ in diam apple	4.9 oz	80	1	0	1	2	3	0	0	0	0	0	0	3	0	0	1	0	0	0

continued

[f] Some nutrients are estimated based on similar items.

Fruits and Fruit Juices

No.	Name/Portion Size		KCAL	CAL	PRO	CAR	FIB	SUG	FAT	SFA	PFA	CHL	SOD	A	C	THI	RIB	B6	CA	IRN	ZN
										NUTRI–UNITS											
1142	Apples,raw,w/o skin 2¾ in diam apple	4.6 oz	70	1	0	1	2	3	0	0	0	0	0	0	2	0	0	1	0	0	0
1143	Apples,dehyd,sulfured,unckd ½ cup	1.8 oz	170	2	0	3	4	6	0	0	0	0	1	0	0	0	1	1	0	1	0
1144	Apples,dehyd,sulf,ckd w sugar ½ cup fruit and liq	4.5 oz	100	1	0	2	2	4	0	0	0	0	0	0	0	0	0	1	0	1	0
1145	Apples,dried,sulfured,unckd ½ cup fruit and liq	1.5 oz	100	1	0	2	3	5	0	0	0	0	0	0	1	0	1	1	0	1	0
1146	Apples,dried,sulf,ckd w/o sugar ½ cup	4.5 oz	70	1	0	1	3	5	0	0	0	0	0	0	0	0	0	1	0	0	0
1147	Apples,dried,sulf,ckd w sugar ½ cup	4.9 oz	120	1	0	2	3	7	0	0	0	0	0	0	0	0	0	1	0	0	0
1148	Apples,frozen,sliced,sweetened ½ cup	2.1 oz	60	1	0	1	1	1	0	0	0	0	0	0	1	0	0	0	0	0	0
1149	Apples,spiced ½ cup	4.0 oz	180	2	0	3	2	5	0	0	0	0	0	0	0	0	0	0	0	1	0
1150	Applsauc,cnd,artif swt or unswt ½ cup	4.3 oz	50	1	0	1	2	2	0	0	0	0	0	0	0	0	0	0	0	0	0
1151	Applesauce,canned,sweetened ½ cup	4.5 oz	100	1	0	2	2	6	0	0	0	0	0	0	1	0	0	0	0	0	0
1152	Applesauce,spiced ½ cup	4.6 oz	120	1	0	2	3	6	0	0	0	0	0	0	0	0	0	0	0	1	0
1153	Apricots,raw 3 med or ⅔ cup halves	3.7 oz	50	0	0	1	1	2	0	0	0	0	0	11	3	0	0	1	0	1	0
1154	Apricots,cnd,sol+liq,artif swt 3 halves+1¾ tbsp liq	3.0 oz	20	0	0	0	1	1	0	0	0	0	0	4	1	0	0	0	0	0	0
1155	Apricots,cnd,sol+liq,w juice 3 halves + 1¾ tbsp liq	3.0 oz	40	0	0	1	1	1	0	0	0	0	0	6	1	0	0	0	0	0	0
1156	Apricots,cnd,sol+liq,light syrp 3 halves+1¾ tbsp liq	3.0 oz	50	1	0	1	1	2	0	0	0	0	0	4	1	0	0	0	0	0	0

1157 Apricots,cnd,sol+liq,heavy syrup 3 halves+1 3/4 tbsp liq	3.0 oz	70	1	0	1	1	3	0	0	0	0	0	4	1	0	0	0	0	0	0
1158 Apricots,cnd,sol+liq,x-hvy syrp 3 halves+1 3/4 tbsp liq	3.0 oz	80	1	0	1	1	3	0	0	0	0	0	5	1	0	0	0	0	1	0
1159 Apricots,dried,ckd w sugar 1/2 cup fruit + liquid	4.8 oz	150	2	0	3	3	6	0	0	0	0	0	12	1	0	0	1	0	2	0
1160 Apricots,dried,ckd w/o sugar 1/2 cup fruit + liquid	4.4 oz	110	1	0	2	3	3	0	0	0	0	0	12	1	0	0	1	0	2	0
1161 Apricots,dried,sulfured,unckd 9 med halves or 1/4 cup	1.1 oz	80	1	0	1	2	3	0	0	0	0	0	9	0	0	1	0	0	2	0
1162 Apricots,dehyd,sulfured,unckd 1/2 cup	1.8 oz	160	2	1	3	5	5	0	0	0	0	0	25	2	0	1	3	1	4	1
1163 Apricots,dehyd,sulf,ckd w sugar 1/2 cup	5.3 oz	190	2	1	3	4	7	0	0	0	0	0	26	4	0	1	2	1	4	1
1164 Apricots,frozen,sweetened 1/2 cup	3.0 oz	80	1	0	1	1	4	0	0	0	0	0	6	3	0	0	1	0	1	0
1165 Avocados,raw,commercial variety 1/2 of 3.1 in avocado	4.0 oz	180	2	1	1	1	0	5	2	2	0	0	3	3	2	2	3	0	1	1
1166 Bananas,raw 1 medium or 4/5 cup slicd	4.2 oz	110	1	0	2	2	4	0	0	0	0	0	0	4	1	1	7	0	0	0
1167 Black/boysenberries,raw 1/2 cup	2.5 oz	40	0	0	1	3	1	0	0	0	0	0	0	5	0	0	0	0	0	0
1168 Blackbrries,cnd,sol+liq,art swt 1/2 cup	4.3 oz	50	0	0	1	2	1	0	0	0	0	0	1	3	0	0	0	1	1	0
1169 Blackbrries,cnd,sol+liq,w juice 1/2 cup	4.4 oz	70	1	0	1	2	2	0	0	0	0	0	1	4	0	0	0	1	1	0
1170 Blackbrries,cnd,sol+liq,lit syr 1/2 cup	4.6 oz	90	1	0	2	2	3	0	0	0	0	0	1	3	0	0	0	1	1	1
1171 Blackbrries,cnd,sol+liq,hvy syr 1/2 cup	4.6 oz	120	1	1	2	5	5	0	0	0	0	0	1	1	0	1	0	1	1	0
1172 Blackberries,froz,unswt 1/2 cup	2.5 oz	50	0	0	1	2	2	0	0	0	0	0	0	1	0	0	0	0	1	0
1173 Blueberries,raw 1/2 cup	2.6 oz	40	0	0	1	3	1	0	0	0	0	0	0	3	0	0	0	0	0	0

continued

Fruits and Fruit Juices

No.	Name/Portion Size		KCAL	CAL	PRO	CAR	FIB	SUG	FAT	SFA	PFA	CHL	SOD	A	C	THI	RIB	B6	CA	IRN	ZN
										NUTRI–UNITS											
1174	Bluebrries,cnd,sol+liq,art swtn 1/2 cup	4.3 oz	50	0	0	1	3	1	0	0	0	0	0	0	3	0	0	0	0	1	0
1175	Bluebrries,cnd,sol+liq,hvy syr 1/2 cup	4.4 oz	110	1	0	2	3	5	0	0	0	0	0	0	0	1	1	0	0	0	0
1176	Blueberries,frozen,unsweetened 1/2 cup	2.9 oz	40	0	0	1	3	1	0	0	0	0	0	0	1	0	0	0	0	0	0
1177	Blueberries,frozen,sweetened 1/2 cup	4.1 oz	90	1	0	2	3	5	0	0	0	0	0	0	0	0	1	1	0	0	0
1178	Boysenbrrys,cnd,sol+liq,hvy syr 1/2 cup	4.3 oz	110	1	0	2	3	1	0	0	0	0	0	0	3	0	0	0	0	1	0
1179	Boysenberries,frozen,unsweetened 1/2 cup	2.2 oz	30	0	0	1	3	1	0	0	0	0	0	0	1	0	0	0	0	1	0
1180	Boysenberries,frozen,sweetened 1/2 cup	2.5 oz	70	1	0	1	3	3	0	0	0	0	0	0	2	0	1	0	0	0	0
1181	Cantaloupe,raw 1/4 cup	4.8 oz	50	0	0	1	1	2	0	0	0	0	0	18	19	1	0	2	0	0	0
1182	Casaba melon,raw 1/10 of 6 3/4 in dia meln	4.9 oz	40	0	0	1	1	2	0	0	0	0	0	0	7	1	0	N	0	1	N
1183	Cherries,maraschino,sol+liq 2 tbsp	1.1 oz	40	0	0	1	0	2	0	0	0	0	0	0	0	0	0	0	0	0	0
1184	Cherries,raw,sweet 1/2 cup	2.6 oz	50	1	0	1	1	2	0	0	0	0	0	1	2	0	1	0	0	0	0
1185	Cherries,sour,cnd+liq,unswt,watr 1/2 cup	4.3 oz	40	0	0	1	1	2	0	0	0	0	0	4	1	0	1	1	0	2	0
1186	Cherries,sour,cnd+liq,lite syrp 1/2 cup	4.4 oz	90	1	0	2	1	4	0	0	0	0	0	4	1	0	1	1	0	2	0
1187	Cherries,sour,cnd+liq,hvy syrp 1/2 cup	4.6 oz	120	1	0	2	1	5	0	0	0	0	0	4	1	0	1	1	0	2	0
1188	Cherries,sour,cnd+liq,xhvy syrp 1/2 cup	4.6 oz	150	1	0	3	1	6	0	0	0	0	0	4	1	0	1	1	0	2	0

1189 Cherries,sour,frozen,unsweetend 1/2 cup	3.7 oz	50	0	0	1	1	2	0	0	0	0	0	4	1	1	0	1	0	1	0
1190 Cherries,sour,frozen,sweetend 1/2 cup	3.9 oz	120	1	0	2	1	5	0	0	0	0	0	2	2	0	1	1	0	1	0
1191 Cherries,swt,cnd,sol+liq, water 1/2 cup	4.3 oz	60	1	0	1	1	3	0	0	0	0	0	1	1	0	1	0	0	0	0
1192 Cherries,swt,cnd+liq,lite syrp 1/2 cup	4.4 oz	80	1	0	2	1	4	0	0	0	0	0	1	2	0	1	0	0	0	0
1193 Cherries,swt,cnd+liq,hvy syrp 1/2 cup	4.6 oz	110	1	0	2	1	5	0	0	0	0	0	1	2	0	1	0	0	1	0
1194 Cherries,swt,cnd+liq,xhvy syrp 1/2 cup	4.6 oz	130	1	0	2	1	6	0	0	0	0	0	1	2	0	1	0	0	1	0
1195 Coconut meat,fresh 2 × 2 × 1/2 in piece	1.6 oz	160	2	0	0	4	0	5	12	0	0	0	0	0	0	0	0	0	1	1
1196 Crabapples,raw 1 1/2 in diam apple	1.1 oz	20	0	0	0	0	1	0	0	0	0	0	0	1	0	0	N	0	0	N
1197 Cranberries,raw 1/2 cup	1.6 oz	20	0	0	0	1	0	0	0	0	0	0	0	2	0	0	0	0	0	0
1198 Cranberry sauce,cnd,sweetened 3 tbsp sauce	1.8 oz	80	1	0	1	0	3	0	0	0	0	0	0	0	0	0	0	0	0	0
1199 Cranberry sauce,home prep,swtnd 3 tbsp sauce	1.8 oz	90	1	0	2	1	4	0	0	0	0	0	0	0	0	0	0	0	0	0
1200 Currants,black or european,raw 1/2 cup	2.4 oz	40	0	0	1	4	1	0	0	0	0	0	1	40	0	0	0	1	1	0
1201 Currants,red or white,raw 1/2 cup	2.4 oz	40	0	0	1	3	1	0	0	0	0	0	0	9	0	0	0	0	1	0
1202 Dates,pitted 5 dates	1.4 oz	110	1	0	2	2	6	0	0	0	0	0	0	0	0	0	1	0	1	0
1203 Dried fruit,mixed 2 oz (approx 1/2 c)	1.9 oz	130	1	0	2	6	7	0	0	0	0	0	5	1	0	1	1	0	2	0
1204 Figs,raw 2 med figs, 2 1/4 in diam	3.5 oz	70	1	0	1	2	4	0	0	0	0	0	1	1	1	1	1	1	0	0
1205 Figs,cnd,sol+liq,water,art swtn 1/3 cup	2.8 oz	40	0	0	1	2	2	0	0	0	0	0	0	0	0	0	1	0	0	0

continued

Fruits and Fruit Juices

No.	Name/Portion Size		KCAL	CAL	PRO	CAR	FIB	SUG	FAT	SFA	PFA	CHL	SOD	A	C	THI	RIB	B6	CA	IRN	ZN
										NUTRI–UNITS											
1206	Figs,cnd,sol+liq,light syrup 1/3 cup	3.0 oz	60	1	0	1	3	3	0	0	0	0	0	0	0	0	0	1	0	0	0
1207	Figs,cnd,sol+liq,heavy syrup 1/3 cup	3.0 oz	80	1	0	1	3	3	0	0	0	0	0	0	0	0	0	1	0	0	0
1208	Figs,cnd,sol+liq,x-heavy syrup 1/3 cup	3.0 oz	90	1	0	2	3	4	0	0	0	0	0	0	0	0	0	1	0	0	0
1209	Figs,dried,uncooked 1/2 cup,chopped	3.0 oz	220	2	1	4	10	12	0	0	0	0	0	0	0	1	1	2	2	2	1
1210	Fruit cocktail,cnd,in juice 1/2 cup,sol+liq	4.3 oz	60	1	0	1	1	3	0	0	0	0	0	2	1	0	0	1	0	0	0
1211	Fruit cocktail,cnd,light syrup 1/2 cup,sol+liq	4.4 oz	70	1	0	1	1	4	0	0	0	0	0	1	1	0	0	1	0	0	0
1212	Fruit cocktail,cnd,heavy syrup 1/2 cup,sol+liq	4.5 oz	90	1	0	2	1	5	0	0	0	0	0	1	1	0	0	1	0	0	0
1213	Fruit cocktail,cnd,xlite syrup 1/2 cup,sol+liq	4.5 oz	60	1	0	1	1	3	0	0	0	0	0	1	1	1	0	1	0	0	0
1214	Fruit salad,cnd,sol+liq,art swt 1/2 cup	4.3 oz	60	1	0	1	1	3	0	0	0	0	0	3	1	0	0	0	0	0	0
1215	Fruit salad,cnd,sol+liq,lit syr 1/2 cup	4.4 oz	70	1	0	1	1	4	0	0	0	0	0	2	1	0	0	0	0	0	0
1216	Fruit salad,cnd,sol+liq,hvy syr 1/2 cup	4.5 oz	90	1	0	2	1	5	0	0	0	0	0	3	1	0	0	0	0	0	0
1217	Fruit salad,cnd+liq,xhvy syrp 1/2 cup	4.5 oz	110	1	0	2	1	6	0	0	0	0	0	3	1	0	0	0	0	0	0
1218	Gooseberries,raw 1/2 cup	2.6 oz	30	0	0	1	2	1	0	0	0	0	0	1	7	0	0	1	0	0	0
1219	Goosebrries,cnd,sol+liq,lit syr 1/2 cup	3.9 oz	80	1	0	1	2	5	0	0	0	0	0	1	4	0	1	0	0	0	0
1220	Goosebrrys,cnd,sol+liq,hvy syr 1/2 cup	3.9 oz	130	1	0	2	2	6	0	0	0	0	0	1	4	2	1	0	0	0	0

1221 Grapefruit,raw,pink or red 1/2 of 4-in diam fruit	4.5 oz	40	0	0	1	1	2	0	0	0	0	0	1	16	1	0	1	0	0	0
1222 Grapefruit,raw,white 1/2 of 4-in diam fruit	4.8 oz	50	0	0	1	1	2	0	0	0	0	0	0	15	1	0	1	0	0	0
1223 Grapefruit segments,cnd,art swt 1/2 cup	4.3 oz	40	0	0	1	1	1	0	0	0	0	0	0	12	0	0	0	0	0	0
1224 Grapefruit segments,cnd,syrup 1/2 cup	4.4 oz	90	1	0	2	1	4	0	0	0	0	0	0	13	1	0	0	0	0	0
1225 Grapes,raw,red,green,blue,white 1/2 cup	2.6 oz	50	0	0	1	0	2	0	0	0	0	0	0	1	1	0	1	0	0	0
1226 Grapes,cnd,thomps,seedless,watr 1/2 cup,sol+liq	4.3 oz	50	0	0	1	0	N	0	0	0	0	0	0	0	1	0	1	0	1	0
1227 Grapes,cnd,thomp,seedls,hvy syr 1/2 cup,sol+liq	4.5 oz	90	1	0	2	0	N	0	0	0	0	0	0	0	1	0	1	0	1	0
1228 Guavas,raw,whole,common 1 medium	3.2 oz	50	0	0	1	2	1	0	0	0	0	0	3	55	1	1	1	0	0	0
1229 Honeydew melon,raw 1/10 of 6 3/4 in dia meln	5.3 oz	50	1	0	1	1	2	0	0	0	0	0	0	12	2	0	1	0	0	N
1230 Kiwi fruit 1 medium	2.7 oz	50	0	0	1	N	N	0	0	0	0	0	1	25	0	0	N	0	0	N
1231 Kumquats,raw 3 medium	2.1 oz	40	0	0	1	1	2	0	0	0	0	0	1	7	1	1	N	1	0	0
1232 Lemons,raw,peeled 1 med 2 1/8 in diam lemon	2.8 oz	20	0	0	1	2	1	0	0	0	0	0	0	14	0	0	1	0	1	0
1233 Lemon peel,raw 1 tbsp grated peel	.2 oz	0	0	0	0	N	0	0	0	0	0	0	0	3	0	0	0	0	0	N
1234 Limes,raw 2 in diam lime	2.4 oz	20	0	0	0	2	0	0	0	0	0	0	0	6	0	0	0	0	0	0
1235 Loganberries,raw 1/2 cup	2.5 oz	50	0	0	1	3	0	0	0	0	0	0	1	6	0	0	0	1	1	0
1236 Loganbrries,cnd,sol+liq,art swt 1/2 cup	3.5 oz	40	0	0	1	4	0	0	0	0	0	0	1	3	0	0	1	0	1	0
1237 Loganberries,cnd,sol+liq, juice 1/2 cup	3.5 oz	50	1	0	1	4	1	0	0	0	0	0	1	4	0	0	1	1	1	0

continued

Fruits and Fruit Juices

No.	Name/Portion Size		KCAL	CAL	PRO	CAR	FIB	SUG	FAT	SFA	PFA	CHL	SOD	A	C	THI	RIB	B6	CA	IRN	ZN
										NUTRI–UNITS											
1238	Loganbrries,cnd,sol+liq,lit syr ½ cup	3.5 oz	70	1	0	1	3	2	0	0	0	0	0	1	3	0	0	1	0	1	0
1239	Loganbrries,cnd,sol+liq,hvy syr ½ cup	3.5 oz	90	1	0	2	3	3	0	0	0	0	0	1	3	0	0	1	0	1	0
1240	Loganbrrys,cnd,sol+liq,xhvy syr ½ cup	3.5 oz	110	1	0	2	3	4	0	0	0	0	0	1	2	0	0	1	0	1	0
1241	Mangos,raw ½ cup, diced or sliced	2.9 oz	50	1	0	1	1	2	0	0	0	0	0	13	8	1	1	1	0	0	0
1242	Nectarines,raw 2½ in diam nectarine	4.9 oz	70	1	0	1	2	4	0	0	0	0	0	4	2	0	1	0	0	0	0
1243	Oranges,peeled,all varieties 2⅝ in diam orange	4.6 oz	60	1	0	1	2	3	0	0	0	0	0	1	23	2	1	1	1	0	0
1244	Orange peel,raw 1 tbsp	.2 oz	0	0	0	0	0	0	0	0	0	0	0	0	3	0	0	0	0	0	N
1245	Papayas,raw ½ of 3.5 in diam fruit	5.4 oz	60	1	0	1	1	3	0	0	0	0	0	2	31	1	1	0	1	0	0
1246	Peaches,raw 2½ in diam peach	3.5 oz	40	0	0	1	2	2	0	0	0	0	0	2	2	0	0	0	0	0	0
1247	Peaches,cnd,sol+liq,artif swtnd ½ cup	4.3 oz	30	0	0	1	1	2	0	0	0	0	0	3	1	0	0	0	0	0	0
1248	Peaches,cnd,sol+liq,in juice ½ cup	4.4 oz	60	1	0	1	1	3	0	0	0	0	0	2	1	0	0	0	0	0	0
1249	Peaches,cnd,sol+liq,lite syrup ½ cup	4.4 oz	70	1	0	1	1	4	0	0	0	0	0	2	1	0	0	0	0	1	0
1250	Peaches,cnd,sol+liq,hvy syrup ½ cup	4.5 oz	90	1	0	2	1	5	0	0	0	0	0	2	1	0	0	0	0	0	0
1251	Peaches,cnd,sol+liq,xhvy syrup ½ cup	4.6 oz	120	1	0	2	1	6	0	0	0	0	0	1	1	0	0	0	0	0	0
1252	Peaches,dehydrated,ckd w sugar ½ cup,sol+liq	4.9 oz	140	1	0	3	1	8	0	0	0	0	0	1	2	0	0	0	0	2	0

1253 Peaches, dried, uncooked	1/4 cup	1.4 oz	100	1	0	2	3	5	0	0	0	0	0	3	1	0	1	0	0	2	0
1254 Peaches,dried,cooked w/o sugar	1/2 cup,sol+liq	4.3 oz	90	1	0	2	1	5	0	0	0	0	0	1	2	0	0	0	0	2	0
1255 Peaches,dried,cooked w sugar	1/2 cup,sol+liq	4.6 oz	130	1	0	2	1	8	0	0	0	0	0	1	1	0	0	0	0	2	0
1256 Peaches,fz.swt,sliced,+ vit c	1/2 cup	4.4 oz	120	1	0	2	2	6	0	0	0	0	0	1	39	0	0	0	0	1	0
1257 Pears,raw,including skin	2.5 in diam × 3.5 in pear	5.9 oz	100	1	0	2	3	5	0	0	0	0	0	0	2	0	1	0	0	0	0
1258 Pears,dried,sulf,unckd	5 halves	3.1 oz	230	2	1	4	6	12	0	0	0	0	0	0	2	0	1	1	1	2	0
1259 Pears,cnd,sol+liq,artif swtnd	1 half + 2 tbsp liq	3.2 oz	30	0	0	0	1	1	0	0	0	0	0	0	0	0	0	0	0	0	0
1260 Pears,cnd,sol+liq,in juice	1 half + 2 tbsp liq	3.2 oz	50	0	0	1	1	2	0	0	0	0	0	0	0	0	0	0	0	0	0
1261 Pears,cnd,sol+liq,light syrup	1 half + 2 tbsp liq	3.3 oz	50	1	0	1	1	3	0	0	0	0	0	0	0	0	0	0	0	0	0
1262 Pears,cnd,sol+liq,heavy syrup	1 half + 2 tbsp liq	3.3 oz	70	1	0	1	1	4	0	0	0	0	0	0	0	0	0	0	0	0	0
1263 Pears,cnd,sol+liq,xheavy syrup	1 half + 2 tbsp liq	3.4 oz	90	1	0	2	1	4	0	0	0	0	0	0	0	0	0	0	0	0	0
1264 Pears,dried,sulfrd,ckd w/o sugr	1/2 cup,sol+liq	4.5 oz	160	2	0	3	4	8	0	0	0	0	0	0	2	0	0	0	0	1	0
1265 Pears,dried,sulf,ckd w sugar	1/2 cup, sol + liq	4.9 oz	200	2	0	4	5	11	0	0	0	0	0	0	2	0	0	0	0	2	0
1266 Persimmons,raw,native	2 1/2 in dia × 3 in high	5.9 oz	210	2	0	4	2	6	0	0	0	0	0	N	37	N	N	N	1	5	N
1267 Pineapple,raw	1/2 cup, diced	2.8 oz	40	0	0	1	1	2	0	0	0	0	0	0	4	1	0	1	0	0	0
1268 Pineapple,cnd,sol+liq,artf swnd	1/2 cup,tidbits	4.3 oz	40	0	0	1	1	2	0	0	0	0	0	0	3	2	0	1	0	1	0
1269 Pineapple,cnd,sol+liq,in juice	1/2 cup, tidbits	4.4 oz	70	1	0	1	1	3	0	0	0	0	0	0	4	2	0	1	0	0	0

continued

Fruits and Fruit Juices

No.	Name/Portion Size		KCAL	CAL	PRO	CAR	FIB	SUG	FAT	SFA	PFA	CHL	SOD	A	C	THI	RIB	B6	CA	IRN	ZN
			NUTRI–UNITS																		
1270	Pineapple,cnd,sol+liq,lite syrp 1/2 cup,all styles	4.4 oz	70	1	0	1	1	4	0	0	0	0	0	0	3	2	0	1	0	1	0
1271	Pineapple,cnd,sol+liq,hvy syrup 1/2 cup,all styles	4.5 oz	100	1	0	2	1	5	0	0	0	0	0	0	3	2	0	1	0	1	0
1272	Pineapple,cnd,sol+liq,xhvy syrp 1/2 cup,all styles	4.6 oz	110	1	0	2	1	6	0	0	0	0	0	0	3	2	0	1	0	1	0
1273	Pineapple,frozen chunks,swtnd 1/2 cup	4.3 oz	110	1	0	2	1	5	0	0	0	0	0	0	3	2	0	1	0	1	0
1274	Plantain(baking banana),raw 1/2 of 2 in diax11 in frt	4.6 oz	160	2	1	3	5	3	0	0	0	0	0	6	8	1	1	4	0	1	0
1275	Plums, raw 1 plum,2 1/8 in dia	2.3 oz	40	0	0	1	1	1	0	0	0	0	0	1	2	0	1	1	0	0	0
1276	Plums,purpl,cnd,sol+liq,art swt 3 plums+2 tbsp liq;2/5 c	3.5 oz	40	0	0	1	1	2	0	0	0	0	0	1	1	0	0	0	0	0	0
1277	Plums,purpl,cnd,sol+liq,lit syr 3 plums+2 tbsp liq;2/5 c	3.6 oz	60	1	0	1	1	3	0	0	0	0	0	1	0	0	0	0	0	1	0
1278	Plums,purp,cnd,sol+liq,hvy syr 3 plums+2 tbsp liq;2/5 c	3.6 oz	90	1	0	2	1	4	0	0	0	0	0	1	0	0	0	0	0	1	0
1279	Plums,purp,cnd,sol+liq,xhvy syr 3 plums+2 tbsp liq;2/5 c	3.6 oz	100	1	0	2	2	5	0	0	0	0	0	1	0	0	0	0	0	1	0
1280	Pomegranate,pulp,raw 3.4 in dia × 2.7 in fruit	5.4 oz	110	1	0	2	2	4	0	0	0	0	0	0	3	1	1	2	0	1	N
1281	Pricklypears,raw 3.5 oz	3.5 oz	40	0	0	1	1	2	0	0	0	0	0	0	5	0	1	N	1	0	N
1282	Prunes,dehy,ckd,sol+liq,w sugar 1/4 cup	2.5 oz	80	1	0	1	5	4	0	0	0	0	0	1	0	0	0	1	0	1	0
1283	Prunes,dried,uncooked,pitted 5 large prunes	1.8 oz	170	2	1	3	7	5	0	0	0	0	0	4	0	1	1	4	1	2	1
1284	Prunes,dried,cooked w/o sugar 3 med+1 tbsp jc or 1/4 c	1.9 oz	60	1	0	1	2	2	0	0	0	0	0	1	1	0	1	1	0	1	0

1285 Prunes,dried,cooked w sugar 3 med+1 tbsp jc or 1/4 c	2.1 oz	70	1	0	1	3	3	0	0	0	0	0	1	1	0	1	1	0	1	0
1286 Raisins,natural,uncooked 2 tbsp raisins	.6 oz	50	1	0	1	1	3	0	0	0	0	0	0	0		0	0	0	0	0
1287 Raspberries,black,raw 1/2 cup	2.5 oz	30	0	0	1	3	1	0	0	0	0	0	0	6		1	0	0	0	0
1288 Raspberries,red,raw 1/2 cup	2.3 oz	40	0	0	1	3	1	0	0	0	0	0	0	5	0	1	0	0	1	0
1289 Raspberrys,blk,cnd,sol+liq,watr 1/2 cup	4.2 oz	60	1	0	1	6	1	0	0	0	0	0	0	2	0	1	1	0	1	0
1290 Raspberrys,red,cnd,sol+liq,watr 1/2 cup	4.2 oz	40	0	0	1	6	1	0	0	0	0	0	0	4	0	1	1	0	1	0
1291 Raspberries,red,frozen,sweetnd 1/2 cup	4.4 oz	130	1	0	2	6	4	0	0	0	0	0	0	7	0	1	0	0	1	0
1292 Rhubarb,raw 1/2 cup, diced	2.1 oz	10	0	0	0	1	0	0	0	0	0	0	0	2	0	0	0	1	0	0
1293 Rhubarb,cooked,sol+liq, w sugar 1/2 cup	4.8 oz	190	2	0	3	2	9	0	0	0	0	0	0	3	0	1	0	2	1	0
1294 Rhubarb,frozen,unswt. 1/2 cup	4.0 oz	20	0	0	0	2	4	0	0	0	0	0	0	2	0	0	0	4	0	0
1295 Rhubarb,frozen,cooked w sugar 1/2 cup	4.8 oz	160	2	0	3	2	9	0	0	0	0	0	0	1	0	0	0	4	0	0
1296 Strawberries,raw 1/2 cup, whole or halves	2.6 oz	20	0	0	0	1	1	0	0	0	0	0	0	14	0	1	0	0	0	0
1297 Strawberries,cnd,sol+liq, water 1/2 cup	4.2 oz	30	0	0	0	1	1	0	0	0	0	0	0	8	0	0	N	0	1	0
1298 Strawberries,frozen,sliced,swtn 1/2 cup	4.5 oz	120	1	0	2	2	7	0	0	0	0	0	0	18	0	1	0	0	1	0
1299 Tangerines,raw 2 3/8 in diam med fruit	3.0 oz	40	0	0	1	1	2	0	0	0	0	0	3	9	1	0	1	0	0	0
1300 Watermelon,raw 2 cups, diced	11.3 oz	100	1	1	2	N	6	0	0	0	0	0	5	10	3	1	5	1	1	0

continued

Fruits and Fruit Juices

No.	Name/Portion Size		KCAL	CAL	PRO	CAR	FIB	SUG	FAT	SFA	PFA	CHL	SOD	A	C	THI	RIB	B6	CA	IRN	ZN
			NUTRI–UNITS																		
Fruit Juices																					
1301	Apple juice,canned or bottled ½ cup; 4 fluid oz	4.4 oz	60	1	0	1	0	3	0	0	0	0	0	0	0	0	0	0	0	1	0
1302	Apple juice,cnd or bottld+vit c ½ cup	4.4 oz	60	1	0	1	0	3	0	0	0	0	0	0	18	0	0	N	0	1	0
1303	Apricot nectar,cnd,40 pct fruit ½ cup	4.4 oz	70	1	0	1	1	3	0	0	0	0	0	7	0	0	0	0	0	1	0
1304	Apricot nectar,cnd,+ vit c ½ cup	4.4 oz	70	1	0	1	1	3	0	0	0	0	0	5	17	0	0	N	0	0	0
1305	Blackberry juice,cnd,unswtnd ½ cup	4.3 oz	50	0	0	1	0	1	0	0	0	0	0	1	4	0	0	0	0	1	0
1306	Cranberry juice cocktail ½ cup	4.5 oz	70	1	0	1	0	4	0	0	0	0	0	0	15	0	0	0	0	0	0
1307	Cranberry juic cocktail w vit c ½ cup	4.5 oz	90	1	0	2	0	4	0	0	0	0	0	0	11	0	0	0	0	1	0
1308	Grapefruit jc,raw,red,pink,whte ½ cup	4.3 oz	50	0	0	1	0	2	0	0	0	0	0	0	16	1	0	1	0	0	0
1309	Grape juice,canned or bottled ½ cup	4.4 oz	80	1	0	1	0	4	0	0	0	0	0	0	0	0	1	1	0	0	0
1310	Grape juice,fz,swt,dilut,vit c ½ cup	4.4 oz	60	1	0	1	0	4	0	0	0	0	0	0	10	0	0	1	0	0	0
1311	Lemon juice,raw 2 tbsp	1.1 oz	10	0	0	0	0	0	0	0	0	0	0	0	5	0	0	0	0	0	0
1312	Lemon juice,cnd or bottld,unswtn 2 tbsp	1.1 oz	10	0	0	0	0	0	0	0	0	0	0	0	2	0	0	0	0	0	0
1313	Lime juice,raw 2 tbsp	1.1 oz	10	0	0	0	0	0	0	0	0	0	0	0	3	0	0	0	0	0	0
1314	Lime juice,cnd or bottld,unswtn 2 tbsp	1.1 oz	10	0	0	0	0	0	0	0	0	0	0	0	1	0	0	0	0	0	0
1315	Orange juice,raw,all varieties ½ cup	4.4 oz	60	1	0	1	0	2	0	0	0	0	0	1	21	1	0	0	0	0	0

1316 Orange juice,cnd,unsweetened 1/2 cup	4.4 oz	50	1	0	1	0	3	0	0	0	0	0	1	14	1	0	1	0	1	0
1317 Orange juic,fz,conc,unswt,dilut 1/2 cup	4.4 oz	60	1	0	1	0	3	0	0	0	0	0	0	16	1	0	1	0	0	0
1318 Peach nectar,cnd,40 prcnt fruit 1/2 cup	4.4 oz	70	1	0	1	1	3	0	0	0	0	0	1	2	0	0	0	0	0	0
1319 Pear Nectar,cnd,40 prcnt fruit 1/2 cup	4.4 oz	80	1	0	1	1	3	0	0	0	0	0	0	0	0	0	0	0	0	0
1320 Pineapple juice,cnd,unsweetened 1/2 cup	4.4 oz	70	1	0	1	0	3	0	0	0	0	0	0	4	1	0	1	0	0	0
1321 Pineapple juice,cnd,+ vit c 1/2 cup	4.4 oz	70	1	0	1	0	3	0	0	0	0	0	0	16	1	0	1	0	0	0
1322 Pineapple,jc,fz,conc,unswt,dil 1/2 cup	4.4 oz	70	1	0	2	0	3	0	0	0	0	0	0	6	1	0	1	0	0	0
1323 Prune juice,canned or bottled 1/2 cup	4.5 oz	90	1	0	2	0	3	0	0	0	0	0	0	2	0	1	3	0	2	0
1324 Prune juice,bottled,+ vit c 1/2 cup	4.5 oz	100	1	0	2	0	4	0	0	0	0	0	1	18	0	0	3	0	6	0
1325 Tangelo juice,raw 1/2 cup	4.4 oz	50	1	0	1	0	2	0	0	0	0	0	2	11	1	0	0	0	0	0
1326 Tangerine juice,raw 1/2 cup	4.4 oz	50	1	0	1	0	2	0	0	0	0	0	2	13	1	0	1	0	0	0
1327 Tangerine juice,cnd,sweetened 1/2 cup	4.4 oz	60	1	0	1	0	3	0	0	0	0	0	2	9	1	0	0	0	0	0
1328 Tangerine jc,fz,conc,swt,dil 1/2 cup	4.4 oz	70	1	0	1	0	3	0	0	0	0	0	3	12	1	0	1	0	0	0
1329 Tomato juice,canned,salted 1/2 cup	4.3 oz	20	0	0	0	1	1	0	0	0	0	4	3	7	1	0	1	0	1	0
1330 Tomato juice,cnd,lo sodium 1/2 cup	4.3 oz	20	0	0	0	0	1	0	0	0	0	0	4	6	1	0	1	0	1	0
1331 Vegetable juice cocktail,cnd 1/2 cup	4.3 oz	20	0	0	0	0	0	0	0	0	0	4	6	11	1	0	2	0	1	0

continued

No.	Name/Portion Size		KCAL	CAL	PRO	CAR	FIB	SUG	FAT	SFA	PFA	CHL	SOD	A	C	THI	RIB	B6	CA	IRN	ZN
									NUTRI–UNITS												
Main Dishes																					
Beans, Seeds and Their Products																					
1332	Adzuki beans,ckd,w salt 1/2 cup5	4.1 oz	150	1	3	2	7	N	0	0	0	0	3	0	0	2	1	1	1	3	3
1333	Baked beans 1/2 cup	4.5 oz	120	1	2	2	7	1	0	0	0	0	5	1	1	3	1	2	1	0	2
1334	Baked beans,canned,w/franks 1/2 cup	4.5 oz	180	2	3	1	7	1	3	3	1	1	6	1	1	1	1	1	1	2	3
1335	Baked beans,cnd,pork+sweet sce 1/2 cup	4.4 oz	140	1	2	2	7	2	1	1	0	1	4	1	1	1	1	1	2	2	3
1336	Baked beans,cnd,pork+tom sce 1/2 cup	4.4 oz	120	1	2	2	7	1	0	0	0	1	6	1	1	1	1	1	1	2	3
1337	Baked beans, homemade w salt 1/2 cup	4.4 oz	190	2	2	2	7	1	2	2	1	0	5	0	0	2	1	1	2	3	1
1338	Black beans,ckd,no salt 1/2 cup	3.0 oz	110	1	2	1	7	0	0	0	0	0	0	0	0	3	1	1	0	2	1
1339	Black bean soup,cnd,dil,salted 1 cup	8.7 oz	120	1	2	1	7	0	0	0	0	0	12	2	0	1	1	1	1	2	2
1340	Blackeyed peas,ckd,no salt 1/2 cup	3.0 oz	100	1	2	1	2	0	0	0	0	0	0	0	0	2	1	1	0	2	1
1341	Falafel 2 2 1/4 in patties	1.2 oz	60	1	1	1	N	0	1	0	1	0	1	0	1	0	0	1	0	1	0
1342	Garbanzo beans,chickpeas,ckd 1/2 cup,salted	2.9 oz	130	1	2	2	7	1	1	0	1	0	2	0	0	1	1	1	1	3	2
1343	Hummus 1/3 cup	2.9 oz	270	3	3	2	N	N	4	2	3	0	2	0	0	2	2	1	1	3	2
1344	Lentils,cooked,no salt 1/2 cup	3.5 oz	120	1	3	1	3	0	0	0	0	0	0	0	0	2	1	2	0	4	2
1345	Lentil soup w ham 1 cup	8.7 oz	140	1	3	1	3	0	1	1	0	0	13	1	1	2	1	2	1	3	1

1346 Lima beans,cooked,no salt ½ cup	3.3 oz	110	1	2	1	7	0	0	0	0	0	0	0	0	2	1	2	0	2	1
1347 Pinto beans,ckd,no salt ½ cup	3.0 oz	120	1	2	2	7	0	0	0	0	0	0	0	1	2	1	1	1	2	1
1348 Red beans,canned,no salt ½ cup	4.5 oz	120	1	2	1	7	0	0	0	0	0	0	0	0	1	1	2	1	3	1
1349 Red beans,cooked w salt ½ cup	4.5 oz	160	2	3	2	8	0	0	0	0	0	3	0	1	3	1	2	1	4	2
1350 Navy,white beans,ckd,no salt ½ cup	3.3 oz	110	1	2	1	6	0	0	0	0	0	0	0	0	1	1	N	1	2	1
1351 Refried beans,canned ½ cup	4.4 oz	140	1	2	2	8	1	0	0	0	0	5	0	3	1	1	1	1	2	2
1352 Split peas,cooked,no salt ½ cup	3.5 oz	120	1	3	1	3	0	0	0	0	0	0	0	0	2	1	0	0	1	1
1353 Soyameat 1 slice	2.3 oz	160	2	3	0	N	0	4	2	6	0	4	0	0	2	1	3	0	1	0
1354 Soybeans,cooked,no salt ½ cup	3.0 oz	150	1	4	1	5	0	2	1	4	0	0	0	0	2	3	2	2	5	1
1355 Tahini,sesame butter 1 tablespoon	.5 oz	90	1	1	0	1	N	2	1	3	0	0	0	0	2	1	0	1	1	1
1356 Tempeh,fermented soybeans ½ cup	2.9 oz	170	2	5	1	N	N	2	1	3	0	0	2	0	1	1	2	2	2	2
1357 Tofu,soybean curd 1 pc (2.5 × 2.8 × 1 in)	4.2 oz	170	2	6	0	N	N	3	1	5	0	0	1	0	3	1	1	16	14	3
1358 Tofu,fried 1 small cube	.5 oz	40	0	1	0	N	N	1	0	1	0	0	0	0	0	0	0	1	1	0
Beef (unsalted except canned or processed)[g]																				
1359 Canned roast beef w juice ½ cup	4.3 oz	240	2	8	0	0	0	5	7	0	7	6	0	0	1	2	4	0	4	10
1360 Chipped or dried beef 1 oz	1.0 oz	50	0	3	0	0	0	0	0	0	1	10	0	1	0	1	1	0	1	2

[g]Add 0.5 nutri-unit of sodium for moderate or 1 nutri-unit for heavy salting per 3 oz serving.

continued

Main Dishes

No.	Name/Portion Size		KCAL	CAL	PRO	CAR	FIB	SUG	FAT	SFA	PFA	CHL	SOD	A	C	THI	RIB	B6	CA	IRN	ZN
										NUTRI–UNITS											
1361	Corned beef,canned 3 oz	3.0 oz	210	2	7	0	0	0	4	5	0	5	9	0	0	0	1	1	0	2	4
1362	Corned beef,cooked 3 oz	3.0 oz	210	2	5	0	0	0	5	5	1	6	10	0	5	0	2	2	0	2	5
1363	Chuck,lean + fat,braised 1 piece (4 × 2.3 × .5 in)	3.0 oz	300	3	7	0	0	0	7	8	1	6	1	0	0	1	2	2	0	3	8
1364	Chuck,lean only,braised 1 piece (4 × 2.3 × .5 in)	3.0 oz	200	2	9	0	0	0	3	3	0	6	1	0	0	1	3	3	0	4	10
1365	Chuck blade,lean + fat,braised 1 piece (4 × 2.3 × .5 in)	3.0 oz	330	3	7	0	0	0	8	10	1	6	1	0	0	1	2	2	0	3	9
1366	Chuck blade,lean only,braised 1 piece (4 × 2.3 × .5 in)	3.0 oz	230	2	8	0	0	0	4	5	0	6	1	0	0	1	3	2	0	3	12
1367	Chuck arm,lean + fat,braised 1 pc (2.5 × 2.5 × .8 in)	3.0 oz	290	3	7	0	0	0	6	8	1	6	1	0	0	1	2	2	0	3	8
1368	Chuck arm,lean only,braised 1 pc (2.5 × 2.5 × .8 in)	3.0 oz	200	2	9	0	0	0	3	3	0	6	1	0	0	1	3	3	0	4	10
1369	Club steak,lean + fat,broiled 1 piece (2 × 4 × .5 in)	3.0 oz	240	2	7	0	0	0	5	6	1	4	1	0	0	1	2	3	0	2	5
1370	Club steak,lean only,broiled 1 piece (2 × 4 × .5 in)	3.0 oz	180	2	7	0	0	0	2	3	0	4	1	0	0	1	2	4	0	2	6
1371	Flank steak,braised 1 pc (2.5 × 2.5 × .8 in)	3.0 oz	220	2	7	0	0	0	4	5	0	4	1	0	0	2	2	3	0	3	7
1372	Porterhouse steak,lean+fat,brl Yield from 1/2 lb w bone	5.3 oz	450	4	12	0	0	0	10	12	1	8	1	0	0	2	4	5	0	4	9
1373	Porterhouse steak,lean only,brl 1 piece (3.5 × 2 × .8 in)	3.0 oz	190	2	7	0	0	0	3	3	0	5	1	0	0	1	2	3	0	3	6
1374	T-bone steak,lean + fat,brl 1 piece (3.5 × 2 × .8 in)	3.0 oz	280	3	6	0	0	0	6	8	1	5	1	0	0	1	2	3	0	2	5
1375	T-bone steak,lean only,brl 1 piece (3.5 × 2 × .8 in)	3.0 oz	180	2	7	0	0	0	3	3	0	5	1	0	0	1	2	3	0	3	6

1376	Tenderloin,lean + fat, brl 1 piece (2.6 × 2.6 × .8 i	3.0 oz	230	2	7	0	0	0	5	6	1	5	1	0	0	1	3	3	0	3	6
1377	Tenderloin, lean only, brl 1 piece (2.6 × 2.6 × .8 i	3.0 oz	180	2	7	0	0	0	2	3	0	5	1	0	0	1	3	4	0	3	6
1378	Sirloin,roundbone,lean+fat,brl 1 piece (2 × 4 × .5 in)	3.0 oz	240	2	7	0	0	0	5	6	1	5	1	0	0	1	3	3	0	3	6
1379	Sirloin,roundbone,lean only,brl 1 piece (2 × 4 × .5 in)	3.0 oz	180	2	8	0	0	0	2	3	0	5	1	0	0	1	3	4	0	3	7
1380	Short ribs,lean + fat,braised 1 serving (2/3 lb raw)	3.0 oz	400	4	6	0	0	0	11	14	1	5	0	0	0	1	1	2	0	2	6
1381	Short ribs,lean only,braised 1 serving,(2/3 lb raw)	3.0 oz	250	3	8	0	0	0	5	6	0	5	0	0	0	1	2	2	0	3	9
1382	Rib,eye,lean + fat, brl 1 piece (2 × 4 × .5 in)	3.0 oz	250	3	7	0	0	0	5	7	1	5	1	0	0	1	2	3	0	2	7
1383	Rib,eye, lean only, brl 1 piece (2 × 4 × .5 in)	3.0 oz	200	2	7	0	0	0	3	4	0	5	1	0	0	1	2	3	0	2	8
1384	Rib roast,whole,lean + fat,rst 1 sl (4.1 × 2.2 × .5 in)	3.0 oz	330	3	6	0	0	0	8	11	1	5	1	0	0	1	2	2	0	2	6
1385	Rib roast,whole,lean only,rst 1 sl (4.1 × 2.2 × .5 in)	3.0 oz	210	2	7	0	0	0	4	5	0	5	1	0	0	1	2	3	0	2	8
1386	Round steak,lean + fat,brl 1 pc (4.1 × 2.2 × .5 in)	3.0 oz	230	2	7	0	0	0	5	6	1	5	1	0	0	1	2	4	0	2	5
1387	Round steak,lean only,brl 1 pc (4.1 × 2.2 × .5 in)	3.0 oz	170	2	7	0	0	0	2	2	0	5	1	0	0	1	2	4	0	3	5
1388	Rump roast,lean + fat 1 pc (4.1 × 2.2 × .5 in)	3.0 oz	220	2	7	0	0	0	4	5	0	5	1	0	0	1	2	3	0	3	7
1389	Rump roast,lean only 1 pc (4.1 × 2.2 × .5 in)	3.0 oz	160	2	8	0	0	0	2	2	0	5	1	0	0	1	3	3	0	3	8
1390	Ground beef, extra lean, broiled 1 patty (3 in diam × 6 in	3.0 oz	220	2	7	0	0	0	4	5	0	6	1	0	0	1	3	3	0	3	7
1391	Ground beef,lean,broiled 1 patty,3 in diam × .6 in	3.0 oz	230	2	6	0	0	0	5	6	1	5	1	0	0	1	2	2	0	2	6
1392	Ground beef,regular,broiled 1 patty,3 in diam × .6 in	3.0 oz	250	2	6	0	0	0	5	6	1	5	1	0	0	0	2	2	0	2	6

[g] Add 0.5 nutri-unit of sodium for moderate or 1 nutri-unit for heavy salting per 3 oz serving.

continued

Main Dishes

No.	Name/Portion Size		KCAL	CAL	PRO	CAR	FIB	SUG	FAT	SFA	PFA	CHL	SOD	A	C	THI	RIB	B6	CA	IRN	ZN
											NUTRI–UNITS										
1393	Brains, simmered 3 oz	3.0 oz	140	1	3	0	0	0	3	2	1	116	1	0	0	1	2	2	0	2	1
1394	Heart,cooked 3 oz	3.0 oz	150	1	8	0	0	0	1	1	1	11	1	0	0	2	15	2	0	7	4
1395	Kidneys, simmered 1/2 cup	2.5 oz	100	1	5	0	0	0	1	1	0	18	1	3	0	2	33	4	0	6	4
1396	Liver,beef,fried 1 sl (6 × 2 × .5 in)	3.0 oz	180	2	7	0	0	0	2	2	1	27	1	123	6	2	41	12	0	6	6
1397	Liver,calf,fried 1 sl (6 × 2 × .5 in)	3.0 oz	220	2	8	0	0	0	3	2	1	25	1	111	10	3	42	8	0	13	7
1398	Sweetbread,beef,braised 3 oz	3.0 oz	270	3	7	0	0	0	6	5	0	26	1	0	0	1	2	3	0	2	N
1399	Sweetbread,calf,braised 3 oz	3.0 oz	140	1	9	0	0	0	1	1	0	26	1	0	0	1	2	4	0	2	N
1400	Tripe,beef 3 oz	3.0 oz	80	1	4	0	0	0	1	2	0	5	0	0	1	0	2	0	0	2	3
Chicken (unsalted except batter dipped)[h]																					
1401	Batter dipped breast 1/2 breast	4.9 oz	360	4	11	1	0	0	6	4	4	8	4	0	0	2	2	6	1	2	2
1402	Batter dipped,deep frd,drumstik 1 drumstick	2.5 oz	190	2	5	0	0	0	3	3	2	4	2	0	0	1	2	2	0	1	2
1403	Batter dipped,deep fried,keel 1 keel	3.4 oz	280	3	8	0	0	0	4	3	2	6	3	0	0	1	1	3	1	1	3
1404	Batter dipped,deep fried,rib 1 rib	2.9 oz	240	2	6	1	0	0	4	4	1	6	2	0	0	1	2	3	1	1	1
1405	Batter dipped,deep fried,thigh 1 thigh	3.0 oz	240	2	6	1	0	0	4	3	3	5	2	0	0	1	2	2	0	1	2
1406	Batter dipped,deep fried,wing 1 wing	1.7 oz	160	2	3	0	0	0	3	3	2	3	2	0	0	1	1	1	0	1	1
1407	Broiled breast,w skin 1/2 breast	3.5 oz	190	2	9	0	0	0	2	2	1	5	1	0	0	1	1	5	0	1	1

1408 Broiled breast,no skin 1/2 breast	3.0 oz	140	1	8	0	0	0	1	1	1	5	1	0	0	1	1	5	0	1	1
1409 Broiled drumstick,w skin 1 drumstick	1.8 oz	110	1	4	0	0	0	2	1	1	3	0	0	0	0	1	2	0	1	2
1410 Broiled drumstick,no skin 1 drumstick	1.6 oz	80	1	4	0	0	0	1	1	1	3	0	0	0	0	1	2	0	1	2
1411 Broiled thigh, w skin 1 thigh	2.2 oz	150	2	5	0	0	0	3	2	2	4	1	0	0	1	2	2	0	1	2
1412 Broiled thigh,no skin 1 thigh	1.8 oz	110	1	4	0	0	0	2	1	1	3	0	0	0	1	1	2	0	1	2
1413 Broiler,one quarter,broiled 1 quarter broiler	3.1 oz	200	2	8	0	0	0	3	2	2	5	1	0	0	1	1	5	0	1	1
1414 Broiler,one half,broiled 1 half broiler	6.2 oz	390	4	16	0	0	0	6	5	4	10	1	1	0	1	2	9	1	2	3
1415 Fried back 1 back from 2.5 lb fryer	1.4 oz	130	1	3	0	0	0	2	2	2	2	0	0	0	1	1	1	0	1	1
1416 Fried breast 1/2 breast (2.5 lb fryer)	2.9 oz	180	2	8	0	0	0	2	2	1	5	1	0	0	1	1	5	0	1	1
1417 Fried drumstick 1 drumstick	1.3 oz	90	1	3	0	0	0	2	1	1	2	0	0	0	0	1	1	0	1	1
1418 Fried neck 1 neck	1.6 oz	150	2	3	0	0	0	3	3	2	3	0	0	0	0	1	1	0	1	2
1419 Fried thigh 1 thigh	1.8 oz	140	1	3	0	0	0	3	2	2	3	1	0	0	1	1	1	0	1	1
1420 Fried wing 1 wing	1.3 oz	120	1	3	0	0	0	2	2	2	2	0	0	0	0	1	1	0	1	1
1421 Roast,light meat,no skin 1 pc (2.5 × 4 × .4 in)	3.0 oz	150	1	8	0	0	0	1	1	1	5	1	0	0	1	1	5	0	1	1
1422 Roast,dark meat,no skin 1/2–2/3 cup	3.0 oz	170	2	7	0	0	0	2	2	2	5	1	0	0	1	2	3	0	1	3
1423 Stewed chicken,w skin 1/2–2/3 cup,chopped	3.0 oz	240	2	7	0	0	0	5	4	3	4	1	0	0	1	2	2	0	1	2

[h] Add 0.5 nutri-unit of sodium for moderate or 1 nutri-unit for heavy salting per 3 oz serving.

continued

Main Dishes

No.	Name/Portion Size		KCAL	CAL	PRO	CAR	FIB	SUG	FAT	SFA	PFA	CHL	SOD	A	C	THI	RIB	B6	CA	IRN	ZN
										NUTRI–UNITS											
1424	Stewed chicken,no skin 1/2–2/3 cup chopped	3.0 oz	200	2	8	0	0	0	3	2	2	5	1	0	0	1	3	3	0	1	2
1425	Oven baked chicken 3.0 oz	3.0 oz	210	2	8	0	0	0	3	2	2	5	1	1	0	0	3	3	0	2	2
1426	Southern fried chicken,salted 3.0 oz	3.0 oz	240	2	6	2	0	0	2	1	1	4	4	1	0	3	3	3	0	2	1
1427	Canned chicken,no skin,salted 1/2 cup	3.6 oz	200	2	7	0	0	0	4	3	2	5	5	1	0	0	2	1	0	1	3
1428	Fried giblets,chicken 3 oz	3.0 oz	240	2	9	0	0	0	3	3	3	25	1	41	2	1	15	5	0	10	7
1429	Fried liver,chicken 1/2 cup	2.5 oz	110	1	5	0	0	0	1	1	0	29	0	46	4	1	14	4	0	7	3
Fish, shellfish (unsalted unless noted)																					
1430	Anchovy,in oil,lightly salted 5 anchovies	.7 oz	40	0	1	0	0	0	1	1	1	1	2	0	0	0	0	0	1	1	0
1431	Bass,baked,stuffed 1 pc w 1/3 cup stuffing	7.2 oz	530	5	10	2	0	N	10	9	2	6	1	0	0	4	2	5	1	2	N
1432	Bass,striped,oven fried 1 pc 3 × 3 × .5 in	3.0 oz	170	2	6	0	0	N	2	2	0	4	1	0	0	1	0	2	0	1	N
1433	Bluefish,broiled or baked 1 pc, 3 × 3 × .5 in	3.0 oz	140	1	7	0	0	0	1	1	1	4	1	0	0	1	1	2	0	1	1
1434	Caviar,sturgeon roe,granular 1 tablespoon	.6 oz	40	0	1	0	0	0	1	0	0	3	4	0	0	0	0	0	1	2	N
1435	Caviar,sturgeon roe,pressed 1 tablespoon	.6 oz	50	1	2	0	0	0	1	0	0	4	4	0	0	0	0	1	1	2	N
1436	Clams,canned,drained 1/2 cup chopped	2.8 oz	80	1	4	0	0	0	1	0	0	3	1	0	0	0	1	1	1	4	1
1437	Cod,broiled 1 fillet, 5 × 2.5 × .8 in	2.3 oz	110	1	6	0	0	0	1	1	1	4	1	0	0	1	1	1	0	1	0
1438	Cod,canned 1/2 cup flaked	2.5 oz	60	1	4	0	0	0	0	0	0	3	1	1	0	1	1	1	0	1	0

1439 Crab,steamed ½ cup	2.8 oz	70	1	4	0	0	0	0	0	0	5	2	7	1	2	1	2	1	1	4
1440 Croaker,baked 1 serving (3 × 3 × .8 in)	3.5 oz	130	1	7	0	0	0	1	1	0	5	1	0	0	2	1	3	1	1	1
1441 Eel,smoked 2 oz	2.0 oz	190	2	3	0	0	0	5	3	0	2	35	4	0	2	2	N	0	0	N
1442 Fish cakes or sticks,fried 3 sticks (4 × 1 × .5 in)	3.0 oz	140	1	4	1	0	0	2	2	2	2	1	0	0	0	1	1	0	0	1
1443 Fish sticks,froz fried,baked 3 sticks (4 × 1 × .5 in)	3.0 oz	150	1	4	0	0	0	2	2	2	3	1	0	0	0	1	N	0	0	1
1444 Flounder,baked 1 fillet, 6 × 2.5 × .3 in	2.0 oz	120	1	5	0	0	0	1	1	0	3	1	0	0	1	1	1	0	1	1
1445 Haddock,fried 1 fillet,6.5 × 3.5 ×.6 in	3.9 oz	180	2	7	0	0	0	2	1	0	5	2	0	1	1	1	2	1	1	0
1446 Haddock,smoked 1 pc (2.5 × 2.5 × .3 in)	3.5 oz	100	1	7	0	0	0	0	0	0	5	62	0	0	1	1	2	0	1	0
1447 Halibut,broiled or baked 1 fillet 6.5 × 2.5 ×.6 in	4.4 oz	210	2	10	0	0	0	3	2	0	5	2	3	0	1	1	N	0	1	2
1448 Herring,pickled,smoked/kippered 1 herring	1.6 oz	100	1	3	0	0	0	2	1	1	3	28	0	0	0	1	0	1	1	0
1449 Lobster,cooked 1 cup	5.3 oz	140	1	9	0	0	0	1	0	0	9	3	0	0	2	1	3	2	1	4
1450 Mackerel,broiled w butter 1 fillet,8.5 × 2.5 ×.5 in	3.7 oz	250	2	7	0	0	0	5	5	1	7	1	2	0	2	3	7	0	1	2
1451 Ocean perch,breaded,fried 1 pc, 3 × 3 × .5 in	3.7 oz	340	3	6	1	0	0	6	3	0	4	2	0	0	1	1	1	1	2	1
1452 Ocean perch,fried 1 pc, 3 × 3 × .5 in	3.1 oz	200	2	5	0	0	0	4	2	0	3	1	0	0	1	1	1	1	1	1
1453 Oysters,cnd,sol+liq w salt 1 can,3.6 oz	3.6 oz	80	1	3	0	0	0	1	0	0	3	4	1	10	0	2	1	1	6	140
1454 Oysters,fried, no salt 4 med,1.75 in diam × 1 in	1.6 oz	110	1	1	1	0	0	2	1	0	1	1	1	4	1	2	0	1	4	96

[i]Add 0.5 nutri-unit of sodium for moderate or 1 nutri-unit for heavy salting per 3 oz. serving.

continued

Main Dishes

No.	Name/Portion Size		KCAL	CAL	PRO	CAR	FIB	SUG	FAT	SFA	PFA	CHL	SOD	A	C	THI	RIB	B6	CA	IRN	ZN
			NUTRI–UNITS																		
1455	Rockfish,oven steamed 1 fillet, 7 × 3.5 × .6 in	4.1 oz	120	1	6	0	0	0	1	0	0	4	1	3	0	1	2	3	0	1	1
1456	Salmon,broil/bake,no salt 1 steak, 6.7 × 2.5 × 1 in	4.5 oz	230	2	11	0	0	0	3	2	2	4	1	1	0	3	1	3	3	2	2
1457	Salmon,chum,cnd,sol+liq,no salt 1/2 cup	3.9 oz	150	2	7	0	0	0	2	0	2	3	1	0	0	0	2	3	5	1	1
1458	Salmon,coho,cnd,sol+liq,w salt 1/2 cup	3.9 oz	170	2	7	0	0	0	2	2	2	3	4	0	0	0	2	3	5	1	1
1459	Salmon,king,cnd,sol+liq,no salt 1/2 cup	3.9 oz	230	2	7	0	0	0	5	4	2	2	0	1	0	0	2	3	3	1	1
1460	Salmon,pink,cnd,sol+liq w salt 1/2 cup	3.9 oz	160	2	7	0	0	0	2	2	2	3	4	0	0	0	2	3	4	1	1
1461	Salmon,red,cnd,sol+liq w salt 1/2 cup	3.9 oz	190	2	7	0	0	0	3	3	2	3	6	1	0	1	2	3	6	1	1
1462	Salmon,smoked 3 oz jar or can	3.0 oz	150	1	6	0	0	0	2	2	0	2	53	0	0	0	3	6	0	1	1
1463	Sardines,canned,drained 8 fish (3 × 1 × .5 in)	3.5 oz	180	2	7	0	0	0	3	3	0	3	62	0	0	0	3	7	0	2	1
1464	Scallops,fried in butter 6 scallops,(.5 oz each)	3.5 oz	190	2	6	1	0	0	3	2	0	3	1	0	0	0	1	1	2	4	2
1465	Scallops,steamed 6 scallops,(.5 oz each)	3.5 oz	110	1	7	0	0	0	0	0	0	4	3	0	0	1	1	1	2	3	2
1466	Shad,baked w butter,bacon 1 piece (3 × 3 × .7 in)	3.5 oz	200	2	7	0	0	0	3	4	1	5	1	0	0	2	3	4	0	1	1
1467	Shrimp,cnd,drained,no salt 10 med (2.5 in long)	1.1 oz	40	0	2	0	0	0	0	0	0	3	0	0	0	0	0	0	1	1	1
1468	Shrimp,canned,drained,salted 3.5 oz serving	3.5 oz	120	1	7	0	0	0	0	0	0	10	1	0	0	0	0	0	2	3	3
1469	Shrimp,french fried 3.5 oz serving	3.5 oz	230	2	6	1	0	0	3	2	0	10	2	0	0	1	1	1	1	2	3

1470 Shrimp,frozen,breaded,raw 3.5 oz serving	3.5 oz	140	1	4	[illegible]	[illegible]	[illegible]	[illegible]	[illegible]	[illegible]	[illegible]	[illegible]	[illegible]	[illegible]	[illegible]	[illegible]	[illegible]	[illegible]	[illegible]	[illegible]
1471 Sturgeon,steamed 3.5 oz serving	3.5 oz	160	2	8	0	0	0	2	2	0	5	1	3	0	1	1	2	1	2	1
1472 Swordfish,broiled 1 piece (4.5 × 2 × 1 in)	4.9 oz	240	2	12	0	0	0	3	3	0	7	2	11	0	1	1	7	1	2	1
1473 Trout,rainbow,broiled 3.5 oz serving	3.5 oz	200	2	7	0	0	0	3	3	1	4	1	1	0	1	2	7	1	1	1
1474 Tuna,baked,no salt 1 steak,6.7 × 2.5 × 1 in	4.5 oz	170	2	10	0	0	0	1	1	0	5	0	0	0	1	2	12	0	2	2
1475 Tuna,canned in oil,drained 1/2 cup	2.8 oz	160	2	7	0	0	0	2	2	1	3	6	0	0	1	1	3	0	2	1
1476 Tuna,oil pak,drnd,50% less salt 1/2 cup	2.8 oz	170	2	6	0	0	0	3	2	1	3	2	0	0	0	1	3	0	1	1
1477 Tuna,watr pak,drn,50% less salt 1/2 cup	2.8 oz	90	1	6	0	0	0	0	0	0	3	2	0	0	0	1	3	0	1	1
1478 Tuna,cnd in water,no salt 3.2 oz can,undrained	3.2 oz	120	1	8	0	0	0	0	0	0	4	0	0	0	0	1	4	0	2	1
1479 Tuna,broil/bake,no salt 1 steak,6.7 × 2.5 × 1 in	4.5 oz	170	2	10	0	0	0	1	1	0	5	0	0	0	1	2	12	0	2	2
Game (unsalted)[j]																				
1480 Beaver,roasted 3 oz	3.0 oz	210	2	8	0	0	0	3	4	2	6	0	0	0	1	4	2	0	1	N
1481 Duck,domestic,flesh only 3 oz	3.0 oz	170	2	6	0	0	0	3	3	1	5	1	0	0	3	5	2	0	3	3
1482 Duck,wild,breast 3 oz	3.0 oz	110	1	5	0	0	0	1	1	0	4	0	0	2	5	3	5	0	4	1
1483 Goose,domestic,roasted 3 oz	3.0 oz	260	3	7	0	0	0	6	5	2	5	1	0	0	1	3	3	0	3	3
1484 Goose,domestic,flesh only,rstd 3 slices (3.5×3×.3 in)	3.5 oz	240	2	9	0	0	0	4	4	1	6	1	0	0	1	5	5	0	3	4

[j] Add 0.5 nutri-unit of sodium for moderate or 1 nutri-unit for heavy salting per serving.

continued

Main Dishes

No.	Name/Portion Size		KCAL	CAL	PRO	CAR	FIB	SUG	FAT	SFA	PFA	CHL	SOD	A	C	THI	RIB	B6	CA	IRN	ZN
										NUTRI–UNITS											
1485	Muskrat,roasted 3 oz	3.0 oz	130	1	7	0	0	0	1	2	1	6	0	0	0	2	2	2	0	1	N
1486	Opossum,roasted 3 oz	3.0 oz	190	2	8	0	0	0	3	3	1	6	0	0	0	1	4	4	0	1	N
1487	Pheasant,raw 3.5 oz	3.5 oz	130	1	7	0	0	0	1	1	0	4	0	1	2	1	2	N	0	1	3
1488	Rabbit,domestic,stewed 3 oz	3.0 oz	180	2	8	0	0	0	3	3	1	5	0	0	0	1	1	2	0	1	4
1489	Raccoon,roasted 3 oz	3.0 oz	220	2	8	0	0	0	4	4	2	6	0	0	0	7	5	2	0	1	4
1490	Venison,raw 3.5 oz	3.5 oz	130	1	6	0	0	0	1	2	0	4	1	0	0	3	6	3	0	2	N
Lamb (unsalted)																					
1491	Lamb chops,loin,lean + fat 1 chop,cut 3/lb	3.5 oz	360	4	7	0	0	0	9	15	1	6	1	0	0	2	3	3	0	1	4
1492	Lamb chops,loin,lean only 1 chop,cut 3/lb	2.3 oz	120	1	6	0	0	0	1	2	0	4	0	0	0	1	2	2	0	1	4
1493	Lamb chops,rib,lean + fat 1 chop,cut 3/lb	3.1 oz	360	4	6	0	0	0	10	16	1	6	0	0	0	1	2	3	0	1	3
1494	Lamb chops,rib,lean only 1 chop,cut 3/lb	2.0 oz	120	1	5	0	0	0	2	3	0	4	0	0	0	1	2	2	0	1	3
1495	Lamb,leg,lean + fat,roasted 2 slices (4 × 2 × .3 in)	3.0 oz	240	2	7	0	0	0	5	8	0	6	1	0	0	2	3	3	0	2	4
1496	Lamb,leg,lean only,roasted 2 slices (4 × 2 × .3 in)	3.0 oz	160	2	8	0	0	0	2	3	0	6	1	0	0	2	3	3	0	2	5
1497	Lamb,shoulder,lean+fat,roasted 3 sl (2.5 × 2.5 × .25 in)	3.0 oz	290	3	6	0	0	0	7	12	1	6	0	0	0	1	2	2	0	1	4
1498	Lamb,shoulder,lean only,roasted 3 sl (2.5 × 2.5 × .25 in)	3.0 oz	170	2	7	0	0	0	3	4	0	6	1	0	0	2	3	3	0	2	5

Pork (unsalted unless processed)[i]																				
1499 Bacon,broiled or fried 2 strips (1 oz each raw)	.5 oz	80	1	1	0	0	0	2	2	1	1	2	0	2	1	0	0	0	0	1
1500 Breakfast strips, cooked 3 (.8 oz) slices	1.2 oz	160	2	3	0	0	0	4	4	2	2	7	0	5	3	1	1	0	1	2
1501 Canadian bacon 1 slice,3.5 in diam × .2	.7 oz	40	0	2	0	0	0	1	1	0	1	3	0	2	2	0	1	0	0	0
1502 Ham,fresh,lean + fat,roasted 1 slice (4 × 2.3 × .5 in)	3.0 oz	230	2	7	0	0	0	5	5	2	5	1	0	0	8	3	2	0	1	3
1503 Ham,fresh,lean only,roasted 1 slice (4 × 2.3 × .5 in)	3.0 oz	190	2	8	0	0	0	3	3	1	5	1	0	0	9	4	3	0	1	3
1504 Ham,cured,extra lean,canned 1 slice (4 × 2.3 × .5 in)	3.0 oz	120	1	6	0	0	0	1	1	0	2	10	0	8	12	2	4	0	1	3
1505 Ham,cured,regular, canned 1 slice (4 × 2.3 × .5 in)	3.0 oz	190	2	5	0	0	0	4	4	1	4	8	0	4	9	3	3	0	1	3
1506 Ham,cured,extra lean,roasted 1 slice (4 × 2.3 × .5 in)	3.0 oz	120	1	5	0	0	0	1	1	0	3	10	0	6	9	2	3	0	1	3
1507 Ham,cured,roasted 1 slice (4 × 2.3 × .5 in)	3.0 oz	150	2	6	0	0	0	2	2	1	3	13	0	6	8	3	3	0	1	3
1508 Ham,cured,country style,bkd 1 slice (4 × 2.3 × .5 in)	3.0 oz	330	3	4	0	0	0	9	10	2	4	7	0	6	8	2	3	0	2	3
1509 Ham,light cure,lean + fat,bkd 1 slice (4 × 2.3 × .5 in)	3.0 oz	250	2	5	0	0	0	6	6	2	5	6	0	6	5	2	3	0	2	4
1510 Ham,light cure,lean only,bkd 1 slice (4 × 2.3 × .5 in)	3.0 oz	160	2	7	0	0	0	2	2	1	5	8	0	4	7	2	3	0	3	5
1511 Pork butt,lean + fat,rst 1 pc (2.5 × 2.5 × .8 in)	3.0 oz	230	2	7	0	0	0	5	5	2	5	1	0	0	8	3	2	0	1	3
1512 Pork butt,lean only,rst 1 pc (2.5 × 2.5 × .8 in)	3.0 oz	190	2	8	0	0	0	3	3	1	5	1	0	0	9	4	3	0	1	3
1513 Pork chop,loin,lean + fat,brl 1 chop,$^1/_3$ lb	2.8 oz	270	3	6	0	0	0	6	7	2	5	1	0	0	9	3	3	0	1	3
1514 Pork chop,loin,lean only,brl 1 chop,trimmed	2.0 oz	140	1	5	0	0	0	3	3	1	4	0	0	0	7	3	3	0	1	2

[i]Add 0.5 nutri-unit of sodium for moderate or 1 nutri-unit for heavy salting per serving.

continued

Main Dishes

No.	Name/Portion Size		KCAL	CAL	PRO	CAR	FIB	SUG	FAT	SFA	PFA	CHL	SOD	A	C	THI	RIB	B6	CA	IRN	ZN
			NUTRI–UNITS																		
1515	Pork loin roast,lean + fat 1 sl (2.5 × 2.5 × .8 in)	3.0 oz	270	3	6	0	0	0	6	7	2	5	1	0	0	8	3	3	0	1	3
1516	Pork loin roast,lean only 1 sl (2.5 × 2.5 × .8 in)	3.0 oz	200	2	7	0	0	0	4	4	1	5	1	0	0	9	4	4	0	1	3
1517	Pork picnic,lean + fat,sim 1 pc (2.5 × 2.5 × .8 in)	3.0 oz	290	3	7	0	0	0	7	7	2	6	1	0	0	6	3	2	0	2	5
1518	Pork picnic,lean only,sim 1 pc (2.5 × 2.5 × .8 in)	3.0 oz	210	2	8	0	0	0	3	3	1	6	1	0	0	7	4	3	0	2	6
1519	Pork picnic,cured,lean + fat,rst 1 pc (2.5 × 2.5 × .8 in)	3.0 oz	240	2	5	0	0	0	5	6	2	3	9	0	0	7	2	2	0	1	3
1520	Pork picnic,cured,lean only,rst .6 cup chopped	3.0 oz	140	1	7	0	0	0	2	2	1	3	10	0	0	8	2	3	0	1	3
1521	Pork spareribs,braised 3 oz serving	3.0 oz	340	3	8	0	0	0	8	9	3	7	1	0	N	5	4	3	1	2	5
1522	Pork and gravy,canned 3 oz serving	3.0 oz	220	2	4	0	0	0	5	5	2	5	1	0	0	6	2	3	0	2	4
1523	Pork w juice,canned,salted 3 oz serving	3.0 oz	190	2	4	0	0	0	4	5	1	5	4	0	0	5	2	4	0	2	4
1524	Pork liver,fried 1 sl (6.5 × 2.5 × .4 in)	3.0 oz	140	1	7	0	0	0	1	1	1	20	0	61	7	3	22	5	0	17	8
1525	Pork tongue,braised 1 slice (3 × 2 × .4 in)	2.1 oz	160	2	4	0	0	0	3	3	1	6	1	0	0	3	4	1	0	3	4
Sausage and Lunchmeat/																					
1526	Bologna,all meat,less salt 1 sl (4 1/2 dia × 1/8 in)	1.0 oz	90	1	1	0	0	0	2	3	0	1	3	0	2	0	0	0	0	1	1
1527	Bologna,beef+pork 1 sl (4 1/2 dia × 1/8 in)	1.0 oz	90	1	1	0	0	0	2	3	1	1	3	0	2	1	0	1	0	0	1
1528	Bologna,turkey 1 sl (4 1/2 dia × 1/8 in)	1.0 oz	60	1	1	0	0	0	1	1	1	2	2	0	0	0	1	1	0	0	1
1529	Braunschweiger 1 sl (3 1/8 dia × 1/8 in)	1.0 oz	100	1	1	0	0	0	3	3	1	3	3	16	1	1	5	1	0	3	1

1530 Capicola 1 sl (4¼ in sq × 1/16)	.7 oz	110	1	1	0	0	0	3	3	1	1	3	0	0	1	0	0	0	1	N
1531 Cervelat,dry 8 sl (1½ dia × ⅛ in)	.8 oz	110	1	2	0	0	0	3	3	0	1	3	0	0	1	1	1	0	1	N
1532 Cervelat,soft 1 sl (4⅜ dia × ⅛ in)	1.0 oz	100	1	1	0	0	0	3	3	0	1	4	0	2	1	1	1	0	1	N
1533 Chopped canned meat 2 tablespoons	1.1 oz	90	1	1	0	0	0	2	2	1	3	4	0	0	1	1	N	0	1	1
1534 Deviled ham,canned 2 tablespoons	1.0 oz	100	1	1	0	0	0	3	3	1	1	3	0	0	1	0	0	0	0	1
1535 Frankfurter,beef 1 frank (5 × ¾ in dia)	1.6 oz	140	1	2	0	0	0	4	5	1	2	5	0	4	0	1	1	0	1	1
1536 Frankfurter,beef and pork 1 frank (5 × ¾ in dia)	1.6 oz	140	1	2	0	0	0	4	4	1	1	5	0	4	1	1	1	0	1	1
1537 Frankfurter,turkey 1 frank (5 × ¾ in dia)	1.6 oz	100	1	2	0	0	0	2	2	2	3	6	0	0	0	1	1	1	1	2
1538 Ham,boiled 1 sl (6¼ × 4 × 1/16 in)	1.0 oz	50	1	2	0	0	0	1	1	0	1	4	0	3	3	1	1	0	0	1
1539 Ham,chopped 1 sl (3 × 2 × ½ in)	1.1 oz	70	1	1	0	0	0	2	2	1	1	4	0	0	2	1	1	0	0	1
1540 Ham,extra lean 1 sl (3 × 2 × ½ in)	1.0 oz	40	0	2	0	0	0	0	0	0	1	4	0	2	3	1	1	0	0	1
1541 Ham,minced 2 tablespoons	1.0 oz	70	1	1	0	0	0	2	2	1	1	3	0	3	3	1	1	0	0	1
1542 Bratwurst,cooked 1 3 oz link	3.0 oz	260	3	4	0	0	0	7	7	2	3	5	0	0	6	2	2	1	1	3
1543 Headcheese 1 sl (4 × 4 × ¼ in)	1.0 oz	60	1	1	0	0	0	1	1	0	2	4	0	2	0	1	1	0	0	0
1544 Knockwurst 1 link (4 × 1⅛ in dia)	2.4 oz	210	2	2	0	0	0	6	6	2	3	7	0	6	3	1	1	0	1	2
1545 Liverwurst 1 sl (3⅛ in dia × ¼)	1.0 oz	90	1	1	0	0	0	2	3	1	3	2	31	0	1	3	1	0	2	1

[j]Add 0.5 nutri-unit of sodium for moderate or 1 nutri-unit for heavy salting per serving.

continued

Main Dishes

No.	Name/Portion Size		KCAL	CAL	PRO	CAR	FIB	SUG	FAT	SFA	PFA	CHL	SOD	A	C	THI	RIB	B6	CA	IRN	ZN
			NUTRI–UNITS																		
1546	Potted chicken,beef,turkey 2 tablespoons	1.0 oz	70	1	2	0	0	0	2	2	0	1	4	0	0	0	1	0	0	0	1
1547	Mortadella 1 sl (5 in dia × 1/16)	.9 oz	80	1	1	0	0	0	2	2	1	1	3	0	2	0	0	0	0	0	1
1548	Salami,dry 2 sl (2 1/2 in dia × 1/8)	.7 oz	80	1	1	0	0	0	2	2	1	1	5	0	0	2	1	1	0	0	1
1549	Salami,cooked 1 sl (4 1/2 in dia × 1/8)	1.0 oz	70	1	1	0	0	0	2	2	0	1	3	0	1	1	1	0	0	1	1
1550	Sausage,brown + serve 3 links (4 × 5/8 in dia)	1.8 oz	200	2	2	0	0	0	6	6	1	2	4	0	0	2	1	1	0	1	2
1551	Sausage,country style 1 oz patty	1.0 oz	100	1	1	0	0	0	3	3	1	1	3	0	0	1	1	1	0	1	1
1552	Sausage,polish 1 link (5 3/8 × 1 in dia)	2.7 oz	240	2	3	0	0	0	6	7	1	3	8	0	5	2	2	1	1	1	3
1553	Sausage,pork 2 links (4 × 7/8 in dia)	1.0 oz	110	1	2	0	0	0	3	3	1	1	4	0	0	3	1	1	0	0	1
1554	Scrapple 1 sl (2 1/2 in sq × 1/2)	1.8 oz	110	1	1	1	0	0	2	2	1	1	5	0	0	1	1	1	0	1	N
1555	Souse 1 sl (3 7/8 in sq × 1/8)	1.0 oz	50	1	1	0	0	0	1	1	0	1	3	0	0	0	0	0	0	1	N
1556	Thuringer 1 sl (4 3/8 in dia × 1/8)	1.0 oz	90	1	1	0	0	0	2	3	0	1	3	0	2	1	1	1	0	1	1
1557	Vienna sausage 2 saus (2 × 7/8 in diam)	1.1 oz	90	1	1	0	0	0	2	3	0	1	3	0	0	0	0	0	0	0	1
Turkey (unsalted unless processed)																					
1558	Canned turkey,salted 1/2 cup	3.5 oz	160	2	7	0	0	0	2	2	1	4	5	0	1	0	2	3	0	2	4
1559	Roast turkey,dark meat 4 pc (2 1/2×1 5/8×1/4 in)	3.0 oz	160	2	7	0	0	0	2	2	1	5	1	0	0	1	2	3	1	2	5

2 sl (4 × 2 × 1/4 in)	3.0 oz																			
1561 Turkey ham 3 oz slice	3.0 oz	120	1	5	0	0	0	2	2	2	0	9	0	0	1	3	3	0	3	2
1562 Turkey roll,salted 3 oz slice	3.0 oz	120	1	5	0	0	0	2	2	2	0	7	0	0	0	1	6	1	1	2
Veal (unsalted)[j]																				
1563 Veal chop,broiled or braised 1 pc (2 1/2 in sq × 3/4)	3.0 oz	200	2	7	0	0	0	3	5	0	6	1	0	0	1	2	3	0	3	4
1564 Veal chuck,braised or pot roast 1 pc (2 1/2 in sq × 3/4)	3.0 oz	200	2	7	0	0	0	3	5	0	6	0	0	0	1	3	3	0	3	4
1565 Veal cutlet,cooked 1 pc (4 × 2 1/3 × 1/2 in)	3.0 oz	180	2	7	0	0	0	3	4	0	6	1	0	0	1	2	3	0	3	4
1566 Veal leg or shoulder 1 pc (4 × 2 1/3 × 1/2 in)	3.0 oz	180	2	7	0	0	0	3	4	0	6	1	0	0	1	2	3	0	3	4
1567 Veal patty 1 patty (3 in dia × 3/4)	3.0 oz	200	2	7	0	0	0	3	4	0	6	2	0	0	1	3	3	0	3	4

Main Dishes, Combination

1568 Blacksea bass,bkd,stuft,no salt 1 pc (3.5 × 4.5 × 1.5 in)	7.2 oz	530	5	10	2	0	0	10	9	2	6	1	0	0	4	2	5	1	2	N
1569 Beans and franks,canned 1 cup	9.0 oz	370	4	6	2	12	2	5	7	0	2	14	1	0	2	2	6	2	5	6
1570 Beans w pork in tomato sauce 1 cup	9.0 oz	310	3	5	3	12	3	2	2	1	1	12	1	2	3	1	3	3	5	6
1571 Beans w pork in sweet sauce 1 cup	9.0 oz	380	4	5	4	12	4	4	4	1	1	10	1	2	2	1	3	3	7	3
1572 Beef meatloaf 2 slices (4 × 3 × 1/2 in)	6.4 oz	320	3	10	1	0	0	5	7	0	12	7	1	1	1	4	5	2	5	8
1573 Beef and vegetable stew,no salt 1 cup	8.6 oz	220	2	5	1	1	1	3	4	0	4	1	10	6	2	2	1	1	3	8
1574 Beef and veg stew,salt added 1 cup	8.6 oz	220	2	5	1	1	1	3	4	0	4	3	10	6	2	2	1	1	3	8

[j] Add 0.5 nutri-unit of sodium for moderate or 1 nutri-unit for heavy salting per serving.

continued

Main Dishes, Combination

No.	Name/Portion Size		KCAL	CAL	PRO	CAR	FIB	SUG	FAT	SFA	PFA	CHL	SOD	A	C	THI	RIB	B6	CA	IRN	ZN
								NUTRI–UNITS													
1575	Beef and vegetable stew,canned 1 cup	8.6 oz	190	2	4	1	1	1	2	2	0	2	10	10	2	1	1	1	1	2	8
1576	Beef liver,onion gravy 1 pc (6.5 × 2.5 × 1/4 in)	3.5 oz	140	1	4	1	0	0	2	1	1	12	4	87	4	2	20	4	0	4	3
1577	Beef potpie,commercial 1 8 oz pie	7.9 oz	430	4	5	3	1	0	7	6	2	3	8	4	0	1	2	3	0	2	3
1578	Beef potpie,home prepared 1/3 of 9 inch pie	7.4 oz	520	5	7	3	1	0	9	8	5	3	6	7	2	4	3	4	1	4	3
1579	Beef stroganoff w rice 2/3 cup on 1/2 cup rice	9.9 oz	370	4	8	2	0	0	4	6	1	6	14	1	1	3	3	4	1	5	6
1580	Beef w mashed potatoes,gravy 3 oz beef,1/2 cup potato	7.4 oz	300	3	7	1	1	0	4	6	0	6	4	1	2	1	3	4	2	3	5
1581	Broccoli cheese casserole 1 cup	8.5 oz	330	3	6	2	3	1	6	9	1	4	10	15	41	2	6	N	8	2	3
1582	Burrito,bean 1 tortilla, 1/2 cup beans	5.9 oz	340	3	3	3	7	0	3	3	3	1	3	7	5	5	2	6	2	3	3
1583	Burrito,beef,medium 8 in tort,1/3 cup filling	5.4 oz	390	4	8	2	7	0	5	7	0	8	3	6	4	3	4	6	1	4	3
1584	Burrito,beef+beans+chili 8 in tort,1/3 cup filling	5.4 oz	360	4	6	3	7	0	3	4	0	1	5	1	5	3	3	5	1	4	2
1585	Burrito,combination 1 large	6.2 oz	400	4	6	3	6	0	5	6	0	5	3	7	5	4	3	4	2	4	2
1586	Burrito,supreme 1 very large	7.9 oz	460	5	6	3	8	0	7	8	0	6	4	14	5	4	4	4	2	4	3
1587	Canneloni 1 cup	8.8 oz	430	4	7	3	2	0	7	12	1	4	12	2	3	14	7	3	6	5	4
1588	Cheese fondue 1 cup	6.2 oz	460	5	8	1	N	3	10	14	3	26	9	6	0	1	7	1	11	2	2
1589	Cheese manicotti w sauce 1 cup	8.5 oz	280	3	8	2	2	1	3	4	0	7	7	6	7	2	5	5	6	2	4

1590 Cheese rarebit,no toast 1/2 cup	4.1 oz	210	2	3	1	0	1	5	8	0	3	4	2	0	1	3	1	6	0	1
1591 Cheese souffle 1 cup	3.4 oz	210	2	3	0	0	1	5	7	1	12	3	3	0	1	3	1	4	1	1
1592 Chicken a la king,no toast 1/2 cup	4.3 oz	230	2	4	0	0	0	5	6	1	6	4	2	2	1	2	2	1	1	1
1593 Chicken and dumplets 1 cup	8.8 oz	220	2	6	1	0	0	3	3	1	4	15	1	1	1	1	1	0	2	0
1594 Chicken and noodles 1 cup	8.3 oz	360	4	9	1	0	0	5	5	3	8	15	2	2	2	2	2	1	3	3
1595 Chicken fried steak w gravy 2 oz steak,1/3 cup gravy	5.6 oz	290	3	6	3	0	0	2	3	0	3	4	0	0	3	4	2	4	3	5
1596 Chicken fricasee 1 cup	8.5 oz	390	4	11	1	0	0	7	6	4	6	4	1	0	1	2	4	0	2	2
1597 Chicken pot pie 1/3 of 9 in diam pie	8.2 oz	550	5	7	3	2	0	9	10	5	5	6	12	2	4	4	7	1	3	1
1598 Chicken pot pie,commercial 1 8 oz pie	7.9 oz	490	5	5	3	1	0	8	6	2	2	9	8	3	3	4	5	0	2	1
1599 Chicken potpie w biscuit top 1 cup	8.4 oz	350	3	5	2	1	0	6	7	2	4	11	7	1	3	2	5	2	2	0
1600 Chili con carne w beans 1 cup	9.0 oz	340	3	6	2	6	1	5	7	0	3	14	1	0	1	2	3	2	5	6
1601 Chili con carne w/o beans 1 cup	8.8 oz	500	5	8	1	0	0	11	16	0	4	13	2	0	1	4	7	2	4	5
1602 Chop suey,home prepared 1 cup	8.8 oz	300	3	8	1	3	0	5	8	1	7	11	2	11	4	4	4	1	5	3
1603 Chop suey,canned 1 cup	8.8 oz	160	2	3	1	5	0	2	2	0	2	14	0	2	2	1	4	2	5	1
1604 Chow mein,no noodles 1 cup	8.8 oz	260	3	10	1	2	0	3	2	3	5	7	1	3	1	3	13	1	3	3
1605 Chow mein,canned,no noodles 1 cup	8.8 oz	100	1	2	1	2	1	0	0	0	1	7	1	4	1	1	3	1	1	1

[j]Add 0.5 nutri-unit of sodium for moderate or 1 nutri-unit for heavy salting per serving.

continued

Main Dishes, Combination

No.	Name/Portion Size		KCAL	CAL	PRO	CAR	FIB	SUG	FAT	SFA	PFA	CHL	SOD	A	C	THI	RIB	B6	CA	IRN	ZN
			NUTRI–UNITS																		
1606	Clam fritters,no salt 3 (2 in diam × 1¾ in)	4.2 oz	370	4	4	3	1	0	5	3	1	10	1	1	0	0	2	1	2	5	1
1607	Crab,deviled 1 cup	8.5 oz	450	5	8	2	1	0	7	6	2	16	21	10	5	3	3	4	2	3	5
1608	Crab imperial 1 cup	7.8 oz	320	3	10	1	1	1	5	8	0	21	16	10	4	2	3	4	3	2	6
1609	Dried beef,creamed 1 cup	8.6 oz	380	4	6	1	0	1	8	12	1	7	18	4	0	2	5	3	5	2	4
1610	Eggplant parmigiana 1 cup	7.8 oz	410	4	3	3	3	0	7	3	2	1	4	4	11	2	1	1	1	2	0
1611	Enchiladas,beef and cheese 2 small	8.9 oz	380	4	5	2	1	0	7	10	2	4	11	5	1	1	3	7	10	2	3
1612	Falafel 1 2¼ in patty	.6 oz	30	0	0	0	N	N	0	0	0	0	0	0	0	0	0	1	0	0	0
1613	Fish,batterfried,tartar sauce 3.5 oz + 1 tbsp sauce	4.1 oz	260	3	5	1	0	0	5	3	8	4	3	0	0	0	1	2	0	1	1
1614	Fz dinner,chicken,potato+veg 11 oz	11.0 oz	540	5	12	2	1	N	8	8	3	10	11	7	4	3	7	7	3	4	4
1615	Fz dinner,meat loaf,potato+peas 11 oz	11.0 oz	410	4	8	2	1	N	6	8	0	6	12	5	4	4	5	6	1	5	6
1616	Fz dinner,turkey,potato+peas 11 oz	11.0 oz	350	3	8	3	1	N	3	3	0	7	12	2	4	3	3	2	2	4	4
1617	Ham croquette 2 (1 in diam × 3 in)	4.6 oz	330	3	7	1	0	0	6	7	2	6	4	1	0	5	3	N	2	1	2
1618	Hamburger goulash 1 cup	7.9 oz	270	3	8	1	2	0	3	4	0	5	6	4	6	2	3	4	1	5	7
1619	Hot turkey sandwich,pot+gravy 1 serving	12.0 oz	370	4	7	4	2	0	2	2	1	3	12	1	2	3	2	5	2	3	6
1620	Hummus ⅓ cup	2.9 oz	270	3	3	2	N	N	4	2	3	0	2	0	0	2	2	1	1	3	2

1621 Lasagna,cheese 1 cup	8.1 oz	320	3	6	3	2	1	2	5	1	2	10	2	2	2	4	3	9	1	4
1622 Lasagna w beef 1 cup	8.5 oz	420	4	8	2	2	0	7	11	0	7	5	6	6	3	5	4	6	4	4
Lean Cuisine—Subgroup[k]																				
1623 Chicken chow mein w rice 11.3 oz	11.1 oz	250	3	5	2	2	0	1	1	1	2	11	2	7	1	1	N	1	2	4
1624 Chicken,glazed w veg + rice 8.5 oz	8.5 oz	270	3	8	2	N	N	2	2	2	4	8	0	1	2	2	N	0	1	N
1625 Cannelloni,beef/pork 9.6 oz	9.6 oz	260	3	6	2	N	N	3	4	0	3	9	10	N	2	4	N	4	2	N
1626 Cannelloni,cheese 9.1 oz	9.1 oz	270	3	7	2	N	N	3	N	N	3	10	4	2	2	2	N	6	1	N
1627 Chicken a l'orange w rice 8 oz	8.0 oz	280	3	8	2	N	N	1	1	1	3	5	2	4	2	2	N	0	1	N
1628 Chicken w veg. w vermicelli 12.7 oz	12.7 oz	260	3	7	2	N	N	2	2	2	3	13	4	10	2	2	N	2	2	N
1629 Chicken cacciatore 10.9 oz	10.9 oz	280	3	7	2	N	N	3	2	2	3	10	2	4	2	2	N	1	2	N
1630 Fish florentine 9 oz	9.0 oz	240	2	8	1	N	N	3	4	4	7	8	3	N	3	3	N	3	1	N
1631 Fish divan filet 12.4 oz	12.4 oz	270	3	10	1	N	N	3	4	4	6	8	3	10	3	4	N	4	1	N
1632 Fish jardiniere filet 11.2 oz	11.3 oz	280	3	9	1	N	N	3	4	4	7	8	4	N	2	3	N	3	1	N
1633 Lasagna, zucchini 11 oz	10.9 oz	270	3	6	2	3	2	2	2	1	2	12	10	5	41	3	5	6	4	5
1634 Linguini w clam sauce 9.6 oz	9.6 oz	260	3	5	2	N	N	2	3	3	3	9	N	N	2	2	N	0	2	N
1635 Meatball stew 10 oz	10.0 oz	250	3	7	1	N	N	3	3	1	4	12	9	2	3	3	N	1	3	N

[k]Some nutrients are estimated based on similar items.

continued

Main Dishes, Combination

No.	Name/Portion Size		KCAL	CAL	PRO	CAR	FIB	SUG	FAT	SFA	PFA	CHL	SOD	A	C	THI	RIB	B6	CA	IRN	ZN
									NUTRI–UNITS												
1636	Oriental beef w veg,rice 8.6 oz	8.6 oz	260	3	6	2	N	N	2	3	1	2	13	3	N	2	2	N	0	2	N
1637	Oriental scallops,veg,rice 11 oz	11.0 oz	220	2	5	2	N	N	1	1	1	1	12	2	3	N	1	N	1	1	N
1638	Salisbury steak,veg 9.5 oz	9.5 oz	270	3	8	1	N	N	4	5	1	6	8	2	2	2	3	N	3	3	N
1639	Spagetti w beef,mushrooms 11.5 oz	11.4 oz	280	3	5	3	3	1	2	2	1	3	14	3	2	3	2	10	1	3	7
1640	Stuffed cabbage w meat 10.8 oz	10.8 oz	210	2	4	1	N	N	3	3	1	3	8	5	2	2	2	N	1	2	N
	Main Dishes, Combination (cont.)																				
1641	Lobster newburg 1 cup	8.8 oz	490	5	14	1	0	0	8	14	0	30	6	0	0	2	3	2	4	3	3
1642	Macaroni,beef+cheese+tom sauce 1 cup	8.0 oz	250	2	5	2	1	0	3	4	0	3	4	6	6	2	3	3	3	4	4
1643	Macaroni w cheese,homestyle 1 cup	7.1 oz	430	4	5	3	1	N	7	8	3	3	11	3	0	3	5	N	7	2	2
1644	Macaroni w cheese,canned 1 cup	8.5 oz	230	2	3	2	1	N	3	4	1	2	7	1	0	2	3	N	4	1	2
1645	Manicotti 1 cup	8.7 oz	340	3	6	3	2	0	3	6	0	2	12	14	15	6	6	5	10	2	4
1646	Meatballs,mushrm gravy,no salt 3 oz meatballs,2 tbsp grv	4.1 oz	440	4	9	0	0	0	11	16	0	7	1	0	0	1	3	5	0	4	7
1647	Meatloaf,lean 2 sl (4 × 3 × 3/8 in)	4.9 oz	250	2	8	1	0	0	3	5	0	9	5	1	0	1	3	4	1	4	7
1648	Omelet,spanish 2 eggs,4 tbsp sauce	5.4 oz	330	3	4	1	0	1	8	8	1	33	3	8	4	1	3	5	2	2	2
1649	Omelet w ham 2 eggs, 1/3 oz ham	4.8 oz	330	3	5	0	0	0	8	12	1	40	4	8	0	1	3	2	1	3	1
1650	Peppers stuffed w beef 1 med pepper	6.5 oz	310	3	7	2	1	0	3	4	1	5	6	2	25	2	4	10	2	4	5

1651 Pinto beans+cheese,no salt 3/5 cup	5.6 oz	170	2	3	1	8	0	1	3	0	2	1	12	3	3	2	2	3	3	2
1652 Pizza,cheese 1/8 of 14 in pizza	2.3 oz	150	2	2	1	1	N	2	2	0	1	5	2	2	1	2	1	3	1	1
1653 Pizza,cheese 1/7 of 10 in pizza	2.0 oz	140	1	2	1	1	N	1	1	0	1	4	1	1	0	1	1	2	1	1
1654 Pizza,cheese+polish sausage 1/8 of 14 in pizza	2.2 oz	160	2	2	1	1	0	2	4	0	1	3	1	1	2	2	1	3	1	0
1655 Pizza,cheese+sausage 1/8 of 14 in pizza	2.4 oz	190	2	3	1	1	N	3	2	1	1	4	1	2	1	1	1	3	1	1
1656 Pollack,creamed 1 cup	8.8 oz	320	3	11	1	0	0	4	7	0	6	3	4	0	1	4	3	1	2	2
1657 Pork,sweet+sour 3/4 cup	7.5 oz	260	3	1	3	N	N	2	2	1	N	15	4	1	1	2	N	0	0	N
1658 Quiche,cheese 1/8 of 8 in quiche	3.5 oz	190	2	2	1	0	1	4	4	2	7	3	1	0	1	2	1	3	1	1
1659 Quiche,chicken 1/8 of 8 in quiche	3.5 oz	220	2	3	1	0	0	5	6	2	9	4	2	0	1	2	2	3	1	1
1660 Quiche lorraine 1/8 of 8 in quiche	3.5 oz	270	3	3	1	1	0	6	7	2	9	5	2	0	2	3	2	3	1	1
1661 Quiche,swiss cheese+crab 1/8 of 8 in quiche	3.5 oz	280	3	4	1	0	0	7	8	2	10	6	4	0	1	2	2	3	1	2
1662 Ratatouille 5 oz	5.0 oz	80	1	1	1	N	N	1	N	N	N	8	2	10	1	0	N	0	1	N
1663 Ravioli,cheese 1 cup	8.6 oz	580	6	2	7	2	N	8	17	1	5	10	7	0	7	3	3	20	1	3
1664 Ravioli,meat 1 cup	8.6 oz	600	6	9	7	2	N	3	4	0	1	8	0	0	8	3	10	1	4	4
1665 Salisbury steak,no salt 1 pc (4 × 3 × 3/8 in)	2.5 oz	160	2	5	1	0	0	2	3	0	3	1	0	0	1	2	2	0	2	4
1666 Salmon rice loaf 1 pc (3.8 × 2.5 × 1.5 in)	6.1 oz	210	2	6	1	0	N	2	2	0	2	5	0	0	2	1	3	2	2	2

continued

Main Dishes, Combination

No.	Name/Portion Size		KCAL	CAL	PRO	CAR	FIB	SUG	FAT	SFA	PFA	CHL	SOD	A	C	THI	RIB	B6	CA	IRN	ZN
			NUTRI–UNITS																		
1667	Shad creole,no rice,no salt ½ cup	4.6 oz	200	2	6	0	0	N	3	4	0	4	1	2	3	2	2	3	0	1	1
1668	Shrimp creole on rice ½ cup on ½ cup rice	8.8 oz	270	3	4	3	2	1	1	2	0	6	12	5	7	2	1	2	1	4	2
1669	Spaghetti,meatballs+tomato sauc 1 cup	8.7 oz	330	3	6	3	2	N	4	3	1	5	10	6	7	3	4	N	2	4	3
1670	Spaghetti,meat sauce+cheese 1 cup	8.1 oz	350	3	8	2	2	N	4	6	0	4	9	5	6	2	4	7	7	4	5
1671	Spaghetti,tomato sauce+cheese 1 cup	8.8 oz	260	3	3	3	3	N	3	2	1	1	10	4	4	3	2	1	2	3	2
1672	Taco,beef+beans+cheese+lettuce 6-in tort, 4 oz filling	5.3 oz	340	3	8	2	1	0	5	7	0	4	1	1	0	2	3	6	4	5	3
1673	Taco,beef+cheese+lettuc+tomato 1 tortilla,2 oz beef	3.8 oz	170	2	4	1	1	0	2	3	0	3	3	2	2	1	2	2	2	2	4
1674	Tamale pie 1 cup	8.0 oz	180	2	5	1	6	0	2	2	0	3	10	6	6	1	2	2	0	3	4
1675	Tostada 1 small	4.9 oz	180	2	3	2	1	0	2	2	0	2	1	13	3	2	2	4	4	3	1
1676	Tostada,beefy 1 large	6.5 oz	290	3	6	1	4	0	4	7	0	6	7	14	4	2	3	3	4	4	6
1677	Tostada,beans+cheese+lett+sauce 1 tortilla,5 oz filling	6.3 oz	220	2	4	2	4	0	3	4	0	2	7	4	4	1	2	4	5	3	2
1678	Turkey a la king ½ cup on 1 sl toast	5.7 oz	210	2	6	1	0	0	2	2	1	3	4	7	2	1	2	2	2	1	4
1679	Turkey and noodles 1 cup	8.3 oz	300	3	11	1	0	0	3	3	1	8	11	2	2	2	3	2	0	3	4
1680	Turkey pot pie,home prepared ⅓ of 9 in pie	8.2 oz	550	5	7	3	1	0	9	9	5	5	6	12	2	4	4	5	1	4	2
1681	Turkey pot pie,frz,commercial 1 8 oz pie	8.0 oz	450	4	4	3	1	0	7	8	2	1	8	8	2	3	2	5	1	2	2

1682 Turkey pot pie,biscuit topping 1 cup	8.3 oz	400	4	9	2	1	0	5	5	3	5	5	16	2	4	3	9	1	3	1
1683 Turkey slice w gravy 3 oz turkey, 1 oz gravy	4.0 oz	160	2	8	0	0	0	1	1	1	5	4	0	0	1	2	2	0	2	3
1684 Tuna and noodles 1 cup	8.3 oz	320	3	7	2	2	0	4	2	4	8	11	1	1	2	2	1	1	3	1
1685 Veal parmigiana 1 cup	7.9 oz	340	3	7	2	5	0	5	9	1	5	15	4	9	2	3	N	2	3	4
1686 Whitefish,baked,stuffed,no salt 1 piece (3 × 3 × 1 inch)	3.5 oz	220	2	5	0	0	0	4	4	0	3	2	8	0	1	1	1	1	1	1

Salads, Relishes, and Salad Dressings

Accompaniment Salads

1687 Carrot and raisin salad,drsg 1/2 cup,1 tbsp m/fat drsg	2.1 oz	110	1	0	1	1	1	2	1	2	0	1	15	1	0	0	0	0	1	0
1688 Coleslaw,w mayo 1/2 cup,1 tbsp hifat drsg	2.1 oz	90	1	0	0	1	0	3	1	4	0	1	0	6	0	0	1	1	0	0
1689 Coleslaw,w mayo type salad drsg 1/2 cup,1/2 tbsp m/fat dr	2.1 oz	60	1	0	0	1	1	1	1	2	0	1	0	6	0	0	1	1	0	0
1690 Coleslaw w apples,creamy drsg 1/2 cup,1 tbsp m/fat drsg	2.1 oz	70	1	0	0	1	1	2	1	3	0	0	0	6	0	0	1	0	0	0
1691 Coleslaw w carrots,mayonnaise 1/2 cup,1.5 tbsp hifat dr	2.1 oz	160	2	0	0	1	0	5	3	7	1	1	1	6	0	0	1	0	0	0
1692 Cottage cheese on pineapple 1/4 cup on 1 med slice	3.4 oz	90	1	2	1	0	2	1	1	0	1	1	0	1	0	1	0	1	0	0
1693 Lettuce wedge 1 cup	3.0 oz	10	0	0	0	1	0	0	0	0	0	0	1	2	1	1	0	0	0	0
1694 Lettce+cucumbr,vinegar-oil drsg 1 cup chunks,1 tbsp drsg	3.5 oz	70	1	0	0	1	0	2	1	3	0	1	1	2	1	1	0	0	1	0
1695 Lettuce and lo fat french drsg 1 cup chopped,1 tbsp drsg	2.9 oz	80	1	0	1	1	2	1	1	1	0	1	1	2	1	0	0	0	0	0
1696 Lettuce and spinach,french drsg 1 cup,2 tbsp m/fat drsg	3.5 oz	180	2	0	1	1	1	5	3	8	0	2	6	4	1	1	2	1	1	0

continued

Salads, Relishes, and Salad Dressings

No.	Name/Portion Size		KCAL	CAL	PRO	CAR	FIB	SUG	FAT	SFA	PFA	CHL	SOD	A	C	THI	RIB	B6	CA	IRN	ZN
										NUTRI–UNITS											
1697	Lettuce and tom,w french drsg 1 cup,1 tbsp m/fat drsg	3.5 oz	70	1	0	0	1	0	2	1	2	0	2	2	4	1	0	1	0	1	0
1698	Gelatin,fruit flavored 1/2 cup	3.9 oz	70	1	1	1	0	3	0	0	0	0	1	0	0	0	0	0	0	0	0
1699	Gelatin w bananas 1/2 cup	3.9 oz	90	1	0	2	0	4	0	0	0	0	0	0	3	0	0	0	0	0	0
1700	Gelatin + carrot salad 1/2 cup	3.9 oz	60	1	0	1	0	2	0	0	0	0	0	3	0	0	0	1	0	0	0
1701	Gelatin w mandarin oranges 1/3 cup gel + 1/6 c frt	3.9 oz	70	1	0	1	0	3	0	0	0	0	0	0	3	0	0	0	0	0	0
1702	Gelatin w mixed fruit 1/2 cup	3.9 oz	70	1	0	1	0	3	0	0	0	0	0	0	1	0	0	0	0	0	0
1703	Gelatin w pears 1/2 cup	3.9 oz	80	1	0	1	0	4	0	0	0	0	0	0	0	0	0	0	0	0	0
1704	Fruit salad,canned,solids + liq 1/2 cup	4.5 oz	90	1	0	2	1	5	0	0	0	0	0	3	1	0	0	0	0	0	0
1705	Fruit salad,canned,artif swtnd 1/2 cup	4.3 oz	40	0	0	1	1	2	0	0	0	0	0	2	1	0	0	0	0	0	0
1706	Fresh fruit w mayo + whip cream 1 cup on let,2 tbsp drsg	6.2 oz	160	2	1	1	1	3	3	6	0	0	0	2	9	1	1	1	1	1	0
1707	Macaroni salad w salad drsg 1/2 cup,2 tbsp drsg	3.4 oz	200	2	1	1	N	0	4	3	5	2	5	1	0	1	1	3	2	1	1
1708	Potato salad w egg + may,fr dr 1/2 cup	4.4 oz	180	2	1	1	1	1	3	2	5	5	6	1	5	1	1	2	0	1	0
1709	Tossed salad,vinegar + oil drsg 1 cup let,cuc,rad + onion	3.5 oz	100	1	0	0	1	1	3	1	4	0	0	3	4	0	0	1	1	1	0
1710	Waldorf salad 3/4 cup,1 tbsp m/fat drsg	3.9 oz	120	1	1	1	2	2	2	1	2	0	2	1	2	1	0	2	0	0	0
Main Dish Salads (see also fast foods)																					
1711	Bean salad,three bean 1/2 cup	2.5 oz	100	1	1	1	2	0	2	1	3	0	1	0	1	0	0	1	0	1	0

1712 Chef salad,bolog,chees,egg,drsg 1 oz each,3 c let,4 tb dr	8.6 oz	580	6	5	1	2	2	16	13	16	15	12	5	3	1	3	2	5	2	3
1713 Chef salad,ham + cheese 1 oz each,2 c let,2 tb dr	6.5 oz	300	3	4	0	1	1	8	7	7	4	8	3	2	2	2	1	4	2	2
1714 Chicken salad 1/2 cup	3.5 oz	130	1	3	0	0	0	2	2	2	6	4	1	1	0	1	1	0	1	2
1715 Lobster salad w tomato slices 1/2 cup sal,1 med tomato	8.8 oz	280	3	8	0	1	0	5	2	7	8	3	0	15	3	2	2	2	3	2
1716 Taco salad,beans + beef 1 cup	5.3 oz	200	2	5	1	5	0	3	4	0	3	2	2	3	1	2	3	3	3	4
1717 Taco salad,beef 1 cup	5.3 oz	340	3	8	1	5	0	6	5	0	5	4	10	1	2	4	3	3	4	5
1718 Tomato stuffed w tuna salad 1/3 c tuna,2 1/2 in tomat	6.0 oz	100	1	1	1	1	1	2	1	2	3	2	5	9	1	1	1	1	1	1
1719 Tossed salad w turkey,sal drsg 1 cup	4.2 oz	130	1	2	0	1	0	3	2	4	1	2	5	3	1	1	1	1	1	0
1720 Tuna apple salad 1 cup	4.2 oz	230	2	5	1	0	0	5	3	6	3	6	1	1	0	1	2	0	2	1
1721 Tuna salad 1/2 cup	3.6 oz	170	2	5	0	0	0	3	2	3	4	7	1	0	1	1	3	0	1	0
Relishes																				
1722 Celery stuffed w peanut butter 1 pc (5 × 3/4 in)	.8 oz	40	0	1	0	0	0	1	0	1	0	1	0	0	0	0	0	0	0	0
1723 Cranberry orange relish 2 tablespoons	1.2 oz	60	1	0	1	0	2	0	0	0	0	0	0	2	0	0	0	0	0	0
1724 Deviled egg 1 egg	2.3 oz	140	1	2	0	0	0	3	2	3	18	4	3	0	1	2	1	1	1	1
1725 Horseradish,prepared 1 tablespoon	.5 oz	10	0	0	0	0	N	0	0	0	0	0	0	0	0	0	0	0	0	0
1726 Mustard,brown 1 tsp	.2 oz	10	0	0	0	N	0	0	0	0	0	1	0	0	0	0	N	0	0	0
1727 Mustard,yellow 1 tsp	.2 oz	0	0	0	0	N	0	0	0	0	0	1	0	0	0	0	N	0	0	0

continued

Salads, Relishes, and Salad Dressings

No.	Name/Portion Size		KCAL	CAL	PRO	CAR	FIB	SUG	FAT	SFA	PFA	CHL	SOD	A	C	THI	RIB	B6	CA	IRN	ZN
			NUTRI–UNITS																		
1728	Olives,green 4 large,whole	.6 oz	20	0	0	0	1	0	1	0	0	0	4	0	0	0	0	0	0	0	0
1729	Olives,ripe 4 medium,whole	.6 oz	30	0	0	0	0	0	1	0	0	0	1	0	0	0	0	0	0	0	0
1730	Peppers,hot green,raw 1 tbsp	.5 oz	10	0	0	0	0	0	0	0	0	0	0	0	12	0	0	0	0	0	0
1731	Peppers,hot green,canned 1 tbsp	.5 oz	0	0	0	0	0	0	0	0	0	0	0	0	3	0	0	0	0	0	0
1732	Peppers,hot,red,raw 1 tbsp	.5 oz	10	0	0	0	0	0	0	0	0	0	0	13	18	0	0	0	0	0	0
1733	Pickled beets 2 tablespoons	.7 oz	10	0	0	0	0	0	0	0	0	0	0	0	0	0	0	0	0	0	0
1734	Pickles,bread + butter 3 tbsp,sliced	1.1 oz	20	0	0	0	0	1	0	0	0	0	2	0	1	0	0	0	0	1	0
1735	Pickles,cucumber,dill or sour 1 med (4 × 1 in diam)	2.5 oz	10	0	0	0	1	0	0	0	0	0	10	0	1	0	0	0	0	1	0
1736	Pickles,cucumber,sweet 1 (2 × 1 in diam)	.5 oz	20	0	0	0	0	1	0	0	0	0	1	0	0	0	0	0	0	0	0
1737	Pimento,canned 1 tbsp	.5 oz	0	0	0	0	0	0	0	0	0	0	0	1	5	0	0	0	0	0	0
1738	Relish,sour 1 tablespoon	.5 oz	0	0	0	0	0	0	0	0	0	0	2	0	0	0	0	0	0	0	0
1739	Relish,sweet 1 tablespoon	.5 oz	20	0	0	0	0	1	0	0	0	0	1	0	0	0	0	0	0	0	0
1740	Tomato catsup 2 tablespoons	1.1 oz	30	0	0	1	0	1	0	0	0	0	3	2	1	0	0	0	0	0	0
Salad Ingredients																					
1741	Alfalfa sprouts 1 oz	1.0 oz	10	0	0	0	0	0	0	0	0	0	0	1	1	0	0	0	0	0	0
1742	Bacon,crisp 1 strip	.2 oz	40	0	1	0	0	0	1	1	0	0	1	0	0	0	0	0	0	0	0

1743 Bean sprouts,mung 1/2 cup	1.8 oz	10	0	0	0	0	0	0	0	0	0	0	0	1	0	0	0	0	0	0
1744 Bean sprouts,soy 1/2 cup	1.9 oz	20	0	1	0	1	0	0	0	0	0	0	0	2	2	1	1	1	1	1
1745 Beef,unsalted 1 oz	1.0 oz	60	1	3	0	0	0	1	1	0	2	0	0	0	0	1	1	0	1	2
1746 Carrot sticks 6 pc (3 × 3/8 in)	1.0 oz	10	0	0	0	1	0	0	0	0	0	0	12	1	0	0	1	0	0	0
1747 Cauliflower 1/4 cup buds	.9 oz	10	0	0	0	0	0	0	0	0	0	0	0	7	0	0	1	0	0	0
1748 Celery sticks 2 pc (5 × 3/4 in)	1.2 oz	10	0	0	0	0	0	0	0	0	0	0	0	1	0	0	0	0	0	0
1749 Cheese 1 oz	1.0 oz	110	1	2	0	0	0	3	5	0	2	2	1	0	0	1	0	4	0	1
1750 Croutons 1/4 cup	.4 oz	40	0	0	1	0	0	0	0	0	0	1	0	0	1	1	0	0	1	0
1751 Cucumber 1/4 cup	.9 oz	0	0	0	0	0	0	0	0	0	0	0	0	1	0	0	0	0	0	0
1752 Egg,hard cooked 1/2 large egg	.9 oz	40	0	1	0	0	0	1	1	0	9	0	1	0	0	1	0	0	1	0
1753 Garbanzo beans 2 tablespoons	.9 oz	40	0	1	0	2	0	0	0	0	0	1	0	0	0	0	0	0	1	1
1754 Ham,boiled 1 oz	1.0 oz	50	1	2	0	0	0	1	1	0	1	4	0	3	3	1	1	0	0	1
1755 Lettuce 1 cup chopped	1.9 oz	10	0	0	0	1	0	0	0	0	0	0	1	1	0	0	0	0	0	0
1756 Mushrooms 1/4 cup	.6 oz	0	0	0	0	0	0	0	0	0	0	0	0	0	0	1	0	0	0	0
1757 Onions,green 1 medium or 3 small	.5 oz	10	0	0	0	0	0	0	0	0	0	0	1	2	0	0	0	0	0	0
1758 Onions,mature 2 tablespoon	.8 oz	10	0	0	0	0	0	0	0	0	0	0	0	1	0	0	0	0	0	0
1759 Pepper,sweet green 1/4 cup sliced	.7 oz	10	0	0	0	0	0	0	0	0	0	0	0	9	0	0	0	0	0	0

continued

Salads, Relishes, and Salad Dressings

No.	Name/Portion Size		KCAL	CAL	PRO	CAR	FIB	SUG	FAT	SFA	PFA	CHL	SOD	A	C	THI	RIB	B6	CA	IRN	ZN
			NUTRI–UNITS																		
1760	Radishes 2 medium	.4 oz	0	0	0	0	0	0	0	0	0	0	0	0	1	0	0	0	0	0	0
1761	Spinach,raw ½ cup leaves	.6 oz	0	0	0	0	0	0	0	0	0	0	0	4	1	0	0	0	0	0	0
1762	Tomato ¼ cup slices	1.6 oz	10	0	0	0	0	0	0	0	0	0	0	2	4	0	0	0	0	0	0
1763	Turkey,unsalted 1 oz	1.0 oz	50	0	3	0	0	0	0	0	0	1	0	0	0	0	0	1	0	0	1
Salad Dressings																					
1764	Blue,roquefort dressing 2 tablespoons	1.1 oz	160	2	0	0	0	0	5	3	7	0	3	0	0	0	0	0	1	0	0
1765	Blue,roquefort,low fat 2 tablespoons	1.1 oz	20	0	0	0	0	0	1	1	0	0	4	0	0	0	0	0	0	0	0
1766	French dressing 2 tablespoons	1.1 oz	140	1	0	0	0	0	4	3	6	1	4	0	0	0	0	0	0	0	0
1767	French dressing,low fat 2 tablespoons	1.1 oz	40	0	0	0	0	0	1	0	1	0	3	0	0	0	0	0	0	0	0
1768	French dressing,low sodium 2 tablespoons	1.1 oz	60	1	0	0	0	0	3	1	4	0	1	0	0	0	0	0	0	0	0
1769	Green goddess 2 tablespoons	1.1 oz	150	2	0	0	0	0	5	2	6	0	3	0	0	0	0	0	0	0	0
1770	Italian dressing 2 tablespoons	1.1 oz	140	1	0	0	0	0	4	2	7	1	2	0	0	0	0	0	0	0	0
1771	Italian dressing,low fat 2 tablespoons	1.1 oz	30	0	0	0	0	0	1	0	1	0	2	0	0	0	0	0	0	0	0
1772	Mayonnaise 2 tablespoons	1.0 oz	200	2	0	0	0	0	7	3	9	1	2	0	0	0	0	0	0	0	0
1773	Mayonnaise,imitation,lo cal 2 tablespoons	1.0 oz	70	1	0	0	0	0	2	1	3	0	1	0	0	0	0	0	0	0	0
1774	Russian dressing 2 tablespoons	1.1 oz	150	2	0	0	0	0	5	2	7	0	3	1	1	0	0	0	0	0	0

1775	Salad dressing,mayo type 2 tablespoons	1.1 oz	120	1	0	1	0	0	3	1	4	1	2	0	0	0	0	0	0	0	0
1776	Sal drsg,mayo type,lo cal,lo sod 2 tablespoons	1.1 oz	40	0	0	0	0	0	1	1	2	1	0	0	0	0	0	0	0	0	0
1777	Vinegar and oil dressing 2 tablespoons	1.1 oz	130	1	0	0	0	0	4	2	6	0	0	0	0	0	0	0	0	0	0
1778	Lemon juice 1 tablespoon	.5 oz	0	0	0	0	0	0	0	0	0	0	0	0	2	0	0	0	0	0	0
1779	Vinegar 1 tablespoon	.5 oz	0	0	0	0	0	0	0	0	0	0	0	0	0	0	0	0	0	0	0
1780	Salad oil,sunflower 1 tablespoon	.5 oz	120	1	0	0	0	0	4	1	8	0	0	0	0	0	0	0	0	0	0
1781	Salad oil,corn 1 tablespoon	.5 oz	120	1	0	0	0	0	4	3	3	0	0	0	0	0	0	0	0	0	0

Sandwiches and Soups

Sandwiches (2 slices white bread unless specified)

1782	Bacon,lettuce and tomato 1 average (3 pc bacon)	5.2 oz	280	3	2	2	2	1	5	4	1	2	6	4	4	2	2	1	1	2	1
1783	Barbequed beef on bun 3 oz barb on 2 oz bun	5.1 oz	350	3	5	2	N	0	5	6	2	4	7	2	1	3	3	3	1	3	0
1784	Barbequed pork on bun 3.5 oz barb, 1.6 oz bun	5.0 oz	370	4	6	2	2	0	6	6	1	2	7	1	2	8	3	3	1	4	0
1785	Barbequed turkey on bun 3 oz barb on 2 oz bun	5.3 oz	290	3	6	3	2	0	1	1	0	3	6	3	2	2	2	8	1	3	0
1786	Bologna and cheese sandwich 1 oz each	3.4 oz	290	3	4	2	1	0	5	7	1	3	9	1	0	2	3	1	4	2	2
1787	Bologna and cheese+but,mayo,let 1 oz bologna,1 oz cheese	5.0 oz	380	4	4	2	1	0	7	9	2	4	10	3	0	2	2	1	5	2	2
1788	Burrito,beef,in sauce 3½ oz filling on tort	5.4 oz	390	4	8	2	7	0	5	7	0	8	3	6	4	3	4	6	1	4	3
1789	Burrito,beef and bean 1 burrito	4.6 oz	300	3	5	3	6	0	3	4	0	1	4	0	4	3	2	5	1	4	2

continued

Sandwiches and Soups

No.	Name/Portion Size		KCAL	CAL	PRO	CAR	FIB	SUG	FAT	SFA	PFA	CHL	SOD	A	C	THI	RIB	B6	CA	IRN	ZN
			NUTRI–UNITS																		
1790	Cheese sandwich,grilled 2 oz cheese	4.2 oz	410	4	5	2	1	0	7	9	2	3	10	4	0	2	3	1	9	2	3
1791	Cheese sandwich,toasted 1 oz cheese,1.5 tsp buttr	2.7 oz	260	3	3	1	1	0	5	7	0	3	6	2	0	1	2	0	4	1	2
1792	Cheeseburger 1 regular burger	4.0 oz	310	3	5	2	1	0	4	5	1	3	8	1	1	3	3	1	3	3	3
1793	Cheeseburger,quarter pounder 1 burger	6.8 oz	520	5	10	2	3	0	9	11	0	6	12	3	1	4	4	2	5	5	8
1794	Chili dog w bun 2 oz dog,2 tbsp chili,bun	4.4 oz	270	3	4	2	0	0	4	3	0	1	10	1	1	2	4	1	2	3	1
1795	Chili dog w bun 1.5 oz dog,1/2 c chili	8.3 oz	510	5	8	3	1	0	7	8	0	4	15	4	3	2	6	2	6	5	4
1796	Corn dog 1 corn dog	3.5 oz	270	3	5	1	2	0	5	5	1	2	9	0	0	1	2	2	0	3	1
1797	Corned beef and cheese on rye 1 oz each	4.1 oz	300	3	6	2	1	0	4	6	0	4	12	1	0	1	2	1	5	3	3
1798	Egg salad sandwich w lettuce 1 average	4.9 oz	380	4	3	2	1	0	7	6	6	15	6	3	0	1	1	1	1	2	1
1799	Fish burger 3 oz breaded fish on bun	4.3 oz	330	3	3	2	1	0	5	5	3	1	4	0	0	2	1	9	1	1	1
1800	Fish burger w tartar sauce 3 oz fish on bun	5.0 oz	430	4	4	3	1	0	7	7	7	2	5	0	0	2	1	2	1	2	2
1801	Fish burger w cheese,chili sce 2 oz fish,1 oz cheese,bun	5.3 oz	430	4	5	3	1	0	7	8	3	3	9	3	1	2	2	11	5	2	2
1802	Fish burger w cheese,tartar sce 2 oz fish, .5 oz ch, bun	4.1 oz	370	4	4	2	1	0	7	7	5	2	5	1	0	1	1	9	3	2	1
1803	French dip sandwich 2 oz bf,2 oz bun,4 oz jus	7.9 oz	340	3	6	3	1	0	4	4	1	4	12	0	0	4	3	4	1	3	1
1804	Ham and cheese sandwich w mayo 1.3 oz ham,.6 oz cheese	3.8 oz	320	3	5	1	1	0	6	6	4	4	9	1	0	4	2	2	4	2	1

1805	Ham salad sandwich 3 oz salad	4.0 oz	320	3	3	2	1	1	5	5	1	2	6	0	1	4	2	N	1	2	2
1806	Ham sandwich w butter,mayo,let 2 oz ham,1 tsp but + mayo	5.0 oz	320	3	6	2	1	0	5	6	3	5	8	1	0	5	1	3	1	3	4
1807	Hamburger,regular 1 hamburger,3.5 oz	3.5 oz	270	3	4	1	1	0	5	7	0	3	5	1	0	3	2	1	2	2	3
1808	Hamburger,quarter pound 1 hamburger,5.8 oz	5.8 oz	420	4	7	2	2	0	5	9	0	5	7	1	1	4	5	3	2	5	7
1809	Hamburger,super 1 hamburger,8.9 oz	8.9 oz	560	6	9	3	3	0	9	11	2	7	9	3	3	5	5	5	5	5	9
1810	Hoagie,small w let,tom + oil 1.5 oz meat,ch/1.5 oz bun	4.6 oz	280	3	4	2	1	0	5	6	1	2	8	2	1	2	2	1	3	2	2
1811	Hot dog on bun w catsup 2 oz dog,1.5 oz bun	3.8 oz	300	3	3	2	1	0	5	6	0	2	9	1	1	2	2	1	1	2	2
1812	Hot dog on bun w catsup+mustard 1.6 oz dog,1.5 oz bun	4.0 oz	260	3	3	2	1	0	4	5	1	2	10	1	1	2	2	1	1	2	1
1813	Hot dog w cheese on bun 1 serving,4 oz	4.0 oz	330	3	5	2	1	0	6	9	1	2	8	1	0	2	2	1	3	2	3
1814	Hot dog,large,on bun 1 serving,6.4 oz	6.4 oz	520	5	6	3	2	0	9	10	2	4	16	0	5	6	5	2	3	5	4
1815	Liverwurst on rye sandwich 1 average	3.2 oz	250	2	3	2	1	1	4	4	1	4	7	7	0	2	4	1	1	3	2
1816	Peanut butter + jelly sandwich 2 tbsp p/b,1 tbsp jelly	3.1 oz	340	3	4	3	1	3	5	3	4	0	4	0	0	1	1	N	1	2	2
1817	Pig in blanket 2 oz dog in blanket	4.4 oz	330	3	3	2	1	0	5	6	1	2	9	0	0	4	4	1	1	2	1
1818	Pita:ham,bologna,pastrami,chees 2 oz meat+ch,2.5 oz pita	4.5 oz	360	4	5	3	1	0	5	6	0	3	11	1	0	2	0	1	3	3	2
1819	Pizzaburger on bun 2 oz bf,.3 oz ch,1 tb sce	5.1 oz	410	4	7	2	1	0	6	9	1	6	5	3	1	3	4	3	2	4	6
1820	Reuben:kraut,beef,cheese on rye 1.75 oz corned beef	6.2 oz	310	3	7	3	2	0	2	4	0	4	18	1	2	1	2	2	3	4	2
1821	Roast beef sandwich w let+pickl 3 oz beef on 1.5 oz bun	5.1 oz	400	4	7	2	1	0	7	10	1	5	4	0	0	2	3	4	1	4	5

continued

Sandwiches and Soups

No.	Name/Portion Size		KCAL	CAL	PRO	CAR	FIB	SUG	FAT	SFA	PFA	CHL	SOD	A	C	THI	RIB	B6	CA	IRN	ZN
			NUTRI–UNITS																		
1822	Submarine:bologna,salami,cheese 3 oz meat+chees,2 oz bun	5.0 oz	440	4	6	2	1	0	7	9	1	4	14	1	0	4	4	1	5	3	2
1823	Sub:turky,past,che,let,tom,drsg 2.5 oz meat+ch,1.5 oz bun	5.1 oz	330	3	7	2	1	0	5	5	2	4	6	2	1	2	3	1	4	2	2
1824	Sub:bol,ham,salam,che,lett,mayo 2 oz meat+cheese,2 oz bun	5.3 oz	410	4	5	2	1	0	7	8	2	3	10	2	2	5	3	1	3	3	3
1825	Tuna sandwich 2.5 oz tuna,1.5 tbsp mayo	4.9 oz	410	4	6	2	1	0	7	5	9	3	8	1	0	1	1	2	1	2	1
1826	Turkey salad sandwich 3 oz salad	5.0 oz	340	3	6	2	1	1	4	4	5	4	5	1	1	2	3	N	1	3	2
1827	Turkey sand w but,mayo,lettuce 2 oz turkey	5.0 oz	310	3	6	2	1	0	4	5	3	5	4	2	0	1	1	5	1	2	2
1828	Turkey sandwich w gravy 1.6 oz turkey,1/2 c gravy	8.5 oz	280	3	6	2	1	0	2	1	1	3	11	0	0	3	2	4	1	3	4
Breads																					
1829	Bun,burger 1 average,1.6 oz	1.6 oz	130	1	1	2	1	1	1	0	0	0	2	0	0	3	2	0	1	1	0
1830	Low sodium bread 2 slices (18 per lb)	1.8 oz	160	2	2	2	1	1	1	0	0	0	0	0	0	2	2	0	1	2	0
1831	Pita bread 1 2.5 oz loaf	2.5 oz	200	2	2	3	1	0	0	1	0	0	2	0	0	7	3	1	1	2	1
1832	Raisin bread 2 slices (18/lb)	1.8 oz	130	1	1	2	1	2	0	0	0	0	2	0	0	3	1	0	1	2	0
1833	Raisin bread,toasted 2 slices (18/lb)	1.5 oz	130	1	1	2	1	2	0	0	0	0	2	0	0	2	1	0	1	2	0
1834	Rye bread 2 slices (18/lb)	1.8 oz	120	1	1	2	1	1	0	0	0	0	3	0	0	2	1	0	1	1	1
1835	Rye bread,toasted 2 slices (18/lb)	1.5 oz	120	1	1	2	1	1	0	0	0	0	3	0	0	2	1	1	1	1	1
1836	Tortilla,white wheat flour 1 8-inch	1.3 oz	90	1	1	1	1	0	0	0	0	0	1	0	0	2	1	0	1	1	0

1837 White bread 2 slices (18/lb)	1.8 oz	140	1	1	2	1	1	0	0	0	0	3	0	0	3	1	0	1	2	0
1838 White bread,toasted 2 slices (18/lb)	1.5 oz	140	1	1	2	1	1	0	0	0	0	3	0	0	2	1	0	1	2	0
1839 Whole wheat bread 2 slices (18/lb)	1.8 oz	120	1	2	2	2	1	0	0	0	0	3	0	0	2	1	1	1	2	1
1840 Whole wheat bread,toasted 2 slices (18/lb)	1.5 oz	120	1	2	2	2	1	0	0	0	0	3	0	0	1	1	1	1	2	1
Meats and Cheeses																				
1841 Beef slice,no salt added 1 oz	1.0 oz	60	1	3	0	0	0	1	1	0	2	0	0	0	0	1	1	0	1	2
1842 Beef slice,salted 1 oz	1.0 oz	60	1	3	0	0	0	1	1	0	2	0	0	0	0	1	1	0	1	2
1843 Bologna 1 sl (4.5 in diam × 1/8)	1.0 oz	90	1	1	0	0	0	2	3	0	1	4	0	0	1	1	1	0	1	1
1844 Bologna,all meat 1 sl (4.5 in diam × 1/8)	1.0 oz	90	1	1	0	0	0	2	3	0	1	3	0	2	1	0	1	0	0	1
1845 Braunschweiger 1 sl (3.1 in diam × 1/4)	1.0 oz	100	1	1	0	0	0	3	3	1	3	3	16	1	1	5	1	0	3	1
1846 Cheese,American process 1 sl (3.5 in sq × 1/8 in)	1.0 oz	90	1	2	0	0	0	2	4	0	1	3	1	0	0	1	0	3	0	1
1847 Cheese,cheddar 1 oz	1.0 oz	110	1	2	0	0	0	3	5	0	2	2	1	0	0	1	0	4	0	1
1848 Cheese,cheddar,low sodium 1 oz (1×1×1.6 in pc)	1.0 oz	110	1	2	0	0	0	3	5	0	2	0	1	0	0	1	0	4	0	1
1849 Cheese,past,proc,low sodium 1 sl (2 1/2 in sq × 1/4)	1.0 oz	100	1	2	0	0	0	3	5	0	2	0	1	0	0	1	0	3	0	1
1850 Cheese,skim American 1 sl (3.5 in sq × 1/8 in)	1.0 oz	60	1	2	0	0	0	1	3	0	0	4	0	0	0	1	0	3	0	1
1851 Cheese,swiss 1 sl (4 in sq × 1/8 in)	1.0 oz	110	1	2	0	0	0	2	4	0	2	1	1	0	0	1	0	5	0	1
1852 Cheese product m/w corn oil 1 sl (3.5 in sq × 1/8 in)	1.0 oz	100	1	2	0	0	0	2	0	2	0	4	1	0	0	1	0	3	0	1

continued

Sandwiches and Soups

No.	Name/Portion Size		KCAL	CAL	PRO	CAR	FIB	SUG	FAT	SFA	PFA	CHL	SOD	A	C	THI	RIB	B6	CA	IRN	ZN
											NUTRI–UNITS										
1853	Chicken,boned,canned 2 tbsp	.9 oz	50	1	2	0	0	0	1	1	0	1	1	0	0	0	0	0	0	0	1
1854	Chicken,white meat,no salt 1 pc (5 × 2 × 1/8 in)	.9 oz	40	0	2	0	0	0	0	0	0	1	0	0	0	0	0	1	0	0	0
1855	Chicken roll,white meat,salted 1 slice,1 oz	1.0 oz	50	0	2	0	0	0	1	1	0	1	2	0	0	0	0	1	0	0	0
1856	Corned beef 1 slice,1 oz	1.0 oz	60	1	2	0	0	0	1	1	0	2	3	0	0	0	1	1	0	1	1
1857	Deviled ham 2 tbsp	1.0 oz	100	1	1	0	0	0	3	3	1	1	3	0	0	1	0	0	0	0	1
1858	Frankfurter 1 frank (5 × 3/4 in diam)	1.6 oz	140	1	2	0	0	0	4	4	0	1	5	0	4	1	1	1	0	1	1
1859	Ham,boiled 1 sl (6.2 × 4 × 1/16 in)	1.0 oz	50	1	2	0	0	0	1	1	0	1	4	0	3	3	1	1	0	0	1
1860	Ham,deviled 2 tbsp	1.0 oz	100	1	1	0	0	0	3	3	1	1	3	0	0	1	0	0	0	0	1
1861	Ham,minced 1 oz	1.0 oz	70	1	1	0	0	0	2	2	0	1	3	0	3	3	1	1	0	0	1
1862	Potted beef 2 tbsp	1.0 oz	70	1	2	0	0	0	2	2	0	1	4	0	0	0	1	0	0	0	1
1863	Refried beans 1/2 cup	4.6 oz	200	2	3	2	10	0	2	2	1	0	5	0	0	2	1	3	1	3	2
1864	Salami,dry 2 sl(2 1/2 in dia × 1/8)	.7 oz	80	1	1	0	0	0	2	2	0	1	4	0	2	2	1	0	0	0	1
1865	Turkey ham 1 sl (3 × 3 × 1/8 in)	1.0 oz	40	0	2	0	0	0	1	1	1	0	3	0	0	0	1	1	0	1	1
1866	Turkey,light,unsalted 1 sl (3 × 3 × 1/8 in)	1.0 oz	50	0	3	0	0	0	0	0	0	1	0	0	0	0	0	1	0	0	1
1867	Turkey roll,light+dark,salted 1 sl (3 × 3 × 1/8 in)	1.0 oz	40	0	2	0	0	0	1	1	1	0	2	0	0	0	0	2	0	0	1

1868 Tuna salad 4 tbsp	1.8 oz	90	1	2	0	0	0	2	1	2	2	3	1	0	0	1	1	0	1	0
Relishes																				
1869 Catsup 1 tbsp	.5 oz	20	0	0	0	0	1	0	0	0	0	2	1	1	0	0	0	0	0	0
1870 Horseradish 1 tbsp	.5 oz	10	0	0	0	0	0	0	0	0	0	0	0	0	0	0	0	0	0	0
1871 Lettuce 1/4 cup shredded,1 leaf	.5 oz	0	0	0	0	0	0	0	0	0	0	0	0	0	0	0	0	0	0	0
1872 Mustard,brown 1 tsp	.2 oz	10	0	0	0	N	0	0	0	0	0	1	0	0	0	0	N	0	0	0
1873 Mustard,yellow 1 tsp	.2 oz	0	0	0	0	N	0	0	0	0	0	1	0	0	0	0	N	0	0	0
1874 Onion 1 tbsp	.4 oz	0	0	0	0	0	0	0	0	0	0	0	0	0	0	0	0	0	0	0
1875 Pickle,sweet 2 tbsp	.5 oz	20	0	0	0	0	1	0	0	0	0	1	0	0	0	0	0	0	0	0
1876 Pickle,sour or dill 2 tbsp	.6 oz	0	0	0	0	0	0	0	0	0	0	2	0	0	0	0	0	0	1	0
1877 Tomato slice 1/4 of 2.6 in tomato	1.1 oz	10	0	0	0	0	0	0	0	0	0	0	1	2	0	0	0	0	0	0
Spreads																				
1878 Butter 2 teaspoons	.4 oz	70	1	0	0	0	0	2	5	0	1	1	1	0	0	0	0	0	0	0
1879 Butter,unsalted 2 teaspoons	.4 oz	70	1	0	0	0	0	2	5	0	1	0	1	0	0	0	0	0	0	0
1880 Honey 1 tablespoon	.7 oz	60	1	0	1	0	3	0	0	0	0	0	0	0	0	0	0	0	0	0
1881 Hummus 1/3 cup	2.9 oz	140	1	1	1	N	N	2	1	2	0	2	0	2	1	1	3	1	1	1
1882 Jam + preserves 1 tablespoon	.7 oz	50	1	0	1	0	3	0	0	0	0	0	0	0	0	0	0	0	0	0

continued

Sandwiches and Soups

No.	Name/Portion Size		KCAL	CAL	PRO	CAR	FIB	SUG	FAT	SFA	PFA	CHL	SOD	A	C	THI	RIB	B6	CA	IRN	ZN
			NUTRI-UNITS																		
1883	Jelly 1 tablespoon	.6 oz	50	0	0	1	0	2	0	0	0	0	0	0	0	0	0	0	0	0	0
1884	Marmalade 1 tablespoon	.7 oz	50	1	0	1	0	3	0	0	0	0	0	0	0	0	0	0	0	0	0
1885	Marg:butter blend,60:40 2 teaspoons	.4 oz	70	1	0	0	0	0	2	2	2	0	1	1	0	0	0	0	0	0	0
1886	Margarine,diet 2 teaspoons	.4 oz	40	0	0	0	0	0	1	1	1	0	1	1	0	0	0	0	0	0	0
1887	Margarine,hard,p/s=1.5 2 teaspoons	.4 oz	70	1	0	0	0	0	2	1	2	0	1	1	0	0	0	0	0	0	0
1888	Margarine,soft,p/s=2.0 2 teaspoons	.4 oz	70	1	0	0	0	0	2	1	3	0	1	1	0	0	0	0	0	0	0
1889	Margarine,liquid oil,p/s=2.5 2 teaspoons	.4 oz	70	1	0	0	0	0	2	1	3	0	1	1	0	0	0	0	0	0	0
1890	Margarine,safflower bar,p/s=2.5 2 teaspoons	.4 oz	70	1	0	0	0	0	2	1	3	0	1	1	0	0	0	0	0	0	0
1891	Margarine,safflowr soft,p/s=4.0 2 teaspoons	.4 oz	70	1	0	0	0	0	2	1	4	0	1	1	0	0	0	0	0	0	0
1892	Margarine,bar,unsalted,p/s=.8 2 teaspoons	.4 oz	70	1	0	0	0	0	2	1	1	0	0	1	0	0	0	0	0	0	0
1893	Margarine,whipped,p/s=2.0 2 teaspoons	.2 oz	40	0	0	0	0	0	1	1	2	0	1	1	0	0	0	0	0	0	0
1894	Margarine,soft,unsalted,p/s=1.5 2 teaspoons	.4 oz	70	1	0	0	0	0	2	1	2	0	0	1	0	0	0	0	0	0	0
1895	Mayonnaise 1 tablespoon	.5 oz	100	1	0	0	0	0	3	1	5	1	1	0	0	0	0	1	0	0	0
1896	Mayonnaise,imitation,lo cal 1 tablespoon	.5 oz	30	0	0	0	0	0	1	0	1	0	1	0	0	0	0	0	0	0	0
1897	Mayo type salad dressing 1 tablespoon	.5 oz	60	1	0	0	0	0	1	1	2	0	1	0	0	0	0	0	0	0	0

1898 Mayo type sal drs,lo cal,lo sod 1 tablespoon	.5 oz	20	0	0	0	0	0	1	0	1	0	0	0	0	0	0	0	0	0	0
1899 P-nut butter,old fashioned 2 tablespoons	1.1 oz	180	2	3	0	2	0	5	4	2	0	1	0	0	0	0	1	0	1	1
1900 P-nut butr,smal amt fat,sug,slt 2 tablespoons	1.1 oz	170	2	2	0	2	0	4	2	4	0	2	0	0	0	0	1	0	1	1
1901 P-nut butr,mod amt fat,sug,salt 2 tablespoons	1.1 oz	180	2	2	0	2	0	5	3	4	0	2	0	0	0	0	1	0	1	1
1902 P-nut butter,no salt 2 tablespoons	1.1 oz	180	2	2	0	2	0	4	2	4	0	0	0	0	0	0	1	0	1	1
Soups[1]																				
1903 Cream of asparagus soup,w water 1 cup	8.5 oz	90	1	1	1	1	1	2	1	2	1	9	1	0	0	1	0	1	1	0
1904 Cream of asparagus soup,w milk 1 cup	8.6 oz	160	2	2	1	1	1	2	3	2	1	10	2	1	1	3	1	3	1	1
1905 Bean w pork soup,w water 1 cup	8.8 oz	170	2	2	2	N	N	2	1	2	0	9	4	0	1	0	0	2	2	1
1906 Beef broth soup,w water 1 cup	8.5 oz	20	0	1	0	0	0	0	0	0	0	8	0	0	0	1	0	0	0	0
1907 Beef noodle soup,w water 1 cup	8.5 oz	80	1	1	1	0	0	1	1	0	0	9	2	0	1	1	0	0	1	2
1908 Beef noodle soup,dehydr,preprd 1 cup	8.5 oz	160	2	3	1	1	0	2	2	1	1	18	5	0	2	1	1	1	2	4
1909 Beef mushrooom soup,w water 1 cup	8.6 oz	70	1	2	0	N	0	1	1	0	0	9	0	2	1	1	0	0	1	2
1910 Black bean soup,cnd,w water 1 cup	8.7 oz	120	1	2	1	7	0	0	0	0	0	12	2	0	1	1	1	1	2	2
1911 Cream of celery soup,w milk 1 cup	8.6 oz	160	2	2	1	1	2	3	4	2	2	10	2	0	1	3	1	4	1	0
1912 Cream of celery soup,w water 1 cup	8.5 oz	90	1	1	1	1	1	2	1	2	1	9	1	0	0	1	0	1	1	0

[1]For soups with "less salt," use part regular soup, part low sodium soup.

continued

Sandwiches and Soups

No.	Name/Portion Size		KCAL	CAL	PRO	CAR	FIB	SUG	FAT	SFA	PFA	CHL	SOD	A	C	THI	RIB	B6	CA	IRN	ZN
											NUTRI–UNITS										
1913	Chedder cheese soup,w water 1 scant cup	7.9 oz	140	1	2	1	N	N	3	5	0	2	9	4	0	0	1	0	3	1	1
1914	Chicken consomme,w water 1 cup	8.5 oz	40	0	1	0	0	0	0	0	0	0	8	0	0	0	1	0	0	1	0
1915	Cream of chicken soup,w milk 1 cup	8.6 oz	190	2	2	1	0	2	3	4	1	2	10	3	0	1	3	1	4	1	1
1916	Cream of chicken soup,w water 1 cup	8.5 oz	120	1	1	1	0	1	2	2	1	1	10	2	0	0	1	0	1	1	1
1917	Chicken corn chowder,w water 1 scant cup	7.9 oz	120	1	1	1	1	0	1	1	1	0	9	3	1	0	1	0	1	1	0
1918	Chicken gumbo soup,w water 1 cup	8.5 oz	60	1	1	1	0	0	0	0	0	0	9	1	2	0	1	1	0	1	0
1919	Chicken noodle soup,w water 1 cup	8.5 oz	70	1	1	1	0	0	1	1	0	0	11	3	0	1	1	0	0	1	1
1920	Chicken noodle soup,dehyd,prep 1 cup	8.5 oz	50	1	1	0	N	N	0	0	0	0	12	0	0	1	1	0	1	1	0
1921	Chicken rice soup,w water 1 cup	8.5 oz	60	1	1	1	0	0	1	0	0	0	8	3	0	0	0	0	0	1	0
1922	Chicken rice soup,dehydr,preprd 1 cup	8.5 oz	60	1	1	1	N	N	0	0	0	0	9	0	0	0	0	0	0	0	0
1923	Chicken-turkey broth 1 cup	8.5 oz	10	0	0	0	0	0	0	0	0	0	7	0	0	0	0	0	0	0	0
1924	Chicken vegetable soup,w water 1 cup	8.6 oz	80	1	1	1	0	1	1	1	1	1	10	11	0	1	1	0	0	1	0
For chili, see number 1600																					
1925	Chunky beef soup 1 scant cup	7.9 oz	160	2	3	1	N	N	1	2	0	1	8	10	2	1	2	1	1	2	3
1926	Chunky chicken soup 1 scant cup	7.9 oz	160	2	4	1	N	N	2	2	1	2	8	5	0	1	2	0	0	2	1
1927	Chunky chili beef soup 1 scant cup	7.9 oz	150	2	2	1	N	N	2	3	0	1	9	5	1	1	1	1	1	2	2

1928 Chunky sirloin burger soup 1 scant cup	7.9 oz	170	2	3	1	2	0	2	2	0	3	10	15	2	1	2	1	1	3	3
1929 Chunky vegetable soup 1 scant cup	7.9 oz	160	2	4	1	N	N	1	1	1	1	10	22	2	1	2	1	0	2	3
1930 Clam chowder,manhatt,w water 1 cup	8.6 oz	80	1	1	1	1	1	1	0	1	0	18	4	1	1	1	1	1	2	1
1931 Clam chowder,n-eng,fz,w milk 1 cup	8.6 oz	160	2	3	1	N	N	2	3	1	1	10	1	1	1	3	1	4	2	1
1932 Clam chowder,n-eng,fz,water 1 cup	8.6 oz	100	1	1	1	N	N	1	0	1	0	9	0	1	0	1	1	1	2	1
1933 French onion soup 1 cup	8.6 oz	40	0	1	0	1	0	1	0	0	0	11	0	0	0	0	0	0	0	0
1934 Gazpacho 1 cup	8.6 oz	60	1	3	0	N	N	1	0	1	0	12	1	1	1	0	1	0	1	0
1935 Green pea soup w milk 1 cup	8.8 oz	240	2	4	2	2	2	2	4	0	1	10	1	1	2	3	1	3	2	2
1936 Green pea soup,w water 1 cup	8.6 oz	160	2	3	2	2	2	1	1	0	0	10	1	1	1	1	1	1	2	2
1937 Green pea soup,dehydr,preprd 1 cup	8.6 oz	120	1	2	1	N	N	0	0	0	0	11	0	0	3	2	0	0	1	1
1938 Green pea soup/ham,fz, water 1 cup	8.6 oz	180	2	3	2	4	2	1	2	1	0	10	2	0	2	1	1	0	2	2
1939 Green pea soup,lo sodium 1 scant cup	7.9 oz	150	1	2	2	2	2	1	0	0	0	0	1	0	1	1	16	1	2	1
1940 Lentil soup w ham 1 cup	8.7 oz	140	1	3	1	N	N	1	1	0	0	13	1	1	2	1	2	1	3	1
1941 Minestrone soup,w water 1 cup	8.6 oz	80	1	1	1	2	1	1	1	1	0	9	10	0	1	1	1	1	1	1
1942 Cream of mushroom soup,w milk 1 cup	8.6 oz	200	2	2	1	0	2	4	5	4	1	11	1	1	1	3	1	4	1	1
1943 Cream of mushroom soup,w water 1 cup	8.5 oz	130	1	1	1	0	0	3	2	4	0	10	0	0	1	1	0	1	1	1
1944 Cream of mushroom soup,lo sod 1 scant cup	7.9 oz	150	1	0	1	0	0	3	2	2	0	0	0	0	1	1	0	1	1	2

[1]For soups with "less salt," use part regular soup, part low sodium soup.

continued

Sandwiches and Soups

No.	Name/Portion Size		KCAL	CAL	PRO	CAR	FIB	SUG	FAT	SFA	PFA	CHL	SOD	A	C	THI	RIB	B6	CA	IRN	ZN
			NUTRI–UNITS																		
1945	Onion soup,w water 1 cup	8.5 oz	60	1	1	1	1	1	1	0	1	0	10	0	0	0	0	0	1	1	1
1946	Onion soup,dehydr,preprd 1 cup	8.5 oz	30	0	0	0	N	N	0	0	0	0	8	0	0	0	1	0	0	0	0
1947	Oyster stew,frozen,w milk 1 cup	8.5 oz	130	1	2	1	0	0	2	4	0	2	10	1	1	1	3	1	3	1	14
1948	Oyster stew,frozen,w water 1 cup	8.5 oz	60	1	1	0	0	0	1	2	0	1	10	0	1	0	0	0	0	1	14
1949	Oyster stew,home prp,2 pts milk 1 cup	8.5 oz	230	2	4	1	0	1	5	6	0	6	8	3	0	2	5	1	5	5	14
1950	Oyster stew,home prp,3 pts milk 1 cup	8.5 oz	210	2	4	1	0	2	4	6	0	5	5	3	0	2	5	2	6	4	14
1951	Cream of potato soup,frz,w milk 1 cup	8.6 oz	150	1	2	1	N	N	2	3	1	1	10	2	0	1	3	1	3	1	1
1952	Cream of potato soup,fz,w water 1 cup	8.6 oz	70	1	1	1	N	N	1	1	0	0	10	1	0	0	0	0	0	1	1
1953	Cream of shrimp soup,w milk 1 cup	8.6 oz	160	2	2	1	N	N	3	5	0	2	10	1	0	1	3	4	3	1	1
1954	Cream of shrimp soup,w water 1 cup	8.6 oz	90	1	1	1	N	N	2	3	0	1	10	1	0	0	0	0	0	1	1
1955	Split pea soup,w water 1 cup	8.6 oz	180	2	3	2	4	2	1	2	1	0	10	2	0	2	1	1	0	2	2
1956	Tomato soup,w milk 1 cup	8.8 oz	160	2	2	2	1	3	2	3	1	1	9	3	23	2	3	2	3	2	1
1957	Tomato soup,w water 1 cup	8.6 oz	90	1	1	1	1	1	1	0	1	0	9	3	22	1	1	1	0	2	0
1958	Tomato soup,lo sodium 1 scant cup	7.9 oz	110	1	1	1	1	1	1	0	0	0	0	3	13	1	1	1	1	1	0
1959	Tom veg soup/noodl,dehy,prep 1 cup	8.5 oz	50	1	1	1	1	0	0	0	0	0	11	1	2	1	1	0	0	1	N

1960	Turkey noodle soup,w water 1 cup	8.5 oz	70	1	1	1	0	0	1	0	0	0	8	1	0	1	1	0	0	1	1
1961	Turkey noodle soup,lo sodium 1 scant cup	7.9 oz	70	1	1	1	0	0	1	0	0	0	0	1	0	1	1	0	0	1	2
1962	Vegetable soup,lo sodium 1 scant cup	7.9 oz	90	1	1	1	1	1	1	0	0	0	0	9	1	1	1	1	0	1	0
1963	Vegetable beef soup,w water 1 cup	8.6 oz	80	1	2	1	1	1	1	1	0	0	10	8	1	0	1	1	0	1	2
1964	Vegetable beef soup,fz,water 1 cup	8.6 oz	90	1	2	1	1	1	1	0	0	2	10	11	0	1	1	1	1	1	N
1965	Vegetable beef soup,lo sodium 1 scant cup	7.9 oz	90	1	1	1	1	1	1	2	0	2	1	11	1	1	1	1	0	1	1
1966	Vegetable beef broth,w water 1 cup	8.6 oz	80	1	1	1	N	N	1	0	1	0	8	8	1	1	1	1	0	1	1
1967	Vegetarian vegtble soup,w water 1 cup	8.6 oz	70	1	1	1	N	N	1	0	1	0	8	12	0	1	1	1	0	1	1

Vegetables (fresh, frozen, canned)

Vegetables (unsalted except canned/mixed dishes)[m]

1968	Alfalfa sprouts,raw 1/2 cup	.6 oz	10	0	0	0	0	0	0	0	0	0	0	0	0	0	0	0	0	0	0
1969	Artichokes,fresh,boiled,draind 3 in diam-medium bud	4.2 oz	50	1	1	1	3	N	0	0	0	0	1	1	3	1	1	1	1	2	1
1970	Asparagus,fresh,ckd,drnd,spears 1/2 cup (1.5–2 in pieces)	2.6 oz	20	0	1	0	1	0	0	0	0	0	0	2	7	1	1	1	0	1	0
1971	Asparagus,cnd,green,drained 1/2 cup (1.5–2 in pieces)	4.2 oz	20	0	1	0	1	0	0	0	0	0	5	3	7	1	1	1	0	2	1
1972	Asparagus,cnd,green,lo sod 1/2 cup (1.5–2 in pieces)	4.2 oz	20	0	1	0	1	0	0	0	0	0	0	2	6	1	1	1	0	1	1
1973	Asparagus,cnd,white,drained 1/2 cup (1.5–2 in pieces)	4.2 oz	30	0	1	0	1	0	0	0	0	0	3	0	6	1	1	2	0	1	1

[m] Add 0.5 nutri-unit sodium for moderate or 1 nutri-unit for heavy salting.

continued

Vegetables (fresh, frozen, canned)

No.	Name/Portion Size		KCAL	CAL	PRO	CAR	FIB	SUG	FAT	SFA	PFA	CHL	SOD	A	C	THI	RIB	B6	CA	IRN	ZN
			NUTRI–UNITS																		
1974	Asparagus,cnd,white,lo sod,drnd 1/2 cup (1.5–2 in pieces)	4.2 oz	20	0	1	0	1	0	0	0	0	0	0	0	6	1	1	2	0	1	1
1975	Asparagus,frzn,boiled,drained 1/2 cup or 4 large spears	2.8 oz	20	0	1	0	1	0	0	0	0	0	0	3	7	1	1	0	0	1	1
1976	Bamboo shoots,raw 1/2 cup in 1 in pieces	2.7 oz	20	0	1	0	1	0	0	0	0	0	0	0	1	2	1	2	0	0	1
1977	Beans,green,fresh/fz,boild,drnd 1/2 cup	2.4 oz	20	0	0	0	1	0	0	0	0	0	0	2	4	1	1	0	1	1	0
1978	Beans,green,canned,drained 1/2 cup	2.4 oz	10	0	0	0	1	0	0	0	0	0	2	1	1	0	0	0	0	1	0
1979	Beans,green,canned,lo sod,drnd 1/2 cup	2.4 oz	20	0	0	0	2	0	0	0	0	0	0	1	1	0	0	0	1	1	0
1980	Beans,green,lightly buttered 1/2 cup	2.4 oz	30	0	0	0	1	0	1	1	0	0	2	2	1	0	0	0	1	1	0
1981	Beans,green,w celery,butter 1/2 cup + 1 tsp butter	2.4 oz	60	1	0	0	1	0	2	3	0	1	1	2	1	0	0	1	1	0	0
1982	Beans,green,w onions 1/2 cup	2.4 oz	30	0	0	0	1	0	1	1	0	0	2	1	1	0	0	1	1	1	0
1983	Beans,green,w peanuts 1/2 cup	2.4 oz	50	1	1	0	2	0	1	1	0	0	2	1	1	0	0	0	1	1	0
1984	Bean sprouts,mung,raw 1 cup	3.7 oz	30	0	1	0	2	0	0	0	0	0	0	0	5	1	2	1	0	1	1
1985	Bean sprouts,mung,boiled,drnd 1/2 cup	2.2 oz	10	0	0	0	1	0	0	0	0	0	0	0	2	0	1	0	0	0	0
1986	Beans,lima,fresh/fz,boiled,drnd 1/2 cup	3.0 oz	110	1	2	1	3	0	0	0	0	0	0	1	3	2	1	2	1	2	1
1987	Beans,lima,canned,drained 1/2 cup	3.0 oz	80	1	1	1	5	0	0	0	0	0	2	1	2	0	0	1	0	2	1
1988	Beans,lima,canned.lo sod,draind 1/2 cup	3.0 oz	80	1	2	1	5	0	0	0	0	0	0	1	2	0	0	1	0	2	1

1989	Beans,yell/wax,fresh/fz,boil,dr ½ cup	2.4 oz	20	0	0	0	2	0	0	0	0	0	0	0	1	1	1	0	0	1	0
1990	Beans,yellow or wax,canned,drnd ½ cup	2.4 oz	20	0	0	0	2	0	0	0	0	0	2	0	1	0	0	0	1	1	0
1991	Beans,yell/wax,cnd,lo sod,drnd ½ cup	2.4 oz	10	0	0	0	1	0	0	0	0	0	0	0	1	0	0	0	0	1	0
1992	Beet Greens,boiled,drained ½ cup	2.6 oz	20	0	1	0	1	0	0	0	0	0	2	15	6	1	2	1	2	2	0
1993	Beets,fresh,boiled,drained ½ cup, diced	3.0 oz	30	0	0	0	1	1	0	0	0	0	0	0	2	0	0	0	0	1	0
1994	Beets,canned,drained ½ cup, whole small	2.8 oz	30	0	0	0	1	1	0	0	0	0	2	0	1	0	0	0	0	2	0
1995	Beets,canned,lo sodium,drained ½ dup diced or sliced	3.0 oz	30	0	0	1	1	1	0	0	0	0	0	0	1	0	0	0	0	1	0
1996	Blackeye/cowpea,immat seeds,ckd ½ cup	2.9 oz	90	1	2	1	3	0	0	0	0	0	0	2	0	1	1	0	0	1	1
1997	Blackeye/cowpeas,young pods,ckd 3 oz,scant cup	3.0 oz	30	0	1	0	4	0	0	0	0	0	0	5	5	1	1	1	1	1	0
1998	Broccoli,fresh spears,ckd,drnd ½ cup of ½ in pieces	2.8 oz	20	0	1	0	2	0	0	0	0	0	0	6	10	1	1	1	1	1	0
1999	Broccoli,fz,choppd,boiled,drnd ½ cup	3.2 oz	30	0	1	0	2	0	0	0	0	0	0	7	12	1	1	1	1	1	0
2000	Broccoli cheese casserole ½ cup	4.2 oz	170	2	3	1	1	1	3	4	1	2	5	8	20	1	3	N	4	1	1
2001	Broccoli w cheese sauce ½ cup + 2 tbsp sauce	3.5 oz	90	1	2	0	2	0	2	3	0	1	2	8	22	1	2	1	4	1	1
2002	Brussels sprout,frsh/fz,ckd,drn ½ cup,4 medium	2.7 oz	30	0	1	0	2	0	0	0	0	0	0	2	16	1	1	1	1	1	0
2003	Cabbage,raw ½ cup shredded/ sliced	1.2 oz	10	0	0	0	1	0	0	0	0	0	0	0	6	0	0	0	0	0	0
2004	Cabbage,cooked ½ cup wedges	3.0 oz	20	0	0	0	1	0	0	0	0	0	0	0	7	1	1	1	1	0	0

continued

[m] Add 0.5 nutri-unit sodium for moderate or 1 nutri-unit for heavy salting.

Vegetables (fresh, frozen, canned)

No.	Name/Portion Size		NUTRI–UNITS KCAL	CAL	PRO	CAR	FIB	SUG	FAT	SFA	PFA	CHL	SOD	A	C	THI	RIB	B6	CA	IRN	ZN
2005	Cabbage,red,raw 1/2 cup shredded/ sliced	1.2 oz	10	0	0	0	1	0	0	0	0	0	0	0	7	0	0	1	0	0	0
2006	Cabbage,savoy,raw 1/2 cup shredded/ sliced	1.2 oz	10	0	0	0	1	0	0	0	0	0	0	1	4	0	0	1	0	0	0
2007	Cabbage,spoon,raw 1/2 cup cut in 1 in pcs	1.2 oz	10	0	0	0	1	0	0	0	0	0	0	4	3	0	0	0	1	0	0
2008	Cabbage,spoon,boiled,drained 1/2 cup cut in 1 in pcs	3.0 oz	10	0	0	0	2	0	0	0	0	0	0	11	4	0	1	2	3	1	0
2009	Carrots,raw 1 in dia × 7.5 in carrot	2.5 oz	30	0	0	1	1	1	0	0	0	0	0	81	2	1	0	1	0	0	0
2010	Carrots,boiled,drained 1/2 cup crosswise slices	2.8 oz	40	0	0	1	2	1	0	0	0	0	1	77	1	0	1	2	0	1	0
2011	Carrots,cooked,drained 1/2 cup sliced	2.8 oz	20	0	0	0	2	1	0	0	0	0	2	47	1	0	0	0	0	1	0
2012	Carrots,canned,lo sod,drained 1/2 cup	2.8 oz	20	0	0	0	2	1	0	0	0	0	2	43	1	0	0	1	0	1	0
2013	Carrots,glazed 1/2 cup	3.5 oz	130	1	0	2	2	4	1	2	0	1	1	30	1	0	0	1	1	2	0
2014	Cauliflower,raw 1 cup sliced florets	3.2 oz	20	0	1	0	2	1	0	0	0	0	0	0	21	1	1	2	1	1	0
2015	Cauliflower,boiled,drained 1/2 cup	2.2 oz	20	0	0	0	1	0	0	0	0	0	0	0	12	1	0	1	0	0	0
2016	Cauliflwr+broccol mix,boild,drd 1/2 cup+1 tsp butter	2.6 oz	70	1	1	0	1	0	2	3	0	1	1	4	13	0	0	1	0	0	0
2017	Celery,raw 1/2 cup chopped, diced	1.9 oz	10	0	0	0	1	0	0	0	0	0	0	0	1	0	0	0	0	0	0
2018	Celery,boiled,drained 1/2 cup diced	2.7 oz	10	0	0	0	1	0	0	0	0	0	0	0	1	0	0	0	1	0	0
2019	Chard,swiss,raw 1 cup	1.1 oz	10	0	0	0	1	0	0	0	0	0	1	4	3	0	0	0	0	1	0

2020 Chard,swiss,boiled,drained ½ cup	3.0 oz	20	0	0	0	3	0	0	0	0	0	2	11	5	0	1	1	1	2	0
2021 Chicory greens,raw 7–10 inner leaves	.9 oz	10	0	0	0	0	0	0	0	0	0	0	0	1	0	0	0	0	0	0
2022 Collards,fresh/fz,boiled,drnd ½ cup	3.0 oz	10	0	0	0	1	0	0	0	0	0	0	8	3	0	0	0	1	0	1
2023 Corn,on cob,ckd,white or yellow 5 in × 1.7 in diam ear	2.7 oz	70	1	1	1	1	0	0	0	0	0	0	1	1	2	1	2	0	1	1
2024 Corn,canned,drained ½ cup	2.9 oz	70	1	1	1	2	0	0	0	0	0	3	1	2	0	1	0	0	1	0
2025 Corn,canned,cream style ½ cup	4.5 oz	90	1	1	2	2	0	0	0	0	0	4	0	2	0	1	1	0	1	1
2026 Corn,canned,cream style,lo sod ½ cup	4.5 oz	90	1	1	2	N	N	0	0	0	0	0	0	2	0	1	1	0	1	1
2027 Corn,fz,kernel,boiled,drained ½ cup	2.9 oz	70	1	1	1	2	0	0	0	0	0	0	1	1	1	1	1	0	0	0
2028 Cress,garden,raw 5 to 8 sprigs	.4 oz	0	0	0	0	0	0	0	0	0	0	0	4	2	0	0	0	0	0	0
2029 Cress,cooked,drained ½ cup	2.4 oz	20	0	0	0	1	0	0	0	0	0	0	21	5	1	1	1	1	1	0
2030 Cucumbers,raw,not pared ½ cup (sliced ⅛ in)	1.8 oz	10	0	0	0	0	0	0	0	0	0	0	0	1	0	0	0	0	0	0
2031 Dandelion greens,boiled,drained ½ cup	3.5 oz	30	0	1	0	2	0	0	N	N	0	0	47	6	2	2	2	3	2	0
2032 Eggplant,boiled,drained ½ cup, diced	3.5 oz	30	0	0	0	2	0	0	0	0	0	0	0	0	1	0	1	0	0	0
2033 Endive,raw ½ cup (small pieces)	.9 oz	0	0	0	0	N	0	0	0	0	0	0	0	1	0	0	0	0	0	0
2034 Fennel,common,leaves,raw 1 oz	1.0 oz	10	0	0	0	1	0	0	0	0	0	0	4	3	0	0	0	1	1	N
2035 Gazpacho 1 cup	8.6 oz	60	1	3	0	N	N	1	0	1	0	12	1	1	1	0	1	0	1	0

continued

[m] Add 0.5 nutri-unit sodium for moderate or 1 nutri-unit for heavy salting.

Vegetables (fresh, frozen, canned)

No.	Name/Portion Size		KCAL	CAL	PRO	CAR	FIB	SUG	FAT	SFA	PFA	CHL	SOD	A	C	THI	RIB	B6	CA	IRN	ZN
									NUTRI–UNITS												
2036	Italian style vegetabls w buttr 1/2 cup	2.4 oz	70	1	1	1	1	0	1	2	0	1	2	13	2	1	0	1	0	1	0
2037	Jerusalem artichokes,raw 4 small (1 1/2 in diam)	3.5 oz	80	1	1	1	N	N	0	0	0	0	0	0	1	3	1	1	0	4	0
2038	Jicama 1/4 cup	1.1 oz	10	0	0	0	N	N	0	0	0	0	0	0	2	0	0	0	0	0	0
2039	Kale,frzn,boiled,drained 1/2 cup	2.3 oz	20	0	1	0	1	0	0	0	0	0	0	17	5	0	1	1	2	1	0
2040	Kohlrabi,boiled,drained 1/2 cup	2.9 oz	20	0	0	0	1	0	0	0	0	0	0	0	15	0	0	1	0	0	0
2041	Leeks,raw 3 to 4 (5 in long each)	3.5 oz	60	1	0	1	2	2	0	0	0	0	0	0	4	1	0	2	1	2	0
2042	Lettuce,raw 1 cup chopped or shredded	1.9 oz	10	0	0	0	1	0	0	0	0	0	0	1	1	0	0	0	0	0	0
2043	Mushrooms,raw 1/2 cup	1.2 oz	10	0	0	0	1	0	0	0	0	0	0	0	0	0	2	0	0	0	0
2044	Mushrooms,canned,solids+liquid 1/2 cup	3.5 oz	20	0	1	0	1	0	0	0	0	0	4	0	1	0	3	1	0	1	1
2045	Mustard greens,fz,boiled,drnd 1/2 cup	2.6 oz	10	0	1	0	2	0	0	0	0	0	0	13	3	0	0	1	2	1	0
2046	Okra,boiled,drained 1/2 cup, crosscut slices	2.8 oz	30	0	0	0	2	0	0	0	0	0	0	2	4	1	1	1	1	0	1
2047	Okra,breaded,oven fried 1/2 cup	3.2 oz	60	1	1	1	2	1	1	0	1	0	0	2	4	1	2	1	2	1	0
2048	Onions,mature,raw 1/4 cup chopped	1.5 oz	10	0	0	0	0	0	0	0	0	0	0	0	1	0	0	1	0	0	0
2049	Onions,mature,cooked 1/2 cup sliced	3.5 oz	30	0	0	0	1	1	0	0	0	0	0	0	2	1	0	2	1	0	0
2050	Onion rings,french frd,veg fat 2 oz	2.0 oz	240	2	1	2	0	0	4	3	3	0	4	0	2	1	2	0	1	1	0

2051 Parsley,raw 1 tbsp chopped	.1 oz	0	0	0	0	0	0	0	0	0	0	0	1	1	0	0	0	0	0	0
2052 Parsnips,cooked,drained 1/2 cup	2.8 oz	70	1	0	1	2	1	0	0	0	0	0	0	3	1	0	1	1	1	0
2053 Peas,edible,podded,ckd,drnd 2 oz	2.0 oz	20	0	1	0	2	0	0	0	0	0	0	0	9	1	1	1	0	1	0
2054 Peas,green,immature,ckd,drnd 1/2 cup	2.8 oz	70	1	1	1	3	1	0	0	0	0	0	2	4	3	1	2	0	1	1
2055 Peas,green,swt,canned,drnd 1/2 cup	3.0 oz	60	1	1	1	2	1	0	0	0	0	2	3	3	1	1	1	0	1	1
2056 Peas,green,swt,cnd,lo sod,drnd 1/2 cup	3.0 oz	60	1	1	1	4	1	0	0	0	0	0	2	2	1	1	0	0	2	1
2057 Peas,green,fz,boiled,drained 1/2 cup	2.8 oz	60	1	1	1	2	1	0	0	0	0	1	2	3	3	1	1	0	1	1
2058 Peas+carrots,fz,boiled,drained 1/2 cup	2.8 oz	40	0	1	1	3	1	0	0	0	0	1	25	2	2	1	1	0	1	0
2059 Peppers,hot,immature,green,raw 1 oz,2 tbsp	1.0 oz	10	0	0	0	0	0	0	0	0	0	0	1	22	0	0	0	0	0	0
2060 Peppers,hot,immature,green,cnd 1 oz (solids+liquids)	1.0 oz	10	0	0	0	0	0	0	0	0	0	0	1	6	0	0	0	0	0	0
2061 Peppers,hot,red,raw,pod-no seed 1 oz,2 tbsp	1.0 oz	20	0	0	0	0	0	0	0	0	0	0	24	34	0	1	0	0	0	N
2062 Peppers,swt,green,immature,raw 1/2 cup sliced	1.4 oz	10	0	0	0	0	0	0	0	0	0	0	1	17	0	0	1	0	0	0
2063 Peppers,swt,green,boiled,drnd 1/2 cup strips	2.4 oz	10	0	0	0	1	0	0	0	0	0	0	1	22	1	1	1	0	0	0
2064 Peppers,sweet,red,mature,raw 1/2 cup sleced	1.4 oz	10	0	0	0	1	0	0	0	0	0	0	7	27	0	0	1	0	0	0
2065 Potatoes,baked in skin,with skin 2.3 in diam × 4.7 in	5.5 oz	170	2	1	3	1	0	0	0	0	0	0	0	7	2	1	5	0	2	1
2066 Potatoes,boild,pared bfore ckng 1/2 cup diced or sliced	2.8 oz	70	1	0	1	1	0	0	0	0	0	0	0	3	1	0	2	0	0	0

[m] Add 0.5 nutri-unit sodium for moderate or 1 nutri-unit for heavy salting.

continued

Vegetables (fresh, frozen, canned)

No.	Name/Portion Size		KCAL	CAL	PRO	CAR	FIB	SUG	FAT	SFA	PFA	CHL	SOD	A	C	THI	RIB	B6	CA	IRN	ZN
			NUTRI–UNITS																		
2067	Potatoes,canned,solids+liquid 3½ oz	3.5 oz	40	0	0	1	1	0	0	0	0	0	3	0	4	0	0	1	1	1	1
2068	Potatoes,french fried,no salt ½ cup	2.4 oz	110	1	1	1	1	0	1	2	0	0	0	0	2	1	0	1	0	1	0
2069	Potatoes,fried from raw,w salt ½ cup	3.0 oz	190	2	1	2	2	0	2	3	1	0	0	0	3	1	0	2	0	1	0
2070	Potatoes,hash-browned,w salt ½ cup	2.6 oz	160	2	1	1	1	0	3	3	1	N	0	0	2	1	0	1	0	1	0
2071	Potatoes,inst,w water,milk,fat ½ cup	3.7 oz	80	1	1	1	1	0	1	1	1	0	2	0	1	0	1	2	1	1	0
2072	Potatoes,inst,flakes,dry,w vitc ½ cup	.8 oz	80	1	1	1	1	0	0	0	0	0	0	0	5	2	0	2	0	0	0
2073	Potatoes,mashed,w milk ½ cup	3.7 oz	80	1	1	1	1	0	0	0	0	0	3	0	2	1	0	2	1	0	0
2074	Potatoes,mashed,w milk+fat ½ cup	3.7 oz	110	1	1	1	1	0	1	1	1	0	3	1	2	1	0	2	1	0	0
2075	Potaotes,scallop/au grat+cheese ½ cup	4.3 oz	160	2	2	1	1	0	3	5	0	2	5	1	4	1	2	2	3	1	1
2076	Potatoes,scallop/au grat,no chs ½ cup	4.3 oz	110	1	1	1	1	0	1	2	0	1	4	1	4	1	1	2	1	1	1
2077	Potato chips 10 chips (2.5 × 1.7 in)	.7 oz	110	1	0	1	1	0	2	2	3	0	1	0	3	0	0	1	0	0	0
2078	Potato sticks ½ cup	.6 oz	90	1	0	1	1	0	2	1	3	0	0	0	3	0	0	1	0	0	0
2079	Potatoes,tator bars 3 oz	3.0 oz	170	2	1	1	2	0	3	2	2	0	3	0	12	1	0	1	0	1	0
2080	Pumpkin,canned ½ cup	4.3 oz	130	1	0	2	N	N	0	0	0	0	3	41	1	0	2	2	1	1	0
2081	Radishes,common,raw 5 med or ¼ cup sliced	1.0 oz	10	0	0	0	0	0	0	0	0	0	0	0	2	0	0	0	0	0	0

2082 Rutabagas,boiled,drained 1/2 cup cubed or sliced	3.0 oz	30	0	0	0	1	0	0	0	0	0	0	0	6	1	0	1	1	0	0
2083 Sauerkraut,cnd,solids+liquid 1/2 cup	4.1 oz	20	0	0	0	2	0	0	0	0	0	8	0	6	0	0	2	1	2	0
2084 Shallot bulbs,raw 1 tbsp chopped	.4 oz	10	0	0	0	0	0	0	0	0	0	0	5	0	0	0	0	0	0	0
2085 Soybeans,immature seeds,ckd 1/2 cup	2.6 oz	90	1	2	1	5	0	1	1	2	0	0	2	4	3	1	1	1	2	N
2086 Soybean sprouts,raw 1/2 cup	1.9 oz	70	1	2	0	1	N	1	0	2	0	0	0	3	2	1	1	1	1	1
2087 Soybean sprouts,cooked 1/2 cup	2.2 oz	80	1	3	0	1	N	1	N	N	0	0	0	3	4	1	1	1	0	2
2088 Spinach,raw 1 cup pieces or leaves	1.1 oz	10	0	0	0	1	0	0	0	0	0	0	9	3	0	1	1	1	1	0
2089 Spinach,fresh/fz,boiled,drained 1/2 cup leaves	3.2 oz	20	0	1	0	2	0	0	0	0	0	1	29	3	1	2	2	2	4	1
2090 Spinach,canned,drained 1/2 cup	3.6 oz	20	0	1	0	2	0	0	0	0	0	0	36	5	0	2	1	3	3	1
2091 Spinach,canned,lo sod,drained 1/2 cup	3.6 oz	30	0	1	0	6	0	0	0	0	0	0	33	5	0	1	1	2	3	1
2092 Squash,summer,all typs,ckd,drnd 1/2 cup sliced	3.2 oz	20	0	0	0	1	1	0	0	0	0	0	1	2	1	0	1	0	0	0
2093 Squash,winter,acorn,baked 1/4 of 4 in squash; 2/5 c	2.8 oz	40	0	0	1	2	0	0	0	0	0	0	1	3	2	0	2	1	1	0
2094 Squash,winter,butternut,baked 1/2 cup mashed	3.6 oz	40	0	0	1	2	1	0	0	0	0	0	29	5	1	0	1	1	1	0
2095 Succotash,frzn,boiled,drained 1/2 cup	3.0 oz	80	1	1	1	2	0	0	0	0	0	0	1	2	1	1	1	0	1	1
2096 Sweet potatoes,baked in skin 1/2 of 5 in × 2.5 in pot	2.0 oz	60	1	0	1	1	1	0	0	0	0	0	50	5	1	1	1	0	0	0
2097 Sweet potatoes,cooked,candied 2 1/2 × 2 in diam piece	3.0 oz	120	1	0	2	1	4	1	1	0	0	1	14	2	0	0	0	0	1	0

[m] Add 0.5 nutri-unit sodium for moderate or 1 nutri-unit for heavy salting.

continued

Vegetables (fresh, frozen, canned)

No.	Name/Portion Size		KCAL	CAL	PRO	CAR	FIB	SUG	FAT	SFA	PFA	CHL	SOD	A	C	THI	RIB	B6	CA	IRN	ZN
			NUTRI–UNITS																		
2098	Sweet potatoes,canned,in syrup 1/2 cup solids+liquids	4.2 oz	130	1	0	2	2	2	0	0	0	0	0	34	4	0	1	1	0	1	0
2099	Sweet potatoes,cnd,dietary pack 1/2 cup solids+liquids	4.2 oz	110	1	1	2	2	2	0	0	0	0	1	38	11	1	1	2	1	1	0
2100	Sweet potatoes,glazed 2 1/2 × 2 in diam piece	2.7 oz	140	1	0	2	2	4	1	1	0	1	1	11	1	0	0	1	0	1	0
2101	Tomatoes,green,raw 1/2 of 3-in diam tomato	3.6 oz	20	0	0	0	1	N	0	0	0	0	0	3	8	1	0	1	0	1	0
2102	Tomatoes,ripe,raw 1/2 of 3-in diam tomato	3.5 oz	20	0	0	0	1	1	0	0	0	0	0	5	6	1	1	0	0	1	0
2103	Tomatoes,ripe,boiled 1/2 cup	4.2 oz	30	0	0	0	1	1	0	0	0	0	0	6	8	1	1	0	0	1	0
2104	Tomatoes,ripe,cnd,solids+liquid 1/2 cup	4.2 oz	30	0	0	1	1	1	0	0	0	0	3	3	5	1	0	0	1	1	0
2105	Tomatoes,ripe,cnd,lo sod,sol+lq 1/2 cup	4.2 oz	20	0	0	0	1	1	0	0	0	0	0	4	7	1	0	1	0	1	0
2106	Tomato juice,canned 1/2 cup	4.3 oz	20	0	0	0	1	1	0	0	0	0	4	3	7	1	0	1	0	1	0
2107	Tomato juice,canned,lo sodium 1/2 cup	4.3 oz	20	0	0	0	0	1	0	0	0	0	0	4	6	1	0	1	0	1	0
2108	Tomato paste,canned 1/4 cup or 4 tbsp	2.3 oz	50	1	1	1	1	2	0	0	0	0	0	6	9	1	1	2	0	2	1

2109 Tomato puree,canned 1/4 cup or 4 tbsp	2.3 oz	30	0	0	0	1	1	0	0	0	0	0	4	8	1	0	1	0	1	0
2110 Tomato puree,canned,lo sodium 1/4 cup or 4 tbsp	2.3 oz	30	0	0	0	1	1	0	0	0	0	0	4	7	1	0	1	0	1	0
2111 Tomato sauce 1/4 cup or 4 tbsp	2.0 oz	20	0	0	0	1	1	0	0	0	0	4	2	3	1	0	1	0	0	0
2112 Turnips,boiled,drained 1/2 cup cubed,1/3 c mashd	2.7 oz	10	0	0	0	1	0	0	0	0	0	0	0	3	0	0	1	0	0	0
2113 Turnip greens,frz,boild,draind 1/3 cup,1/4 of 10 oz pkg	1.9 oz	10	0	0	0	1	0	0	0	0	0	0	0	1	0	0	0	0	1	0
2114 Vegetables,mixed,boiled,drained 1/2 cup	3.2 oz	40	0	1	1	3	1	0	0	0	0	1	42	2	1	1	1	0	1	0
2115 Vegetable juice cocktail,canned 1/2 cup	4.3 oz	20	0	0	0	0	N	0	0	0	0	4	6	11	1	0	2	0	1	0
2116 Water chestnuts,chinese,raw 4 chestnuts	.9 oz	30	0	0	0	0	N	0	0	0	0	0	0	0	0	1	1	0	0	0
2117 Watercress Whole,1 cup (10 sprigs)	1.2 oz	0	0	0	0	0	0	0	0	0	0	0	7	5	0	0	0	1	0	0
2118 Yams,candied 3 3/4 in × 2 in dia piece	4.3 oz	220	2	0	3	2	6	2	4	0	1	1	21	3	0	0	1	0	1	0
2119 Zucchini,raw 1/2 cup sliced	3.2 oz	10	0	0	0	1	1	0	0	0	0	0	1	3	1	0	1	0	0	0
2120 Zucchini,ckd or boiled 1/2 cup sliced	3.2 oz	10	0	0	0	1	0	0	0	0	0	0	1	1	0	0	1	0	0	0

[m] Add 0.5 nutri-unit sodium for moderate or 1 nutri-unit for heavy salting.

Menu Items with Maximum Quantities of Nutrients

Menu Items with Maximum Quantity of Protein

No.	Name/Portion Size		KCAL	NUTRI-UNITS PRO
1138	Wendy's triple burger w cheese 1 serving, 14 oz	14.1 oz	1040	22
1061	Kentucky Fried,orig,3 pieces 3 pieces, 7.5 oz	7.6 oz	360	21
1137	Wendy's triple burger 1 serving, 12 oz	12.7 oz	840	20
1071	McDonalds chicken mcnuggets 1 serving, 20 pc	13.1 oz	900	19
1062	KFC extra crispy dinner 2 pc,pot,gravy,slaw,roll	15.4 oz	950	16
1068	Kentucky Fr Chick,orig dinner 2 pc,pot,gravy,slaw,roll	15.0 oz	830	16
1414	Broiler,one half,broiled 1 half broiler	6.2 oz	390	16
1136	Wendy's double burger w cheese 1 serving, 11.5 oz	11.5 oz	800	15
1641	Lobster newburg 1 cup	8.8 oz	490	14
1135	Wendy's double burger 1 serving, 10 oz	10.1 oz	670	14
1614	Fz dinner,chicken,potato+veg 11 oz	11.0 oz	540	12
1472	Swordfish,broiled 1 piece (4.5 × 2 × 1 in)	4.9 oz	240	12
1372	Porterhouse steak,lean+fat,brl Yield from 1/2 lb w bone	5.3 oz	450	12
1114	Arbys sub (no dressing) 1 serving, 9.5 oz	10.1 oz	480	11
1596	Chicken fricasee 1 cup	8.5 oz	390	11
1679	Turkey and noodles 1 cup	8.3 oz	300	11

No.	Name/Portion Size		KCAL	NUTRI-UNITS PRO
1094	Pizza H,thin,super,supreme 1/4 of 13 in pizza	6.3 oz	520	9
1100	Pizza H,thick,super,pork w mush 1/4 of 13 in pizza	6.0 oz	500	9
1112	Arbys super roast beef sandwich 1 serving, 9.5 oz	10.3 oz	620	9
1632	Fish jardiniere filet 11.2 oz	11.3 oz	280	9
1407	Broiled breast,w skin 1/2 breast	3.5 oz	190	9
1101	Pizza H,thick,supreme 1/4 of 13 in pizza	6.0 oz	480	9
1111	Arbys beef and cheddar sandwich 1 serving, 6 oz	6.3 oz	480	9
1113	Arbys ham+cheese sandwich 1 serving, 8.25 oz	8.7 oz	480	9
1123	J in b jumbo burger w cheese 1 serving,8.7 oz	8.7 oz	570	9
1484	Goose,domestic,flesh only,rstd 3 slices (3.5×3×.3 in)	3.5 oz	240	9
1664	Ravioli,meat 1 cup	8.6 oz	600	9
1809	Hamburger,super 1 hamburger,8.9 oz	8.9 oz	560	9
1070	McDonalds chicken mcnuggets 1 serving, 9 pc	5.9 oz	400	9
1119	Burger King,whopper 1 serving, 10 oz	10.0 oz	610	9
1646	Meatballs,mushrm gravy,no salt 3 oz meatballs,2 tbsp grv	4.1 oz	440	9
1364	Chuck,lean only,braised 1 piece (4 × 2.3 × .5 in)	3.0 oz	200	9

1401	Batter dipped breast 1/2 breast	4.9 oz	360	11
1656	Pollack,creamed 1 cup	8.8 oz	320	11
1456	Salmon,broil/bake,no salt 1 steak, 6.7 × 2.5 × 1 in	4.5 oz	230	11
1102	Pizza H,super,supreme 1/4 of 13 in pizza	7.1 oz	590	11
1134	Wendy's single burger w cheese 1 serving, 8.5 oz	8.5 oz	580	10
1431	Bass,baked,stuffed 1 pc w 1/3 cup stuffing	7.2 oz	530	10
1568	Blacksea bass,bkd,stuft,no salt 1 pc (3.5 × 4.5 × 1.5 in)	7.2 oz	530	10
1572	Beef meatloaf 2 slices (4 × 3 × 1/2 in)	6.4 oz	320	10
1608	Crab imperial 1 cup	7.8 oz	320	10
1447	Halibut,broiled or baked 1 fillet 6.5 × 2.5 ×.6 in	4.4 oz	210	10
1474	Tuna,baked,no salt 1 steak,6.7 × 2.5 × 1 in	4.5 oz	170	10
1479	Tuna,broil/bake,no salt 1 steak,6.7 × 2.5 × 1 in	4.5 oz	170	10
1096	Pizza H,thick,superstyle,cheese 1/4 of 13 in pizza	6.0 oz	450	10
1130	McD quarter pounder w cheese 1 serving, 6.8 oz	6.8 oz	520	10
1604	Chow mein,no noodles 1 cup	8.8 oz	260	10
1631	Fish divan filet 12.4 oz	12.4 oz	270	10
1793	Cheeseburger,quarter pounder 1 burger	6.8 oz	520	10
1368	Chuck arm,lean only,braised 1 pc (2.5 × 2.5 × .8 in)	3.0 oz	200	9
1449	Lobster,cooked 1 cup	5.3 oz	140	9
1594	Chicken and noodles 1 cup	8.3 oz	360	9
1399	Sweetbread,calf,braised 3 oz	3.0 oz	140	9
1428	Fried giblets 3 oz	3.0 oz	240	9
1682	Turkey pot pie,biscuit topping 1 cup	8.3 oz	400	9
1518	Pork picnic,lean only,sim 1 pc (2.5 × 2.5 × .8 in)	3.0 oz	210	8
1607	Crab,deviled 1 cup	8.5 oz	450	8
1098	Pizza H,thick,suprstyl,pepproni 1/4 of 13 in pizza	6.0 oz	490	8
1099	Pizza H,thick,pork w mushroom 1/4 of 13 in pizza	5.3 oz	430	8
1627	Chicken a l'orange w rice 8 oz	8.0 oz	280	8
1630	Fish florentine 9 oz	9.0 oz	240	8
1672	Taco,beef+beans+cheese+lettuce 6-in tort, 4 oz filling	5.3 oz	340	8
1408	Broiled breast,no skin 1/2 breast	3.0 oz	140	8
1795	Chili dog w bun 1.5 oz dog,1/2 c chili	8.3 oz	510	8
1366	Chuck blade,lean only,braised 1 piece (4 × 2.3 × .5 in)	3.0 oz	230	8
1421	Roast,light meat,no skin 1 pc (2.5 × 4 × .4 in)	3.0 oz	150	8

continued

Menu Items with Maximum Quantity of Protein *(continued)*

No.	Name/Portion Size		KCAL	NUTRI-UNITS PRO
1616	Fz dinner,turkey,potato+peas 11 oz	11.0 oz	350	8
1010	Jack in Box scrambled eggs 1 serving, 9.4 oz	9.4 oz	390	8
1088	Pizza H,thin,superstyle,cheese 1/4 of 13 in pizza	5.3 oz	410	8
1092	Pizza H,thin,super,pork w mushr 1/4 of 13 in pizza	5.3 oz	450	8
1133	Wendy's single burger 1 serving, 7 oz	7.1 oz	470	8
1381	Short ribs,lean only,braised 1 serving,(2/3 lb raw)	3.0 oz	250	8
1424	Stewed chicken,no skin 1/2–2/3 cup chopped	3.0 oz	200	8
1425	Oven baked chicken 3.0 oz	3.0 oz	210	8
1579	Beef stroganoff w rice 2/3 cup on 1/2 cup rice	9.9 oz	370	8
1588	Cheese fondue 1 cup	6.2 oz	460	8
1602	Chop suey,home prepared 1 cup	8.8 oz	300	8
1622	Lasagna w beef 1 cup	8.5 oz	420	8
1624	Chicken,glazed w veg + rice 8.5 oz	8.5 oz	270	8
1670	Spaghetti,meat sauce+cheese 1 cup	8.1 oz	350	8
1717	Taco salad,beef 1 cup	5.3 oz	340	8
1379	Sirloin,roundbone,lean only,brl 1 piece (2 × 4 × .5 in)	3.0 oz	180	8
1618	Hamburger goulash 1 cup	7.9 oz	270	8
1638	Salisbury steak,veg 9.5 oz	9.5 oz	270	8
1097	Pizza H,thick,pepperoni 1/4 of 13 in pizza	5.3 oz	450	8
1359	Canned roast beef w juice 1/2 cup	4.3 oz	240	8
1480	Beaver,roasted 3 oz	3.0 oz	210	8
1489	Raccoon,roasted 3 oz	3.0 oz	220	8
1503	Ham,fresh,lean only,roasted 1 slice (4 × 2.3 × .5 in)	3.0 oz	190	8
1512	Pork butt,lean only,rst 1 pc (2.5 × 2.5 × .8 in)	3.0 oz	190	8
1521	Pork spareribs,braised 3 oz serving	3.0 oz	340	8
1583	Burrito,beef,medium 8 in tort,1/3 cup filling	5.4 oz	390	8
1788	Burrito,beef,in sauce 3 1/2 oz filling on tort	5.4 oz	390	8
1370	Club steak,lean only,broiled 1 piece (2 × 4 × .5 in)	3.0 oz	180	8
1389	Rump roast,lean only 1 pc (4.1 × 2.2 × .5 in)	3.0 oz	160	8
1390	Ground beef, extra lean, broiled 1 patty (3 in diam × 6 in	3.0 oz	220	8
1394	Heart,cooked 3 oz	3.0 oz	150	8
1440	Croaker,baked 1 serving (3 × 3 × .8 in)	3.5 oz	130	8

1413	Broiler,one quarter,broiled	1 quarter broiler	3.1 oz	200	8
1416	Fried breast	1/2 breast (2.5 lb fryer)	2.9 oz	180	8
1478	Tuna,cnd in water,no salt	3.2 oz can,undrained	3.2 oz	120	8
1486	Opossum,roasted	3 oz	3.0 oz	190	8
1601	Chili con carne w/o beans	1 cup	8.8 oz	500	8
1683	Turkey slice w gravy	3 oz turkey, 1 oz gravy	4.0 oz	160	8
1108	Arbys chicken breast sandwich	1 serving, 7.25 oz	7.2 oz	550	8
1471	Sturgeon,steamed	3.5 oz serving	3.5 oz	160	8
1560	Roast turkey,light meat	2 sl (4 × 2 × 1/4 in)	3.0 oz	130	8
1589	Cheese manicotti w sauce	1 cup	8.5 oz	280	8
1647	Meatloaf,lean	2 sl (4 × 3 × 3/8 in)	4.9 oz	250	8
1715	Lobster salad w tomato slices	1/2 cup sal,1 med tomato	8.8 oz	280	8
1064	Kentucky Fried,keel,orig	1 serving, 3.4 oz	3.4 oz	280	8
1397	Liver,calf,fried	1 sl (6 × 2 × .5 in)	3.0 oz	220	8
1403	Batter dipped,deep fried,keel	1 keel	3.4 oz	280	8
1488	Rabbit,domestic,stewed	3 oz	3.0 oz	180	8
1615	Fz dinner,meat loaf,potato+peas	11 oz	11.0 oz	410	8
1496	Lamb,leg,lean only,roasted	2 slices (4 × 2 × .3 in)	3.0 oz	160	8
1559	Roast turkey,dark meat	4 pc (2 1/2×1 5/8×1/4 in)	3.0 oz	160	8
1685	Veal parmigiana	1 cup	7.9 oz	340	8
1095	Pizza H,thick,cheese	1/4 of 13 in pizza	5.3 oz	390	7
1373	Porterhouse steak,lean only,brl	1 piece (3.5 × 2 × .8 in)	3.0 oz	190	7
1375	T-bone steak,lean only,brl	1 piece (3.5 × 2 × .8 in)	3.0 oz	180	7
1377	Tenderloin, lean only, brl	1 piece (2.6 × 2.6 × .8 i	3.0 oz	180	7
1387	Round steak,lean only,brl	1 pc (4.1 × 2.2 × .5 in)	3.0 oz	170	7
1468	Shrimp,canned,drained,salted	3.5 oz serving	3.5 oz	120	7
1650	Peppers stuffed w beef	1 med pepper	6.5 oz	310	7
1680	Turkey pot pie,home prepared	1/3 of 9 in pie	8.2 oz	550	7
1820	Reuben:kraut,beef,cheese on rye	1.75 oz corned beef	6.2 oz	310	7
1125	McDonalds big mac	1 serving, 6.6 oz	6.6 oz	520	7
1129	McDonalds quarter pounder	1 serving, 5.8 oz	5.8 oz	420	7
1383	Rib,eye, lean only, brl	1 piece (2 × 4 × .5 in)	3.0 oz	200	7
1457	Salmon,chum,cnd,sol+liq,no salt	1/2 cup	3.9 oz	150	7
1487	Pheasant,raw	3.5 oz	3.5 oz	130	7

Menu Items with Maximum Quantity of Sugar

No.	Name/Portion Size		KCAL	NUTRI-UNITS SUG
183	Malt, chocolate, large 1 21-oz serving	20.7 oz	840	19
999	Dairy Queen choclate malt,large 1 large, 20.7 oz	20.7 oz	840	19
862	Banana split w soft serve 1 banana split	13.5 oz	540	18
1030	Dairy Queen banana split 1 serving, 13.5 oz	13.5 oz	540	18
1001	Dairy Queen misty freeze 1 serving, 14.5 oz	14.5 oz	500	17
1000	Dairy Queen misty float 1 serving, 14.3 oz	14.3 oz	440	17
996	Dairy Queen freeze 1 serving, 14 oz	14.0 oz	520	17
684	Condensed milk,sweetened,canned 1/2 cup	5.4 oz	490	17
883	Sundae,deluxe,soft serve 1 sundae	9.5 oz	570	16
1042	Dairy Queen fiesta sundae 1 serving, 9.5 oz	9.5 oz	570	16
879	Parfait,soft serve 1 parfait	10.0 oz	460	16
1044	Dairy Queen parfait 1 serving, 10 oz	10.0 oz	460	16
1040	DQ chocolate sundae,large 1 serving, 8.7 oz	8.7 oz	400	14
182	Malt, chocolate, medium 1 15-oz serving	14.7 oz	600	13
998	Dairy Queen choclate malt,med 1 medium, 14.7 oz	14.7 oz	600	13
869	Hot fudge brownie w soft serve 1 serving	9.4 oz	560	13

No.	Name/Portion Size		KCAL	NUTRI-UNITS SUG
1005	McDonalds chocolate shake 1 serving, 10.2 oz	10.2 oz	360	10
1007	McDonalds vanilla shake 1 serving, 10.2 oz	10.2 oz	320	10
1295	Rhubarb,frozen,cooked w sugar 1/2 cup	4.8 oz	160	9
1049	McDonalds sundae,caramel 1 serving, 5.8 oz	5.8 oz	330	9
1050	McDonalds sundae,hot fudge 1 serving, 5.8 oz	5.8 oz	310	9
1051	McDonalds sundae,strawberry 1 serving, 5.8 oz	5.8 oz	290	9
1293	Rhubarb,cooked,sol+liq, w sugar 1/2 cup	4.8 oz	190	9
964	Raisin pie m/w lard 1/6 of 9 in diam pie	5.5 oz	420	9
965	Raisin pie m/w veg fat 1/6 of 9 in diam pie	5.5 oz	420	9
159	Fruit flavored soft drinks 1 1/2 cup or 12 oz can	13.1 oz	170	9
700	Yogurt,fruit,part skim milk 8 oz container	8.0 oz	230	9
918	Yogurt,part skim,fruit flavors 1 8-oz container	8.0 oz	230	8
1252	Peaches,dehydrated,ckd w sugar 1/2 cup,sol+liq	4.9 oz	140	8
1025	McD hot cakes,butter and syrup 1 serving, 7.3 oz	7.3 oz	480	8
948	Lemon meringue pie m/w lard 1/6 of 9 in diam pie	4.9 oz	360	8
949	Lemon meringue pie m/w veg fat 1/6 of 9 in diam pie	4.9 oz	360	8

994	Burger King shake,vanilla 1 medium, 14 oz	14.0 oz	330	13
180	Ice cream float 1 14-oz serving	14.0 oz	330	12
995	Dairy Queen float 1 serving, 14 oz	14.0 oz	330	12
1258	Pears,dried,sulf,unckd 5 halves	3.1 oz	230	12
1037	DQ choc dipped cone,large 1 cone, 8.3 oz	8.3 oz	450	12
1209	Figs,dried,uncooked 1/2 cup,chopped	3.0 oz	220	12
1003	Jack in Box strawberry shake 1 serving, 11.6 oz	11.6 oz	380	11
1002	Jack in Box chocolate shake 1 serving, 11 oz	11.2 oz	370	11
1004	Jack in Box vanilla shake 1 serving, 11 oz	11.1 oz	340	11
1265	Pears,dried,sulf,ckd w sugar 1/2 cup, sol + liq	4.9 oz	200	11
1008	Wendy's frosty 1 serving, 8.8 oz	8.8 oz	390	11
882	Sundae,chocolate,soft serve med 1 sundae	6.5 oz	300	10
1039	DQ chocolate sundae,medium 1 serving, 6.5 oz	6.5 oz	300	10
195	Shake, strawberry 1 10-oz serving	10.3 oz	350	10
1006	McDonalds strawberry shake 1 serving, 10.3 oz	10.3 oz	350	10
194	Shake,chocolate 1 10-oz serving	10.2 oz	370	10
196	Shake, vanilla 1 10-oz serving	10.2 oz	320	10
939	Chocolate meringue pie w lard 1/6 of 9 in diam pie	5.4 oz	380	8
940	Chocolate meringue pie/veg fat 1/6 of 9 in diam pie	5.4 oz	380	8
954	Pecan pie m/w lard 1/6 of 9 in diam pie	4.8 oz	570	8
955	Pecan pie m/w veg fat 1/6 of 9 in diam pie	4.8 oz	570	8
1264	Pears,dried,sulfrd,ckd w/o sugr 1/2 cup,sol+liq	4.5 oz	160	8
863	Cone,choc dipped,soft serve,med 1 cone	5.5 oz	300	8
933	Cherry pie m/w lard 1/6 of 9 in diam pie	5.5 oz	410	8
934	Cherry pie m/w veg fat 1/6 of 9 in diam pie	5.5 oz	410	8
950	Mince pie m/w lard 1/6 of 9 in diam pie	5.5 oz	430	8
951	Mince pie m/w veg fat 1/6 of 9 in diam pie	5.5 oz	430	8
1036	DQ choc dipped cone,medium 1 cone, 5.5 oz	5.5 oz	300	8
1255	Peaches,dried,cooked w sugar 1/2 cup,sol+liq	4.6 oz	130	8
181	Malt, chocolate, small 1 8-oz serving	8.5 oz	340	8
866	Cone,soft serve,large 1 cone	7.5 oz	340	8
997	Dairy Queen choclate malt,small 1 small, 8.5 oz	8.5 oz	340	8
1034	Dairy Queen cone,large 1 serving, 7.5 oz	7.5 oz	340	8
966	Rhubarb pie m/w lard 1/6 of 9 in diam pie	5.5 oz	400	8

continued

Menu Items with Maximum Quantity of Sugar *(continued)*

No.	Name/Portion Size		KCAL	NUTRI-UNITS SUG
967	Rhubarb pie m/w veg fat 1/6 of 9 in diam pie	5.5 oz	400	8
977	Butterscotch topping 3 tablespoons	1.8 oz	160	8
156	Cola soft drinks 1 1/2 cup or 12 oz can	13.0 oz	140	7
1147	Apples,dried,sulf,ckd w sugar 1/2 cup	4.9 oz	120	7
145	Tea, iced w sugar, cnd 1 1/2 cup or 12 oz	12.7 oz	140	7
921	Apple pie m/w lard 1/6 of 9 in diam pie	5.5 oz	400	7
922	Apple pie m/w veg fat 1/6 of 9 in diam pie	5.5 oz	400	7
1163	Apricots,dehyd,sulf,ckd w sugar 1/2 cup	5.3 oz	190	7
978	Cherry topping 3 tablespoons	1.8 oz	150	7
927	Blackberry pie m/w lard 1/6 of 9 in diam pie	5.5 oz	380	7
928	Blackberry pie m/w veg fat 1/6 of 9 in diam pie	5.5 oz	380	7
929	Blueberry pie m/w lard 1/6 of 9 in diam pie	5.5 oz	380	7
930	Blueberry pie m/w veg fat 1/6 of 9 in diam pie	5.5 oz	380	7
946	Lemon chiffon m/w lard 1/6 of 9 in diam pie	3.8 oz	340	7
947	Lemon chiffon pie m/w veg fat 1/6 of 9 in diam pie	3.8 oz	340	7
165	Grape drink, canned, w vit c 1 8-oz cup	8.8 oz	140	7

No.	Name/Portion Size		KCAL	NUTRI-UNITS SUG
701	Yogurt,lo fat,van,coffee,lemon 8 oz container	8.0 oz	190	6
709	Caramel cake,icing,m/w butter 1/16 of 9-in 2-layer cake	2.8 oz	290	6
710	Caramel cake,icing,m/w veg fat 1/16 of 9-in 2-layer cake	2.8 oz	300	6
952	Peach pie m/w lard 1/6 of 9 in diam pie	5.5 oz	400	6
953	Peach pie m/w veg fat 1/6 of 9 in diam pie	5.5 oz	400	6
956	Pineapple pie m/w lard 1/6 of 9 in diam pie	5.5 oz	400	6
957	Pineapple pie m/w veg fat 1/6 of 9 in diam pie	5.5 oz	400	6
736	Honey spice cake w icing 1/16 of 9-in 2-layer cake	2.7 oz	270	6
752	White cake,icing,m/w butter 1/16 of 9-in 2-layer cake	2.8 oz	280	6
753	White cake,icing,m/w veg fat 1/16 of 9-in 2-layer cake	2.8 oz	290	6
1194	Cherries,swt,cnd+liq,xhvy syrp 1/2 cup	4.6 oz	130	6
931	Butterscotch pie m/w lard 1/6 of 9 in diam pie	5.4 oz	410	6
932	Butterscotch pie m/w veg fat 1/6 of 9 in diam pie	5.4 oz	410	6
2118	Yams,candied 3 3/4 in × 2 in dia piece	4.3 oz	220	6
161	Cherry flav drink, w vit c 1 8-oz cup	8.8 oz	120	6
163	Fruit flav drnk,powd,dil,w vitc 1 8-oz cup	8.8 oz	120	6

889	Charlotte russe,whip crm fillng 4 lady fingrs+1/3 c filln	4.0 oz	330	7
1203	Dried fruit,mixed 2 oz (approx 1/2 c)	1.9 oz	130	7
990	Strawberry topping 3 tablespoons	1.8 oz	140	7
1031	Dairy Queen buster bar 1 serving, 5.3 oz	5.3 oz	390	7
1298	Strawberries,frozen,sliced,swtn 1/2 cup	4.5 oz	120	7
937	Chocolate chiffon pie w lard 1/6 of 9 in diam pie	3.8 oz	350	7
938	Chocolate chiffon pie w veg fat 1/6 of 9 in diam pie	3.8 oz	350	7
1159	Apricots,dried,ckd w sugar 1/2 cup fruit + liquid	4.8 oz	150	7
1188	Cherries,sour,cnd+liq,xhvy syrp 1/2 cup	4.6 oz	150	7
1251	Peaches,cnd,sol+liq,xhvy syrup 1/2 cup	4.6 oz	120	7
179	Egg nog, non-alcoholic 1 8-oz glass	8.7 oz	340	6
336	Egg nog,non alcoholic 1 8-oz glass	8.7 oz	340	6
798	Marshmallows 1 cup,not pkd (.5 in dia)	1.6 oz	150	6
960	Pineapple custard pie m/w lard 1/6 of 9 in diam pie	5.4 oz	330	6
961	Pineapp custard pie m/w veg fat 1/6 of 9 in diam pie	5.4 oz	330	6
1143	Apples,dehyd,sulfured,unckd 1/2 cup	1.8 oz	170	6
1220	Goosebrrys,cnd,sol+liq,hvy syr 1/2 cup	3.9 oz	130	6

714	Chocolate cake,icing,m/w butter 1/16 of 9-in 2-layer cake	2.6 oz	270	6
715	Chocolate cake,icng,m/w veg fat 1/16 of 9-in 2-layer cake	2.6 oz	280	6
756	Yellow cake,icing,m/w butter 1/16 of 9-in 2-layer cake	2.6 oz	260	6
757	Yellow cake,icing,m/w veg fat 1/16 of 9-in 2-layer cake	2.6 oz	270	6
958	Pineapple chiffon pie m/w lard 1/6 of 9 in diam pie	3.8 oz	310	6
959	Pineapple chiffon m/w veg fat 1/6 of 9 in diam pie	3.8 oz	310	6
160	Ginger ale or swt quinine soda 1 1/2 cup or 12 oz can	12.9 oz	110	6
367	French toast,butter + syrup 2 sl tst,2 tsp,2 tbsp	5.4 oz	430	6
368	French toast,soft marg. + syrup 2 sl tst,2 tsp,2 tbsp	5.4 oz	430	6
748	Strawbr shortck+1 tbsp whip top 3×4 in pc+0.4 cup berries	4.3 oz	290	6
771	Candied fruit,all types 10 cherries or pieces	1.2 oz	120	6
844	Strawberry shortcake w whp top 3×4 in ck/.4 cup berries	4.3 oz	290	6
1038	DQ chocolate sundae,small 1 serving, 3.7 oz	3.7 oz	170	6
1266	Persimmons,raw,native 2 1/2 in dia × 3 in high	5.9 oz	210	6
740	Pineapple upsidedown cake 4 × 2.5 in piece	3.8 oz	310	6
935	Cherry pie,frozen,baked 1/6 of 8 in diam pie	3.4 oz	280	6
962	Pumpkin pie m/w lard 1/6 of 9 in diam pie	5.4 oz	320	6

Menu Items with Maximum Quantity of Fat

No.	Name/Portion Size		KCAL	NUTRI-UNITS FAT
1138	Wendy's triple burger w cheese 1 serving, 14 oz	14.1 oz	1040	20
1071	McDonalds chicken mcnuggets 1 serving, 20 pc	13.1 oz	900	17
1062	KFC extra crispy dinner 2 pc,pot,gravy,slaw,roll	15.4 oz	950	16
1712	Chef salad,bolog,chees,egg,drsg 1 oz each,3 c let,4 tb dr	8.6 oz	580	16
1137	Wendy's triple burger 1 serving, 12 oz	12.7 oz	840	15
1136	Wendy's double burger w cheese 1 serving, 11.5 oz	11.5 oz	800	14
1068	Kentucky Fr Chick,orig dinner 2 pc,pot,gravy,slaw,roll	15.0 oz	830	14
1018	McDonalds biscuit+sausage,egg 1 serving, 6.2 oz	6.2 oz	590	12
1135	Wendy's double burger 1 serving, 10 oz	10.1 oz	670	12
1601	Chili con carne w/o beans 1 cup	8.8 oz	500	11
1380	Short ribs,lean + fat,braised 1 serving (2/3 lb raw)	3.0 oz	400	11
1646	Meatballs,mushrm gravy,no salt 3 oz meatballs,2 tbsp grv	4.1 oz	440	11
1134	Wendy's single burger w cheese 1 serving, 8.5 oz	8.5 oz	580	10
1022	McDonalds sausage mcmuffin+egg 1 serving, 5.8 oz	5.8 oz	520	10
1431	Bass,baked,stuffed 1 pc w 1/3 cup stuffing	7.2 oz	530	10
1568	Blacksea bass,bkd,stuft,no salt 1 pc (3.5 × 4.5 × 1.5 in)	7.2 oz	530	10
1010	Jack in Box scrambled eggs 1 serving, 9.4 oz	9.4 oz	390	9
1491	Lamb chops,loin,lean + fat 1 chop,cut 3/lb	3.5 oz	360	9
1814	Hot dog,large,on bun 1 serving,6.4 oz	6.4 oz	520	9
1114	Arbys sub (no dressing) 1 serving, 9.5 oz	10.1 oz	480	9
1130	McD quarter pounder w cheese 1 serving, 6.8 oz	6.8 oz	520	9
1793	Cheeseburger,quarter pounder 1 burger	6.8 oz	520	9
1649	Omelet w ham 2 eggs, 1/3 oz ham	4.8 oz	330	9
1112	Arbys super roast beef sandwich 1 serving, 9.5 oz	10.3 oz	620	8
1384	Rib roast,whole,lean + fat,rst 1 sl (4.1 × 2.2 × .5 in)	3.0 oz	330	8
490	Egg,spanish omelet 2 eggs,4 tbsp sauce	5.4 oz	330	8
668	Egg,spanish omelet,salted 2 eggs,4 tbsp sauce	5.4 oz	330	8
1014	Jack in Box pancakes 1 serving, 8.2 oz	8.2 oz	630	8
1648	Omelet,spanish 2 eggs,4 tbsp sauce	5.4 oz	330	8
1614	Fz dinner,chicken,potato+veg 11 oz	11.0 oz	540	8
1641	Lobster newburg 1 cup	8.8 oz	490	8
1663	Ravioli,cheese 1 cup	8.6 oz	580	8

1372	Porterhouse steak,lean+fat,brl Yield from 1/2 lb w bone	5.3 oz	450	10
1588	Cheese fondue 1 cup	6.2 oz	460	10
1016	McDonalds biscuit+bacon,egg,chee 1 serving, 5.1 oz	5.1 oz	480	10
1123	J in B jumbo burger w cheese 1 serving,8.7 oz	8.7 oz	570	10
1493	Lamb chops,rib,lean + fat 1 chop,cut 3/lb	3.1 oz	360	10
954	Pecan pie m/w lard 1/6 of 9 in diam pie	4.8 oz	570	9
955	Pecan pie m/w veg fat 1/6 of 9 in diam pie	4.8 oz	570	9
1119	Burger King,whopper 1 serving, 10 oz	10.0 oz	610	9
1125	McDonalds big mac 1 serving, 6.6 oz	6.6 oz	520	9
1597	Chicken pot pie 1/3 of 9 in diam pie	8.2 oz	550	9
1680	Turkey pot pie,home prepared 1/3 of 9 in pie	8.2 oz	550	9
1017	McDonalds biscuit+sausage 1 serving, 4.3 oz	4.3 oz	470	9
1578	Beef potpie,home prepared 1/3 of 9 inch pie	7.4 oz	520	9
1809	Hamburger,super 1 hamburger,8.9 oz	8.9 oz	560	9
1508	Ham,cured,country style,bkd 1 slice (4 × 2.3 × .5 in)	3.0 oz	330	9
183	Malt, chocolate, large 1 21-oz serving	20.7 oz	840	9
999	Dairy Queen choclate malt,large 1 large, 20.7 oz	20.7 oz	840	9
1021	McDonalds sausage mcmuffin 1 serving, 4.1 oz	4.1 oz	430	8
1108	Arbys chicken breast sandwich 1 serving, 7.25 oz	7.2 oz	550	8
1365	Chuck blade,lean + fat,braised 1 piece (4 × 2.3 × .5 in)	3.0 oz	330	8
1094	Pizza H,thin,super,supreme 1/4 of 13 in pizza	6.3 oz	520	8
1102	Pizza H,super,supreme 1/4 of 13 in pizza	7.1 oz	590	8
1124	J in B moby jack sandwich 1 serving,5 oz	5.0 oz	460	8
1133	Wendy's single burger 1 serving, 7 oz	7.1 oz	470	8
1521	Pork spareribs,braised 3 oz serving	3.0 oz	340	8
1598	Chicken pot pie,commercial 1 8 oz pie	7.9 oz	490	8
1713	Chef salad,ham + cheese 1 oz each,2 c let,2 tb dr	6.5 oz	300	8
1609	Dried beef,creamed 1 cup	8.6 oz	380	8
1011	J in B omelette,double cheese 1 serving, 5.8 oz	5.9 oz	420	8
1070	McDonalds chicken mcnuggets 1 serving, 9 pc	5.9 oz	400	8
1611	Enchiladas,beef and cheese 2 small	8.9 oz	380	8
1790	Cheese sandwich,grilled 2 oz cheese	4.2 oz	410	7
1800	Fish burger w tartar sauce 3 oz fish on bun	5.0 oz	430	7
1075	Fish,batter fried 2 pieces, 4.8 oz	4.8 oz	370	7

continued

Menu Items with Maximum Quantity of Fat *(continued)*

No.	Name/Portion Size		KCAL	NUTRI-UNITS FAT
1587	Canneloni 1 cup	8.8 oz	430	7
1787	Bologna and cheese+but,mayo,let 1 oz bologna,1 oz cheese	5.0 oz	380	7
1798	Egg salad sandwich w lettuce 1 average	4.9 oz	380	7
1821	Roast beef sandwich w let+pickl 3 oz beef on 1.5 oz bun	5.1 oz	400	7
1822	Submarine:bologna,salami,cheese 3 oz meat+chees,2 oz bun	5.0 oz	440	7
1622	Lasagna w beef 1 cup	8.5 oz	420	7
1681	Turkey pot pie,frz,commercial 1 8 oz pie	8.0 oz	450	7
1610	Eggplant parmigiana 1 cup	7.8 oz	410	7
1825	Tuna sandwich 2.5 oz tuna,1.5 tbsp mayo	4.9 oz	410	7
1012	J in b omelette,ham and cheese 1 serving, 6 oz	6.1 oz	430	7
1013	J in b omelette,ranchero 1 serving, 6.9 oz	6.9 oz	410	7
1060	Jack in Box onion rings 1 serving, 3 oz	3.0 oz	350	7
1497	Lamb,shoulder,lean+fat,roasted 3 sl (2.5 × 2.5 × .25 in)	3.0 oz	290	7
1824	Sub:bol,ham,salam,che,lett,mayo 2 oz meat+cheese,2 oz bun	5.3 oz	410	7
1127	McDonalds filet of fish 1 serving, 4.6 oz	4.6 oz	400	7
1363	Chuck,lean + fat,braised 1 piece (4 × 2.3 × .5 in)	3.0 oz	300	7

No.	Name/Portion Size		KCAL	NUTRI-UNITS FAT
182	Malt, chocolate, medium 1 15-oz serving	14.7 oz	600	6
998	Dairy Queen choclate malt,med 1 medium, 14.7 oz	14.7 oz	600	6
1111	Arbys beef and cheddar sandwich 1 serving, 6 oz	6.3 oz	480	6
1113	Arbys ham+cheese sandwich 1 serving, 8.25 oz	8.7 oz	480	6
1374	T-bone steak,lean + fat,brl 1 piece (3.5 × 2 × .8 in)	3.0 oz	280	6
1581	Broccoli cheese casserole 1 cup	8.5 oz	330	6
1615	Fz dinner,meat loaf,potato+peas 11 oz	11.0 oz	410	6
1819	Pizzaburger on bun 2 oz bf,.3 oz ch,1 tb sce	5.1 oz	410	6
54	Macadamia nuts 1 oz (12 nuts)	1.0 oz	200	6
367	French toast,butter + syrup 2 sl tst,2 tsp,2 tbsp	5.4 oz	430	6
368	French toast,soft marg. + syrup 2 sl tst,2 tsp,2 tbsp	5.4 oz	430	6
369	French toast w soft margarine 2 slices w 2 tsp marg	4.0 oz	330	6
1367	Chuck arm,lean + fat,braised 1 pc (2.5 × 2.5 × .8 in)	3.0 oz	290	6
1515	Pork loin roast,lean + fat 1 sl (2.5 × 2.5 × .8 in)	3.0 oz	270	6
1552	Sausage,polish 1 link (5 3/8 × 1 in dia)	2.7 oz	240	6
1599	Chicken potpie w biscuit top 1 cup	8.4 oz	350	6

1586	Burrito,supreme 1 very large	7.9 oz	460	7
1607	Crab,deviled 1 cup	8.5 oz	450	7
1031	Dairy Queen buster bar 1 serving, 5.3 oz	5.3 oz	390	7
1577	Beef potpie,commercial 1 8 oz pie	7.9 oz	430	7
1596	Chicken fricasee 1 cup	8.5 oz	390	7
1643	Macaroni w cheese,homesyyle 1 cup	7.1 oz	430	7
1772	Mayonnaise 2 tablespoons	1.0 oz	200	7
1795	Chili dog w bun 1.5 oz dog,1/2 c chili	8.3 oz	510	7
1801	Fish burger w cheese,chili sce 2 oz fish,1 oz cheese,bun	5.3 oz	430	7
1542	Bratwurst,cooked 1 3 oz link	3.0 oz	260	7
1661	Quiche,swiss cheese+crab 1/8 of 8 in quiche	3.5 oz	280	7
1802	Fish burger w cheese,tartar sce 2 oz fish, .5 oz ch, bun	4.1 oz	370	7
883	Sundae,deluxe,soft serve 1 sundae	9.5 oz	570	7
1042	Dairy Queen fiesta sundae 1 serving, 9.5 oz	9.5 oz	570	7
1517	Pork picnic,lean + fat,sim 1 pc (2.5 × 2.5 × .8 in)	3.0 oz	290	7
869	Hot fudge brownie w soft serve 1 serving	9.4 oz	560	6
1513	Pork chop,loin,lean + fat,brl 1 chop,1/3 lb	2.8 oz	270	6
1083	Taco Bell enchirito 1 serving, 7.5 oz	7.5 oz	380	6
1660	Quiche lorraine 1/8 of 8 in quiche	3.5 oz	270	6
1027	Arby's apple turnover 1 turnover, 3 oz	3.0 oz	290	6
1098	Pizza H,thick,suprstyl,pepproni 1/4 of 13 in pizza	6.0 oz	490	6
1451	Ocean perch,breaded,fried 1 pc, 3 × 3 × .5 in	3.7 oz	340	6
378	Pancakes w hard marg. + syrup 3 4-in cks,1 tbsp,2 tbsp	6.2 oz	370	6
1398	Sweetbread,beef,fried 3 oz	3.0 oz	270	6
1617	Ham croquette 2 (1 in diam × 3 in)	4.6 oz	330	6
1717	Taco salad,beef 1 cup	5.3 oz	340	6
1804	Ham and cheese sandwich w mayo 1.3 oz ham,.6 oz cheese	3.8 oz	320	6
1813	Hot dog w cheese on bun 1 serving,4 oz	4.0 oz	330	6
63	Pecans dried 24 halves (4 tablespoons)	1.0 oz	190	6
941	Coconut custard pie m/w lard 1/6 of 9 in diam pie	5.4 oz	360	6
942	Coconut custard pie m/w veg fat 1/6 of 9 in diam pie	5.4 oz	360	6
1028	Arby's blueberry turnover 1 turnover, 3 oz	3.0 oz	320	6
1029	Arby's cherry turnover 1 turnover, 3 oz	3.0 oz	300	6
1090	Pizza H,thin,suprstyle,pepproni 1/4 of 13 in pizza	5.3 oz	430	6

Menu Items with Maximum Quantity of Saturated Fat

No.	Name/Portion Size		KCAL	NUTRI-UNITS SFA
1138	Wendy's triple burger w cheese 1 serving, 14 oz	14.1 oz	1040	29
1137	Wendy's triple burger 1 serving, 12 oz	12.7 oz	840	21
1136	Wendy's double burger w cheese 1 serving, 11.5 oz	11.5 oz	800	19
1663	Ravioli,cheese 1 cup	8.6 oz	580	17
1135	Wendy's double burger 1 serving, 10 oz	10.1 oz	670	17
1493	Lamb chops,rib,lean + fat 1 chop,cut 3/lb	3.1 oz	360	16
183	Malt, chocolate, large 1 21-oz serving	20.7 oz	840	16
999	Dairy Queen choclate malt,large 1 large, 20.7 oz	20.7 oz	840	16
1601	Chili con carne w/o beans 1 cup	8.8 oz	500	16
1646	Meatballs,mushrm gravy,no salt 3 oz meatballs,2 tbsp grv	4.1 oz	440	16
1491	Lamb chops,loin,lean + fat 1 chop,cut 3/lb	3.5 oz	360	15
1123	J in B jumbo burger w cheese 1 serving,8.7 oz	8.7 oz	570	14
1588	Cheese fondue 1 cup	6.2 oz	460	14
1125	McDonalds big mac 1 serving, 6.6 oz	6.6 oz	520	14
1134	Wendy's single burger w cheese 1 serving, 8.5 oz	8.5 oz	580	14
1071	McDonalds chicken mcnuggets 1 serving, 20 pc	13.1 oz	900	14

No.	Name/Portion Size		KCAL	NUTRI-UNITS SFA
1809	Hamburger,super 1 hamburger,8.9 oz	8.9 oz	560	11
182	Malt, chocolate, medium 1 15-oz serving	14.7 oz	600	11
998	Dairy Queen choclate malt,med 1 medium, 14.7 oz	14.7 oz	600	11
1130	McD quarter pounder w cheese 1 serving, 6.8 oz	6.8 oz	520	11
1793	Cheeseburger,quarter pounder 1 burger	6.8 oz	520	11
1017	McDonalds biscuit+sausage 1 serving, 4.3 oz	4.3 oz	470	11
1018	McDonalds biscuit+sausage,egg 1 serving, 6.2 oz	6.2 oz	590	11
1021	McDonalds sausage mcmuffin 1 serving, 4.1 oz	4.1 oz	430	11
883	Sundae,deluxe,soft serve 1 sundae	9.5 oz	570	11
1042	Dairy Queen fiesta sundae 1 serving, 9.5 oz	9.5 oz	570	11
869	Hot fudge brownie w soft serve 1 serving	9.4 oz	560	11
1133	Wendy's single burger 1 serving, 7 oz	7.1 oz	470	11
1622	Lasagna w beef 1 cup	8.5 oz	420	11
1010	Jack in Box scrambled eggs 1 serving, 9.4 oz	9.4 oz	390	11
1384	Rib roast,whole,lean + fat,rst 1 sl (4.1 × 2.2 × .5 in)	3.0 oz	330	11
862	Banana split w soft serve 1 banana split	13.5 oz	540	10

1380	Short ribs,lean + fat,braised 1 serving (2/3 lb raw)	3.0 oz	400	14
1641	Lobster newburg 1 cup	8.8 oz	490	14
1119	Burger King,whopper 1 serving, 10 oz	10.0 oz	610	13
1059	Dairy Queen onion rings 1 serving, 3 oz	3.0 oz	300	13
1712	Chef salad,bolog,chees,egg,drsg 1 oz each,3 c let,4 tb dr	8.6 oz	580	13
1609	Dried beef,creamed 1 cup	8.6 oz	380	12
1587	Canneloni 1 cup	8.8 oz	430	12
1031	Dairy Queen buster bar 1 serving, 5.3 oz	5.3 oz	390	12
1016	McDonalds biscuit+bacon,egg,chee 1 serving, 5.1 oz	5.1 oz	480	12
1022	McDonalds sausage mcmuffin+egg 1 serving, 5.8 oz	5.8 oz	520	12
1195	Coconut meat,fresh 2 × 2 × 1/2 in piece	1.6 oz	160	12
1372	Porterhouse steak,lean+fat,brl Yield from 1/2 lb w bone	5.3 oz	450	12
1062	KFC extra crispy dinner 2 pc,pot,gravy,slaw,roll	15.4 oz	950	12
1649	Omelet w ham 2 eggs, 1/3 oz ham	4.8 oz	330	12
1497	Lamb,shoulder,lean+fat,roasted 3 sl (2.5 × 2.5 × .25 in)	3.0 oz	290	12
1060	Jack in Box onion rings 1 serving, 3 oz	3.0 oz	350	12
1068	Kentucky Fr Chick,orig dinner 2 pc,pot,gravy,slaw,roll	15.0 oz	830	12

1030	Dairy Queen banana split 1 serving, 13.5 oz	13.5 oz	540	10
1114	Arbys sub (no dressing) 1 serving, 9.5 oz	10.1 oz	480	10
1112	Arbys super roast beef sandwich 1 serving, 9.5 oz	10.3 oz	620	10
1821	Roast beef sandwich w let+pickl 3 oz beef on 1.5 oz bun	5.1 oz	400	10
1365	Chuck blade,lean + fat,braised 1 piece (4 × 2.3 × .5 in)	3.0 oz	330	10
1597	Chicken pot pie 1/3 of 9 in diam pie	8.2 oz	550	10
1611	Enchiladas,beef and cheese 2 small	8.9 oz	380	10
1814	Hot dog,large,on bun 1 serving,6.4 oz	6.4 oz	520	10
1508	Ham,cured,country style,bkd 1 slice (4 × 2.3 × .5 in)	3.0 oz	330	10
1787	Bologna and cheese+but,mayo,let 1 oz bologna,1 oz cheese	5.0 oz	380	10
1822	Submarine:bologna,salami,cheese 3 oz meat+chees,2 oz bun	5.0 oz	440	10
1680	Turkey pot pie,home prepared 1/3 of 9 in pie	8.2 oz	550	9
648	Ricotta 1/2 cup	4.4 oz	220	9
1431	Bass,baked,stuffed 1 pc w 1/3 cup stuffing	7.2 oz	530	9
1568	Blacksea bass,bkd,stuft,no salt 1 pc (3.5 × 4.5 × 1.5 in)	7.2 oz	530	9
1083	Taco Bell enchirito 1 serving, 7.5 oz	7.5 oz	380	9
1819	Pizzaburger on bun 2 oz bf,.3 oz ch,1 tb sce	5.1 oz	410	9

continued

Menu Items with Maximum Quantity of Saturated Fat *(continued)*

No.	Name/Portion Size		KCAL	NUTRI-UNITS SFA
1008	Wendy's frosty 1 serving, 8.8 oz	8.8 oz	390	9
1521	Pork spareribs,braised 3 oz serving	3.0 oz	340	9
1790	Cheese sandwich,grilled 2 oz cheese	4.2 oz	410	9
179	Egg nog, non-alcoholic 1 8-oz glass	8.7 oz	340	9
336	Egg nog,non alcoholic 1 8-oz glass	8.7 oz	340	9
1080	Taco Bell beefy tostada 1 serving, 6.5 oz	6.5 oz	320	9
1129	McDonalds quarter pounder 1 serving, 5.8 oz	5.8 oz	420	9
1685	Veal parmigiana 1 cup	7.9 oz	340	9
1808	Hamburger,quarter pound 1 hamburger,5.8 oz	5.8 oz	420	9
1013	J in B omelette,ranchero 1 serving, 6.9 oz	6.9 oz	410	9
1813	Hot dog w cheese on bun 1 serving,4 oz	4.0 oz	330	9
1075	Fish,batter fried 2 pieces, 4.8 oz	4.8 oz	370	9
1581	Broccoli cheese casserole 1 cup	8.5 oz	330	9
1037	DQ choc dipped cone,large 1 cone, 8.3 oz	8.3 oz	450	8
1041	Dairy Queen dilly bar 1 serving, 3 oz	3.0 oz	240	8
1614	Fz dinner,chicken,potato+veg 11 oz	11.0 oz	540	8
1661	Quiche,swiss cheese+crab 1/8 of 8 in quiche	3.5 oz	280	8
1676	Tostada,beefy 1 large	6.5 oz	290	8
1795	Chili dog w bun 1.5 oz dog,1/2 c chili	8.3 oz	510	8
1801	Fish burger w cheese,chili sce 2 oz fish,1 oz cheese,bun	5.3 oz	430	8
1367	Chuck arm,lean + fat,braised 1 pc (2.5 × 2.5 × .8 in)	3.0 oz	290	8
1602	Chop suey,home prepared 1 cup	8.8 oz	300	8
787	Chocolate chips,semisweet 1/4 cup	1.5 oz	210	8
1578	Beef potpie,home prepared 1/3 of 9 inch pie	7.4 oz	520	8
684	Condensed milk,sweetened,canned 1/2 cup	5.4 oz	490	8
889	Charlotte russe,whip crm fillng 4 lady fingrs+1/3 c filln	4.0 oz	330	8
1011	J in B omelette,double cheese 1 serving, 5.8 oz	5.9 oz	420	8
1079	Taco Bell beef burrito 1 serving, 6.5 oz	6.5 oz	400	8
1111	Arbys beef and cheddar sandwich 1 serving, 6 oz	6.3 oz	480	8
1807	Hamburger,regular 1 hamburger,3.5 oz	3.5 oz	270	8
1591	Cheese souffle 1 cup	3.4 oz	210	7
1660	Quiche lorraine 1/8 of 8 in quiche	3.5 oz	270	7

1615	Fz dinner,meat loaf,potato+peas 11 oz	11.0 oz	410	8
1363	Chuck,lean + fat,braised 1 piece (4 × 2.3 × .5 in)	3.0 oz	300	8
490	Egg,spanish omelet 2 eggs,4 tbsp sauce	5.4 oz	330	8
668	Egg,spanish omelet,salted 2 eggs,4 tbsp sauce	5.4 oz	330	8
1081	Taco Bell burrito supreme 1 serving, 8.7 oz	8.7 oz	420	8
1648	Omelet,spanish 2 eggs,4 tbsp sauce	5.4 oz	330	8
1102	Pizza H,super,supreme 1/4 of 13 in pizza	7.1 oz	590	8
1495	Lamb,leg,lean + fat,roasted 2 slices (4 × 2 × .3 in)	3.0 oz	240	8
1586	Burrito,supreme 1 very large	7.9 oz	460	8
1681	Turkey pot pie,frz,commercial 1 8 oz pie	8.0 oz	450	8
1824	Sub:bol,ham,salam,che,lett,mayo 2 oz meat+cheese,2 oz bun	5.3 oz	410	8
1643	Macaroni w cheese,homesyyle 1 cup	7.1 oz	430	8
941	Coconut custard pie m/w lard 1/6 of 9 in diam pie	5.4 oz	360	8
1608	Crab imperial 1 cup	7.8 oz	320	8
652	Cream,half + half 1/2 cup	4.3 oz	160	8
1374	T-bone steak,lean + fat,brl 1 piece (3.5 × 2 × .8 in)	3.0 oz	280	8
1590	Cheese rarebit,no toast 1/2 cup	4.1 oz	210	8

1599	Chicken potpie w biscuit top 1 cup	8.4 oz	350	7
269	Bread stuffing,prepared dry 1/2 cup	2.5 oz	250	7
939	Chocolate meringue pie w lard 1/6 of 9 in diam pie	5.4 oz	380	7
996	Dairy Queen freeze 1 serving, 14 oz	14.0 oz	520	7
367	French toast,butter + syrup 2 sl tst,2 tsp,2 tbsp	5.4 oz	430	7
1113	Arbys ham+cheese sandwich 1 serving, 8.25 oz	8.7 oz	480	7
1517	Pork picnic,lean + fat,sim 1 pc (2.5 × 2.5 × .8 in)	3.0 oz	290	7
1542	Bratwurst,cooked 1 3 oz link	3.0 oz	260	7
1800	Fish burger w tartar sauce 3 oz fish on bun	5.0 oz	430	7
1124	J in B moby jack sandwich 1 serving,5 oz	5.0 oz	460	7
1617	Ham croquette 2 (1 in diam × 3 in)	4.6 oz	330	7
1513	Pork chop,loin,lean + fat,brl 1 chop,1/3 lb	2.8 oz	270	7
1569	Beans and franks,canned 1 cup	9.0 oz	370	7
1583	Burrito,beef,medium 8 in tort,1/3 cup filling	5.4 oz	390	7
1788	Burrito,beef,in sauce 3 1/2 oz filling on tort	5.4 oz	390	7
1791	Cheese sandwich,toasted 1 oz cheese,1.5 tsp buttr	2.7 oz	260	7
942	Coconut custard pie m/w veg fat 1/6 of 9 in diam pie	5.4 oz	360	7

Menu Items with Maximum Quantity of Polyunsaturated Fat

No.	Name/Portion Size		KCAL	NUTRI-UNITS PFA
46	Butternuts 8–10 nuts	1.0 oz	170	11
78	Walnuts,english 20 halves (4 tablespoons)	1.0 oz	180	10
73	Sunflower seed,oil rst,salt 3 tablespoons	1.0 oz	170	10
77	Walnuts,black 20 halves (4 tablespoons)	1.0 oz	170	10
1772	Mayonnaise 2 tablespoons	1.0 oz	200	9
1825	Tuna sandwich 2.5 oz tuna,1.5 tbsp mayo	4.9 oz	410	9
74	Sunflower seed,dry rst,salt 3 tablespoons	1.0 oz	160	8
75	Sunflower seed,dry rst,nosalt 3 tablespoons	1.0 oz	160	8
1613	Fish,batterfried,tartar sauce[a] 3.5 oz + 1 tbsp sauce	4.1 oz	260	8
1780	Salad oil,sunflower 1 tablespoon	.5 oz	120	8
1696	Lettuce and spinach,french drsg 1 cup,2 tbsp m/fat drsg	3.5 oz	180	8
1691	Coleslaw w carrots,mayonnaise 1/2 cup,1.5 tbsp hifat dr	2.1 oz	160	7
1774	Russian dressing 2 tablespoons	1.1 oz	150	7
1715	Lobster salad w tomato slices 1/2 cup sal,1 med tomato	8.8 oz	280	7
1713	Chef salad,ham + cheese 1 oz each,2 c let,2 tb dr	6.5 oz	300	7
1764	Blue,roquefort dressing 2 tablespoons	1.1 oz	160	7
69	Pop't wheat,no salt 1 ounce	1.0 oz	150	6
1070	McDonalds chicken mcnuggets[a] 1 serving, 9 pc	5.9 oz	400	5
1578	Beef potpie,home prepared 1/3 of 9 inch pie	7.4 oz	520	5
1802	Fish burger w cheese,tartar sce[a] 2 oz fish, .5 oz ch, bun	4.1 oz	370	5
1357	Tofu,soybean curd 1 pc (2.5 × 2.8 × 1 in)	4.2 oz	170	5
319	Mayonnaise 1 tablespoon	.5 oz	100	5
1895	Mayonnaise 1 tablespoon	.5 oz	100	5
44	Beechnuts 1 oz	1.0 oz	160	5
1826	Turkey salad sandwich 3 oz salad	5.0 oz	340	5
1075	Fish,batter fried[a] 2 pieces, 4.8 oz	4.8 oz	370	5
368	French toast,soft marg. + syrup 2 sl tst,2 tsp,2 tbsp	5.4 oz	430	5
1680	Turkey pot pie,home prepared 1/3 of 9 in pie	8.2 oz	550	5
369	French toast w soft margarine 2 slices w 2 tsp marg	4.0 oz	330	5
954	Pecan pie m/w lard 1/6 of 9 in diam pie	4.8 oz	570	5
1114	Arbys sub (no dressing) 1 serving, 9.5 oz	10.1 oz	480	5
1597	Chicken pot pie 1/3 of 9 in diam pie	8.2 oz	550	5

1770	Italian dressing 2 tablespoons	1.1 oz	140	7	1707	Macaroni salad w salad drsg 1/2 cup,2 tbsp drsg	3.4 oz	200	5
1800	Fish burger w tartar sauce[a] 3 oz fish on bun	5.0 oz	430	7	1708	Potato salad w egg + may,fr dr 1/2 cup	4.4 oz	180	5
65	Pinenuts,pinon 4 tablespoons	1.0 oz	160	7	61	Peanuts,roasted + salted 3 tablespoons	1.0 oz	170	5
1124	J in b moby jack sandwich 1 serving,5 oz	5.0 oz	460	7	62	Peanuts,roasted,no salt 3 tablespoons	1.0 oz	170	5
329	Tahini,sesame butter 2 tablespoons	1.1 oz	180	6	1628	Chicken w veg. w vermicelli 12.7 oz	12.7 oz	260	5
1798	Egg salad sandwich w lettuce 1 average	4.9 oz	380	6	1632	Fish jardiniere filet 11.2 oz	11.3 oz	280	5
1777	Vinegar and oil dressing 2 tablespoons	1.1 oz	130	6	1066	Kentucky Fried,thigh,orig 1 serving, 3.4 oz	3.4 oz	270	4
45	Brazilnuts 8 medium nuts	1.0 oz	180	6	1108	Arbys chicken breast sandwich 1 serving, 7.25 oz	7.2 oz	550	4
1127	McDonalds filet of fish[a] 1 serving, 4.6 oz	4.6 oz	400	6	58	Nuts'n stuff, no salt 1 ounce	1.0 oz	150	4
1720	Tuna apple salad 1 cup	4.2 oz	230	6	1709	Tossed salad,vinegar + oil drsg 1 cup let,cuc,rad + onion	3.5 oz	100	4
1766	French dressing 2 tablespoons	1.1 oz	140	6	1768	French dressing,low sodium 2 tablespoons	1.1 oz	60	4
1353	Soyameat 1 slice	2.3 oz	160	6	1775	Salad dressing,mayo type 2 tablespoons	1.1 oz	120	4
1769	Green goddess 2 tablespoons	1.1 oz	150	6	63	Pecans dried 24 halves (4 tablespoons)	1.0 oz	190	4
955	Pecan pie m/w veg fat 1/6 of 9 in diam pie	4.8 oz	570	6	1014	Jack in Box pancakes 1 serving, 8.2 oz	8.2 oz	630	4
53	Hickorynuts 30 small nuts	1.0 oz	180	6	71	Soy nuts no salt 1/3 cup	1.3 oz	160	4
68	Pop't wheat,seasoned 1 ounce	1.0 oz	150	6	72	Soy nuts with salt 1/3 cup	1.3 oz	160	4

[a]Fried in corn, cottonseed, or soy oil.

continued

Menu Items with Maximum Quantity of Polyunsaturated Fat *(continued)*

No.	Name/Portion Size		KCAL	NUTRI-UNITS PFA
1942	Cream of mushroom soup,w milk 1 cup	8.6 oz	200	4
60	Peanuts,dry roasted,w salt 3 tablespoons	1.0 oz	160	4
64	Pecans dry roasted 24 halves (4 tablespoons)	1.0 oz	190	4
312	Margarine,safflwr,soft,p/s=4.0 2 teaspoons	.4 oz	70	4
622	Margarine,saffl,soft,p/s=4.0 1 large pat,2 teaspoons	.4 oz	70	4
1015	McDonalds biscuit w spread 1 serving, 3 oz	3.0 oz	330	4
1016	McDonalds biscuit+bacon,egg,chee 1 serving, 5.1 oz	5.1 oz	480	4
1017	McDonalds biscuit+sausage 1 serving, 4.3 oz	4.3 oz	470	4
1018	McDonalds biscuit+sausage,egg 1 serving, 6.2 oz	6.2 oz	590	4
1596	Chicken fricasee 1 cup	8.5 oz	390	4
1630	Fish florentine 9 oz	9.0 oz	240	4
1631	Fish divan filet 12.4 oz	12.4 oz	270	4
1719	Tossed salad w turkey,sal drsg 1 cup	4.2 oz	130	4
1816	Peanut butter + jelly sandwich 2 tbsp p/b,1 tbsp jelly	3.1 oz	340	4
1891	Margarine,safflowr soft,p/s=4.0 2 teaspoons	.4 oz	70	4
256	Potato chips,unsalted 10 chips (2.5 × 1.8 in)	.7 oz	110	4
419	Granola, homemade 1 oz (1/4 cup)	1.0 oz	140	4
1069	McDonalds chicken mcnuggets 1 serving, 6 pc	3.9 oz	270	4
1138	Wendy's triple burger w cheese 1 serving, 14 oz	14.1 oz	1040	4
711	Carrot cake w cream cheese icng 2.75 in sq × 1.5 in piece	2.3 oz	230	4
928	Blackberry pie m/w veg fat 1/6 of 9 in diam pie	5.5 oz	380	4
56	Mixed nuts,oil roasted,w salt 1 oz (3 tablespoons)	1.0 oz	170	3
57	Mixed nuts,oil roasted,no salt 1 oz (3 tablespoons)	1.0 oz	170	3
492	Egg substitute 1/4 cup	2.1 oz	100	3
669	Egg substitute 1/4 cup (4 tbsp)	2.1 oz	100	3
922	Apple pie m/w veg fat 1/6 of 9 in diam pie	5.5 oz	400	3
930	Blueberry pie m/w veg fat 1/6 of 9 in diam pie	5.5 oz	380	3
934	Cherry pie m/w veg fat 1/6 of 9 in diam pie	5.5 oz	410	3
951	Mince pie m/w veg fat 1/6 of 9 in diam pie	5.5 oz	430	3
953	Peach pie m/w veg fat 1/6 of 9 in diam pie	5.5 oz	400	3

244	Hushpuppies[a] 1 1/2 oz	1.6 oz	150	4
327	P-nut butr,mod amt fat,sug,salt 2 tablespoons	1.1 oz	180	4
1058	Hush puppies 1 serving, 3 pieces	1.6 oz	150	4
1354	Soybeans,cooked,no salt 1/2 cup	3.0 oz	150	4
1401	Batter dipped breast,chicken[a] 1/2 breast	4.9 oz	360	4
1901	P-nut butr,mod amt fat,sug,salt 2 tablespoons	1.1 oz	180	4
326	P-nut butr,smal amt fat,sug,slt 2 tablespoons	1.1 oz	180	4
328	P-nut butter,no salt 2 tablespoons	1.1 oz	180	4
1684	Tuna and noodles 1 cup	8.3 oz	320	4
1688	Coleslaw,w mayo 1/2 cup,1 tbsp hifat drsg	2.1 oz	90	4
1900	P-nut butr,smal amt fat,sug,slt 2 tablespoons	1.1 oz	170	4
1902	P-nut butter,no salt 2 tablespoons	1.1 oz	180	4
1414	Broiler,one half,broiled 1 half broiler	6.2 oz	390	4
1804	Ham and cheese sandwich w mayo 1.3 oz ham,.6 oz cheese	3.8 oz	320	4
1943	Cream of mushroom soup,w water 1 cup	8.5 oz	130	4
11	Potato chips 10 chips (2 1/2 × 1 3/4)	.7 oz	110	4
255	Potato chips 10 chips (2.5 × 1.8 in)	.7 oz	110	4
957	Pineapple pie m/w veg fat 1/6 of 9 in diam pie	5.5 oz	400	3
965	Raisin pie m/w veg fat 1/6 of 9 in diam pie	5.5 oz	420	3
967	Rhubarb pie m/w veg fat 1/6 of 9 in diam pie	5.5 oz	400	3
1009	Jack in Box breakfast jack 1 serving, 4.3 oz	4.3 oz	380	3
1113	Arbys ham+cheese sandwich 1 serving, 8.25 oz	8.7 oz	480	3
2077	Potato chips 10 chips (2.5 × 1.7 in)	.7 oz	110	3
294	Spanish rice,hi fat 1/2 cup	3.5 oz	230	3
378	Pancakes w hard marg. + syrup 3 4-in cks,1 tbsp,2 tbsp	6.2 oz	370	3
1057	Wendys french fries,salted 1 serving, 4.2 oz	4.2 oz	330	3
1355	Tahini,sesame butter 1 tablespoon	.5 oz	90	3
1356	Tempeh,fermented soybeans 1/2 cup	2.9 oz	170	3
1423	Stewed chicken,w skin 1/2–2/3 cup,chopped	3.0 oz	240	3
1588	Cheese fondue 1 cup	6.2 oz	460	3
1711	Bean salad,three bean 1/2 cup	2.5 oz	100	3
1889	Margarine,liquid oil,p/s=2.5 2 teaspoons	.4 oz	70	3
1343	Hummus 1/3 cup	2.9 oz	270	3
1620	Hummus 1/3 cup	2.9 oz	270	3

[a]Fried in corn, cottonseed, or soy oil

Menu Items with Maximum Quantity of Cholesterol

No.	Name/Portion Size		KCAL	NUTRI-UNITS CHL
1393	Brains,simmered 3 oz	3.0 oz	140	116
1010	Jack in Box scrambled eggs 1 serving, 9.4 oz	9.4 oz	390	57
1649	Omelet w ham 2 eggs, 1/3 oz ham	4.8 oz	330	32
1641	Lobster newburg 1 cup	8.8 oz	490	30
1429	Fried liver, chicken 1/2 cup	2.5 oz	110	29
1396	Liver,beef,fried 1 sl (6 × 2 × .5 in)	3.0 oz	180	27
1398	Sweetbread,beef,fried 3 oz	3.0 oz	270	26
1399	Sweetbread,calf,braised 3 oz	3.0 oz	140	26
1588	Cheese fondue 1 cup	6.2 oz	460	26
1428	Fried giblets 3 oz	3.0 oz	240	25
1648	Omelet,spanish 2 eggs,4 tbsp sauce	5.4 oz	330	25
1397	Liver,calf,fried 1 sl (6 × 2 × .5 in)	3.0 oz	220	25
1011	J in b omelette,double cheese 1 serving, 5.8 oz	5.9 oz	420	25
1012	J in b omelette,ham and cheese 1 serving, 6 oz	6.1 oz	430	24
1013	J in b omelette,ranchero 1 serving, 6.9 oz	6.9 oz	410	23
367	French toast,butter + syrup 2 sl tst,2 tsp,2 tbsp	5.4 oz	430	15
1019	McDonalds egg mcmuffin 1 serving, 4.7 oz	4.7 oz	310	15
1712	Chef salad,bolog,chees,egg,drsg 1 oz each,3 c let,4 tb dr	8.6 oz	580	15
1137	Wendy's triple burger 1 serving, 12 oz	12.7 oz	840	14
485	Egg,fried,low fat 1 large	1.6 oz	80	14
486	Egg,hard cooked 1 large	1.8 oz	80	14
487	Egg,omelet 1 large egg	2.3 oz	100	14
489	Egg,poached 1 large	1.8 oz	80	14
491	Egg,scrambled 1 large	2.3 oz	100	14
672	Egg yolk,no salt 1 large	.6 oz	60	14
366	French toast,plain 2 slices bread + egg mix	3.7 oz	260	13
368	French toast,soft marg. + syrup 2 sl tst,2 tsp,2 tbsp	5.4 oz	430	13
369	French toast w soft margarine 2 slices w 2 tsp marg	4.0 oz	330	13
946	Lemon chiffon m/w lard 1/6 of 9 in diam pie	3.8 oz	340	13
892	Cream puff w custard filling 3 1/2 in dia × 2 in puff	4.6 oz	300	13

1608	Crab imperial 1 cup	7.8 oz	320	21
1524	Pork liver,fried 1 sl (6.5 × 2.5 × .4 in)	3.0 oz	140	20
1022	McDonalds sausage mcmuffin+egg 1 serving, 5.8 oz	5.8 oz	520	19
1018	McDonalds biscuit+sausage,egg 1 serving, 6.2 oz	6.2 oz	590	19
1068	Kentucky Fr Chick,orig dinner 2 pc,pot,gravy,slaw,roll	15.0 oz	830	19
1023	McD scrambled eggs 1 serving, 2.7 oz	2.7 oz	140	18
1395	Kidneys,simmered 1/2 cup	2.5 oz	100	18
1724	Deviled egg 1 egg	2.3 oz	140	15
1016	McDonalds biscuit+bacon,egg,chee 1 serving, 5.1 oz	5.1 oz	480	18
1062	KFC extra crispy dinner 2 pc,pot,gravy,slaw,roll	15.4 oz	950	18
1071	McDonalds chicken mcnuggets 1 serving, 20 pc	13.1 oz	900	17
1607	Crab,deviled 1 cup	8.5 oz	450	16
488	Egg,omelet,with ham 1 large egg,1/2 tbsp ham	2.4 oz	160	16
665	Egg,omelet,with ham,salted 1 large egg,1/2 tbsp ham	2.4 oz	160	16
1798	Egg salad sandwich w lettuce 1 average	4.9 oz	380	15
889	Charlotte russe,whip crm fillng 4 lady fingrs+1/3 c filln	4.0 oz	330	15
1138	Wendy's triple burger w cheese 1 serving, 14 oz	14.1 oz	1040	15
1107	McDonalds shrimp salad 1 serving,9.3 oz	9.3 oz	100	13
1576	Beef liver,onion gravy 1 pc (6.5 × 2.5 × 1/4 in)	3.5 oz	140	12
947	Lemon chiffon pie m/w veg fat 1/6 of 9 in diam pie	3.8 oz	340	12
1061	Kentucky Fried,orig,3 pieces 3 pieces, 7.5 oz	7.6 oz	360	12
1009	Jack in Box breakfast jack 1 serving, 4.3 oz	4.3 oz	380	12
1572	Beef meatloaf 2 slices (4 × 3 × 1/2 in)	6.4 oz	320	12
1591	Cheese souffle 1 cup	3.4 oz	210	12
958	Pineapple chiffon pie m/w lard 1/6 of 9 in diam pie	3.8 oz	310	11
941	Coconut custard pie m/w lard 1/6 of 9 in diam pie	5.4 oz	360	11
944	Custard pie m/w lard 1/6 of 9 in diam pie	5.4 oz	330	11
959	Pineapple chiffon m/w veg fat 1/6 of 9 in diam pie	3.8 oz	310	11
1394	Heart,cooked 3 oz	3.0 oz	150	11
747	Sponge cake 1/12 of 10-in tube cake	2.3 oz	200	11
945	Custard pie m/w veg fat 1/6 of 9 in diam pie	5.4 oz	330	11
942	Coconut custard pie m/w veg fat 1/6 of 9 in diam pie	5.4 oz	360	10
1136	Wendy's double burger w cheese 1 serving, 11.5 oz	11.5 oz	800	10
1606	Clam fritters,no salt 3 (2 in diam × 1 3/4 in)	4.2 oz	370	10

continued

Menu Items with Maximum Quantity of Cholesterol *(continued)*

No.	Name/Portion Size		KCAL	NUTRI-UNITS CHL
1614	Fz dinner,chicken,potato+veg 11 oz	11.0 oz	540	10
937	Chocolate chiffon pie w lard 1/6 of 9 in diam pie	3.8 oz	350	10
1468	Shrimp,canned,drained,salted 3.5 oz serving	3.5 oz	120	10
1469	Shrimp,french fried 3.5 oz serving	3.5 oz	230	10
1414	Broiler,one half,broiled 1 half broiler	6.2 oz	390	10
179	Egg nog, non-alcoholic 1 8-oz glass	8.7 oz	340	10
245	Spoon bread 1/2 cup	4.2 oz	230	10
1066	Kentucky Fried,thigh,orig 1 serving, 3.4 oz	3.4 oz	270	10
1661	Quiche,swiss cheese+crab 1/8 of 8 in quiche	3.5 oz	280	10
938	Chocolate chiffon pie w veg fat 1/6 of 9 in diam pie	3.8 oz	350	10
893	Custard,baked 1/2 cup	4.7 oz	150	9
948	Lemon meringue pie m/w lard 1/6 of 9 in diam pie	4.9 oz	360	9
857	Eclair,custard fill,choc icing 5 × 2 × 1¾ in eclair	3.5 oz	240	9
894	Eclair w custd fillng,choc icng 5 × 2 × 1¾ in eclair	3.5 oz	240	9
1119	Burger King,whopper 1 serving, 10 oz	10.0 oz	610	8
1070	McDonalds chicken mcnuggets 1 serving, 9 pc	5.9 oz	400	8
1472	Swordfish,broiled 1 piece (4.5 × 2 × 1 in)	4.9 oz	240	8
1359	Canned roast beef w juice 1/2 cup	4.3 oz	240	7
1105	McDonalds garden salad 1 serving,7.2 oz	7.2 oz	90	7
1646	Meatballs,mushrm gravy,no salt 3 oz meatballs,2 tbsp grv	4.1 oz	440	7
1658	Quiche,cheese 1/8 of 8 in quiche	3.5 oz	190	7
1450	Mackerel,broiled w butter 1 fillet,8.5 × 2.5 ×.5 in	3.7 oz	250	7
902	Lemon refrigerator dessert 1/2 cup	3.9 oz	230	7
1622	Lasagna w beef 1 cup	8.5 oz	420	7
1521	Pork spareribs,braised 3 oz serving	3.0 oz	340	7
890	Cheesecake,plain 1/8 of 8 in diam cake	3.0 oz	250	7
891	Cheesecake w cherry topping, fz 1/8 of 8 in diam cake	3.0 oz	220	7
943	Coconut custard pie,frozen 1/6 of 8 in diam pie	3.5 oz	250	7

1647	Meatloaf,lean 2 sl (4 × 3 × 3/8 in)	4.9 oz	250	9
1752	Egg,hard cooked 1/2 large egg	.9 oz	40	7
1660	Quiche lorraine 1/8 of 8 in quiche	3.5 oz	270	9
949	Lemon meringue pie m/w veg fat 1/6 of 9 in diam pie	4.9 oz	360	9
1449	Lobster,cooked 1 cup	5.3 oz	140	9
1659	Quiche,chicken 1/8 of 8 in quiche	3.5 oz	220	9
1372	Porterhouse steak,lean+fat,brl Yield from 1/2 lb w bone	5.3 oz	450	8
888	Bread pudding w raisins 3/4 cup	6.3 oz	340	8
1583	Burrito,beef,medium 8 in tort,1/3 cup filling	5.4 oz	390	8
1788	Burrito,beef,in sauce 3 1/2 oz filling on tort	5.4 oz	390	8
743	Pound cake,cherry sc,whip toppn 3.5 × 3 × 1 in pc + sauce	3.2 oz	260	8
1401	Batter dipped breast 1/2 breast	4.9 oz	360	8
1679	Turkey and noodles 1 cup	8.3 oz	300	8
1594	Chicken and noodles 1 cup	8.3 oz	360	8
1684	Tuna and noodles 1 cup	8.3 oz	320	8
1715	Lobster salad w tomato slices 1/2 cup sal,1 med tomato	8.8 oz	280	8
1470	Shrimp,frozen,breaded,raw 3.5 oz serving	3.5 oz	140	7
1135	Wendy's double burger 1 serving, 10 oz	10.1 oz	670	7
1602	Chop suey,home prepared 1 cup	8.8 oz	300	7
1616	Fz dinner,turkey,potato+peas 11 oz	11.0 oz	350	7
1630	Fish florentine 9 oz	9.0 oz	240	7
1632	Fish jardiniere filet 11.2 oz	11.3 oz	280	7
1809	Hamburger,super 1 hamburger,8.9 oz	8.9 oz	560	7
962	Pumpkin pie m/w lard 1/6 of 9 in diam pie	5.4 oz	320	7
1123	J in b jumbo burger w cheese 1 serving,8.7 oz	8.7 oz	570	7
925	Banana custard pie m/w lard 1/6 of 9 in diam pie	5.4 oz	340	7
1065	Kentucky Fried,rib,orig 1 serving, 2.9 oz	2.9 oz	240	7
1404	Batter dipped,deep fried,rib 1 rib	2.9 oz	240	7
1491	Lamb chops,loin,lean + fat 1 chop,cut 3/lb	3.5 oz	360	7
1518	Pork picnic,lean only,sim 1 pc (2.5 × 2.5 × .8 in)	3.0 oz	210	7
1589	Cheese manicotti w sauce 1 cup	8.5 oz	280	7
1609	Dried beef,creamed 1 cup	8.6 oz	380	7

Menu Items with Maximum Quantity of Sodium

No.	Name/Portion Size		KCAL	NUTRI-UNITS SOD
1446	Haddock,smoked 1 pc (2.5 × 2.5 × .3 in)	3.5 oz	100	62
1463	Sardines,canned,drained 8 fish (3 × 1 × .5 in)	3.5 oz	180	62
1462	Salmon,smoked 3 oz jar or can	3.0 oz	150	53
1441	Eel,smoked 2 oz	2.0 oz	190	35
1448	Herring,pickled,smoked/kippered 1 herring	1.6 oz	100	28
1068	Kentucky Fr Chick,orig dinner 2 pc,pot,gravy,slaw,roll	15.0 oz	830	23
1607	Crab,deviled 1 cup	8.5 oz	450	21
1062	KFC extra crispy dinner 2 pc,pot,gravy,slaw,roll	15.4 oz	950	19
1138	Wendy's triple burger w cheese 1 serving, 14 oz	14.1 oz	1040	19
1908	Beef noodle soup,dehydr,preprd 1 cup	8.5 oz	160	18
1930	Clam chowder,manhatt,w water 1 cup	8.6 oz	80	18
1820	Reuben:kraut,beef,cheese on rye 1.75 oz corned beef	6.2 oz	310	18
1071	McDonalds chicken mcnuggets 1 serving, 20 pc	13.1 oz	900	18
1609	Dried beef,creamed 1 cup	8.6 oz	380	18
1111	Arbys beef and cheddar sandwich 1 serving, 6 oz	6.3 oz	480	17
1113	Arbys ham+cheese sandwich 1 serving, 8.25 oz	8.7 oz	480	17

No.	Name/Portion Size		KCAL	NUTRI-UNITS SOD
1569	Beans and franks,canned 1 cup	9.0 oz	370	14
1822	Submarine:bologna,salami,cheese 3 oz meat+chees,2 oz bun	5.0 oz	440	14
1114	Arbys sub (no dressing) 1 serving, 9.5 oz	10.1 oz	480	14
1600	Chili con carne w beans 1 cup	9.0 oz	340	14
1601	Chili con carne w/o beans 1 cup	8.8 oz	500	13
1345	Lentil soup w ham 1 cup	8.7 oz	140	13
1940	Lentil soup w ham 1 cup	8.7 oz	140	13
1018	McDonalds biscuit+sausage,egg 1 serving, 6.2 oz	6.2 oz	590	13
1016	McDonalds biscuit+bacon,egg,chee 1 serving, 5.1 oz	5.1 oz	480	13
1507	Ham,cured,roasted 1 slice (4 × 2.3 × .5 in)	3.0 oz	150	13
1636	Oriental beef w veg,rice 8.6 oz	8.6 oz	260	13
1083	Taco Bell enchirito 1 serving, 7.5 oz	7.5 oz	380	13
1108	Arbys chicken breast sandwich 1 serving, 7.25 oz	7.2 oz	550	13
1616	Fz dinner,turkey,potato+peas 11 oz	11.0 oz	350	13
1628	Chicken w veg. w vermicelli 12.7 oz	12.7 oz	260	13
1668	Shrimp creole on rice ½ cup on ½ cup rice	8.8 oz	270	13

1014	Jack in Box pancakes		630	17
	1 serving, 8.2 oz	8.2 oz		
1608	Crab imperial		320	16
	1 cup	7.8 oz		
1814	Hot dog,large,on bun		520	16
	1 serving,6.4 oz	6.4 oz		
1795	Chili dog w bun		510	15
	1.5 oz dog,1/2 c chili	8.3 oz		
1123	J in b jumbo burger w cheese		570	15
	1 serving,8.7 oz	8.7 oz		
1094	Pizza H,thin,super,supreme		520	15
	1/4 of 13 in pizza	6.3 oz		
1593	Chicken and dumplets		220	15
	1 cup	8.8 oz		
1594	Chicken and noodles		360	15
	1 cup	8.3 oz		
1639	Spagetti w beef,mushrooms		280	15
	11.5 oz	11.4 oz		
1657	Pork,sweet+sour		260	15
	3/4 cup	7.5 oz		
1685	Veal parmigiana		340	15
	1 cup	7.9 oz		
1579	Beef stroganoff w rice		370	14
	2/3 cup on 1/2 cup rice	9.9 oz		
1112	Arbys super roast beef sandwich		620	14
	1 serving, 9.5 oz	10.3 oz		
1136	Wendy's double burger w cheese		800	14
	1 serving, 11.5 oz	11.5 oz		
1092	Pizza H,thin,super,pork w mushr		450	14
	1/4 of 13 in pizza	5.3 oz		
1102	Pizza H,super,supreme		590	14
	1/4 of 13 in pizza	7.1 oz		
1603	Chop suey,canned		160	14
	1 cup	8.8 oz		
1587	Canneloni		430	12
	1 cup	8.8 oz		
1619	Hot turkey sandwich,pot+gravy		370	12
	1 serving	12.0 oz		
1615	Fz dinner,meat loaf,potato+peas		410	12
	11 oz	11.0 oz		
1137	Wendy's triple burger		840	12
	1 serving, 12 oz	12.7 oz		
1645	Manicotti		340	12
	1 cup	8.7 oz		
1920	Chicken noodle soup,dehyd,prep		50	12
	1 cup	8.5 oz		
1130	McD quarter pounder w cheese		520	12
	1 serving, 6.8 oz	6.8 oz		
1793	Cheeseburger,quarter pounder		520	12
	1 burger	6.8 oz		
1090	Pizza H,thin,suprstyle,pepproni		430	12
	1/4 of 13 in pizza	5.3 oz		
1091	Pizza H,thin,pork w mushroom		380	12
	1/4 of 13 in pizza	4.6 oz		
1093	Pizza H,thin,supreme		400	12
	1/4 of 13 in pizza	5.3 oz		
1098	Pizza H,thick,suprstyl,pepproni		490	12
	1/4 of 13 in pizza	6.0 oz		
1100	Pizza H,thick,super,pork w mush		500	12
	1/4 of 13 in pizza	6.0 oz		
1339	Black bean soup,cnd,dil,salted		120	12
	1 cup	8.7 oz		
1637	Oriental scallops,veg,rice		220	12
	11 oz	11.0 oz		
1712	Chef salad,bolog,chees,egg,drsg		580	12
	1 oz each,3 c let,4 tb dr	8.6 oz		
1910	Black bean soup,cnd,w water		120	12
	1 cup	8.7 oz		

continued

Menu Items with Maximum Quantity of Sodium *(continued)*

No.	Name/Portion Size		KCAL	NUTRI-UNITS SOD
1570	Beans w pork in tomato sauce 1 cup	9.0 oz	310	12
2035	Gazpacho 1 cup	8.6 oz	60	12
1633	Lasagna, zucchini 11 oz	10.9 oz	270	12
1797	Corned beef and cheese on rye 1 oz each	4.1 oz	300	12
1017	McDonalds biscuit+sausage 1 serving, 4.3 oz	4.3 oz	470	12
1140	Clam chowder(potato base) 1 serving, 8 oz	8.8 oz	220	12
1635	Meatball stew 10 oz	10.0 oz	250	12
1803	French dip sandwich 2 oz bf,2 oz bun,4 oz jus	7.9 oz	340	12
1933	French onion soup 1 cup	8.6 oz	40	11
1623	Chicken chow mein w rice 11.3 oz	11.1 oz	250	11
1599	Chicken potpie w biscuit top 1 cup	8.4 oz	350	11
1013	J in b omelette,ranchero 1 serving, 6.9 oz	6.9 oz	410	11
1088	Pizza H,thin,superstyle,cheese 1/4 of 13 in pizza	5.3 oz	410	11
1818	Pita:ham,bologna,pastrami,chees 2 oz meat+ch,2.5 oz pita	4.5 oz	360	11
1919	Chicken noodle soup,w water 1 cup	8.5 oz	70	11
1937	Green pea soup,dehydr,preprd 1 cup	8.6 oz	120	11
1663	Ravioli,cheese 1 cup	8.6 oz	580	10
1824	Sub:bol,ham,salam,che,lett,mayo 2 oz meat+cheese,2 oz bun	5.3 oz	410	10
1025	McD hot cakes,butter and syrup 1 serving, 7.3 oz	7.3 oz	480	10
1904	Cream of asparagus soup,w milk 1 cup	8.6 oz	160	10
1915	Cream of chicken soup,w milk 1 cup	8.6 oz	190	10
1935	Green pea soup w milk 1 cup	8.8 oz	240	10
1506	Ham,cured,extra lean,roasted 1 slice (4 × 2.3 × .5 in)	3.0 oz	120	10
1928	Chunky sirloin burger soup 1 scant cup	7.9 oz	170	10
1943	Cream of mushroom soup,w water 1 cup	8.5 oz	130	10
1947	Oyster stew,frozen,w milk 1 cup	8.5 oz	130	10
1953	Cream of shrimp soup,w milk 1 cup	8.6 oz	160	10
1575	Beef and vegetable stew,canned 1 cup	8.6 oz	190	10
1669	Spaghetti,meatballs+tomato sauc 1 cup	8.7 oz	330	10
1089	Pizza H,thin,pepperoni 1/4 of 13 in pizza	4.6 oz	370	10
1096	Pizza H,thick,superstyle,cheese 1/4 of 13 in pizza	6.0 oz	450	10
1099	Pizza H,thick,pork w mushroom 1/4 of 13 in pizza	5.3 oz	430	10

1643	Macaroni w cheese,homesyyle 1 cup	7.1 oz	430	11
1959	Tom veg soup/noodl,dehy,prep 1 cup	8.5 oz	50	11
1134	Wendy's single burger w cheese 1 serving, 8.5 oz	8.5 oz	580	11
1679	Turkey and noodles 1 cup	8.3 oz	300	11
1139	Wendy's chili w beans 1 serving, 8 oz	8.8 oz	230	11
1614	Fz dinner,chicken,potato+veg 11 oz	11.0 oz	540	11
1684	Tuna and noodles 1 cup	8.3 oz	320	11
1828	Turkey sandwich w gravy 1.6 oz turkey,1/2 c gravy	8.5 oz	280	11
1942	Cream of mushroom soup,w milk 1 cup	8.6 oz	200	11
1520	Pork picnic,cured,lean only,rst .6 cup chopped	3.0 oz	140	11
1602	Chop suey,home prepared 1 cup	8.8 oz	300	11
1611	Enchiladas,beef and cheese 2 small	8.9 oz	380	11
1945	Onion soup,w water 1 cup	8.5 oz	60	11
1951	Cream of potato soup,frz,w milk 1 cup	8.6 oz	150	11
1009	Jack in Box breakfast jack 1 serving, 4.3 oz	4.3 oz	380	10
1022	McDonalds sausage mcmuffin+egg 1 serving, 5.8 oz	5.8 oz	520	10
1629	Chicken cacciatore 10.9 oz	10.9 oz	280	10
1101	Pizza H,thick,supreme 1/4 of 13 in pizza	6.0 oz	480	10
1735	Pickles,cucumber,dill or sour 1 med (4 × 1 in diam)	2.5 oz	10	10
1812	Hot dog on bun w catsup+mustard 1.6 oz dog,1.5 oz bun	4.0 oz	260	10
1911	Cream of celery soup,w milk 1 cup	8.6 oz	160	10
1929	Chunky vegetable soup 1 scant cup	7.9 oz	160	10
1952	Cream of potato soup,fz,w water 1 cup	8.6 oz	70	10
1790	Cheese sandwich,grilled 2 oz cheese	4.2 oz	410	10
1135	Wendy's double burger 1 serving, 10 oz	10.1 oz	670	10
1787	Bologna and cheese+but,mayo,let 1 oz bologna,1 oz cheese	5.0 oz	380	10
1931	Clam chowder,n-eng,fz,w milk 1 cup	8.6 oz	160	10
1938	Green pea soup/ham,fz, water 1 cup	8.6 oz	180	10
1948	Oyster stew,frozen,w water 1 cup	8.5 oz	60	10
1954	Cream of shrimp soup,w water 1 cup	8.6 oz	90	10
1955	Split pea soup,w water 1 cup	8.6 oz	180	10
1012	J in b omelette,ham and cheese 1 serving, 6 oz	6.1 oz	430	10
1077	Jack in Box taco,super 1 serving, 5 oz	5.1 oz	290	10

Menu Items with Maximum Quantity of Vitamin A

No.	Name/Portion Size		KCAL	NUTRI-UNITS A
1396	Liver,beef,fried 1 sl (6 × 2 × .5 in)	3.0 oz	180	123
1397	Liver,calf,fried 1 sl (6 × 2 × .5 in)	3.0 oz	220	111
1576	Beef liver,onion gravy 1 pc (6.5 × 2.5 × 1/4 in)	3.5 oz	140	87
2009	Carrots,raw 1 in dia × 7.5 in carrot	2.5 oz	30	81
2010	Carrots,boiled,drained 1/2 cup crosswise slices	2.8 oz	40	77
1524	Pork liver,fried 1 sl (6.5 × 2.5 × .4 in)	3.0 oz	140	61
173	Carrot juice 1/2 cup	4.3 oz	30	54
2096	Sweet potatoes,baked in skin 1/2 of 5 in × 2.5 in pot	2.0 oz	60	50
2011	Carrots,cooked,drained 1/2 cup sliced	2.8 oz	20	47
2031	Dandelion greens,boiled,drained 1/2 cup	3.5 oz	30	47
1429	Fried liver 1/2 cup	2.5 oz	110	46
2012	Carrots,canned,lo sod,drained 1/2 cup	2.8 oz	20	43
2114	Vegetables,mixed,boiled,drained 1/2 cup	3.2 oz	40	42
2080	Pumpkin,canned 1/2 cup	4.3 oz	130	41
1428	Fried giblets 3 oz	3.0 oz	240	41
2099	Sweet potatoes,cnd,dietary pack 1/2 cup solids+liquids	4.2 oz	110	38
460	Total 1 oz (7/8 cup)	1.0 oz	100	20
1181	Cantaloupe,raw 1/4 cup	4.8 oz	50	18
2039	Kale,frzn,boiled,drained 1/2 cup	2.3 oz	20	17
1682	Turkey pot pie,biscuit topping 1 cup	8.3 oz	400	16
1529	Braunschweiger 1 sl (3 1/8 dia × 1/8 in)	1.0 oz	100	16
1845	Braunschweiger 1 sl (3.1 in diam × 1/4)	1.0 oz	100	16
1581	Broccoli cheese casserole 1 cup	8.5 oz	330	15
962	Pumpkin pie m/w lard 1/6 of 9 in diam pie	5.4 oz	320	15
963	Pumpkin pie m/w veg fat 1/6 of 9 in diam pie	5.4 oz	320	15
1687	Carrot and raisin salad,drsg 1/2 cup,1 tbsp m/fat drsg	2.1 oz	110	15
1992	Beet greens,boiled,drained 1/2 cup	2.6 oz	20	15
970	Sweetpotato pie m/w lard 1/6 of 9 in diam pie	5.4 oz	320	15
971	Sweetpotato pie m/w veg fat 1/6 of 9 in diam pie	5.4 oz	320	15
1928	Chunky sirloin burger soup 1 scant cup	7.9 oz	170	15
2097	Sweet potatoes,cooked,candied 2 1/2 × 2 in diam piece	3.0 oz	120	14
1586	Burrito,supreme 1 very large	7.9 oz	460	14

2090	Spinach,canned,drained 1/2 cup	3.6 oz	20	36
2098	Sweet potatoes,canned,in syrup 1/2 cup solids+liquids	4.2 oz	130	34
2091	Spinach,canned,lo sod,drained 1/2 cup	3.6 oz	30	33
88	Carrot sticks 6 strips (3×3/8 in)	1.0 oz	10	32
1545	Liverwurst 1 sl (3 1/8 in dia × 1/4)	1.0 oz	90	31
2013	Carrots,glazed 1/2 cup	3.5 oz	130	31
2089	Spinach,fresh/fz,boiled,drained 1/2 cup leaves	3.2 oz	20	30
2094	Squash,winter,butternut,baked 1/2 cup mashed	3.6 oz	40	29
1163	Apricots,dehyd,sulf,ckd w sugar 1/2 cup	5.3 oz	190	26
1162	Apricots,dehyd,sulfured,unckd 1/2 cup	1.8 oz	160	25
2058	Peas+carrots,fz,boiled,drained 1/2 cup	2.8 oz	40	25
2061	Peppers,hot,red,raw,pod-no seed 1 oz,2 tbsp	1.0 oz	20	24
1929	Chunky vegetable soup 1 scant cup	7.9 oz	160	23
2118	Yams,candied 3 3/4 in × 2 in dia piece	4.3 oz	220	21
2029	Cress,cooked,drained 1/2 cup	2.4 oz	20	21
433	Most 1 oz (1/2 cup)	1.0 oz	90	20
442	Product 19 1 oz (1 cup)	1.0 oz	110	20
1645	Manicotti 1 cup	8.7 oz	340	14
1676	Tostada,beefy 1 large	6.5 oz	290	14
2045	Mustard greens,fz,boiled,drnd 1/2 cup	2.6 oz	10	13
2036	Italian style vegetabls w buttr 1/2 cup	2.4 oz	70	13
1732	Peppers,hot,red,raw 1 tbsp	.5 oz	10	13
1241	Mangos,raw 1/2 cup, diced or sliced	2.9 oz	50	13
429	King vitamin 1 oz (3/4 cup)	1.0 oz	110	13
1132	Taco Bell bellbeefer w cheese 1 serving, 4.8 oz	4.8 oz	280	13
1675	Tostada 1 small	4.9 oz	180	13
1597	Chicken pot pie 1/3 of 9 in diam pie	8.2 oz	550	12
1680	Turkey pot pie,home prepared 1/3 of 9 in pie	8.2 oz	550	12
1746	Carrot sticks 6 pc (3 × 3/8 in)	1.0 oz	10	12
1967	Vegetarian vegtble soup,w water 1 cup	8.6 oz	70	12
1131	Taco Bell bellbeefer 1 serving, 4.3 oz	4.3 oz	220	12
1160	Apricots,dried,ckd w/o sugar 1/2 cup fruit + liquid	4.4 oz	110	12
1159	Apricots,dried,ckd w sugar 1/2 cup fruit + liquid	4.8 oz	150	12
1472	Swordfish,broiled 1 piece (4.5 × 2 × 1 in)	4.9 oz	240	12

continued

Menu Items with Maximum Quantity of Vitamin A *(continued)*

No.	Name/Portion Size		KCAL	NUTRI-UNITS A
2100	Sweet potatoes,glazed 2½ × 2 in diam piece	2.7 oz	140	11
1153	Apricots,raw 3 med or ⅔ cup halves	3.7 oz	50	11
1965	Vegetable beef soup,lo sodium 1 scant cup	7.9 oz	90	11
1924	Chicken vegetable soup,w water 1 cup	8.6 oz	80	11
1964	Vegetable beef soup,fz,water 1 cup	8.6 oz	90	11
2020	Chard,swiss,boiled,drained ½ cup	3.0 oz	20	11
1607	Crab,deviled 1 cup	8.5 oz	450	11
2008	Cabbage,spoon,boiled,drained ½ cup cut in 1 in pcs	3.0 oz	10	11
1625	Cannelloni,beef/pork 9.6 oz	9.6 oz	260	10
1633	Lasagna, zucchini 11 oz	10.9 oz	270	10
1925	Chunky beef soup,lo sodium 1 scant cup	7.9 oz	160	10
1717	Taco salad,beef 1 cup	5.3 oz	340	10
1573	Beef and vegetable stew,no salt 1 cup	8.6 oz	220	10
1574	Beef and veg stew,salt added 1 cup	8.6 oz	220	10
1608	Crab imperial 1 cup	7.8 oz	320	10
1575	Beef and vegetable stew,canned 1 cup	8.6 oz	190	10

No.	Name/Portion Size		KCAL	NUTRI-UNITS A
2000	Broccoli cheese casserole ½ cup	4.2 oz	170	8
2022	Collards,fresh/fz,boiled,drnd ½ cup	3.0 oz	10	8
1614	Fz dinner,chicken,potato+veg 11 oz	11.0 oz	540	7
1663	Ravioli,cheese 1 cup	8.6 oz	580	7
1678	Turkey a la king ½ cup on 1 sl toast	5.7 oz	210	7
2064	Peppers,sweet,red,mature,raw ½ cup sleced	1.4 oz	10	7
1599	Chicken potpie w biscuit top 1 cup	8.4 oz	350	7
1815	Liverwurst on rye sandwich 1 average	3.2 oz	250	7
1999	Broccoli,fz,choppd,boiled,drnd ½ cup	3.2 oz	30	7
1578	Beef potpie,home prepared ⅓ of 9 inch pie	7.4 oz	520	7
1439	Crab,steamed ½ cup	2.8 oz	70	7
1585	Burrito,combination 1 large	6.2 oz	400	7
1303	Apricot nectar,cnd,40 pct fruit ½ cup	4.4 oz	70	7
1582	Burrito,bean 1 tortilla, ½ cup beans	5.9 oz	340	7
2117	Watercress Whole,1 cup (10 sprigs)	1.2 oz	0	7
2103	Tomatoes,ripe,boiled ½ cup	4.2 oz	30	7

1941	Minestrone soup,w water 1 cup	8.6 oz	80	10
1962	Vegetable soup,lo sodium 1 scant cup	7.9 oz	90	9
1161	Apricots,dried,sulfured,unckd 9 med halves or 1/4 cup	1.1 oz	80	9
1635	Meatball stew 10 oz	10.0 oz	250	9
192	Ovaltine mix,dry 1 serving package	.7 oz	80	9
347	Ovaltine mix, dry 1 serving package	.7 oz	80	9
2088	Spinach,raw 1 cup pieces or leaves	1.1 oz	10	9
1966	Vegetable beef broth,w water 1 cup	8.6 oz	80	9
2001	Broccoli w cheese sauce 1/2 cup + 2 tbsp sauce	3.5 oz	90	8
1598	Chicken pot pie,commercial 1 8 oz pie	7.9 oz	490	8
490	Egg,spanish omelet 2 eggs,4 tbsp sauce	5.4 oz	330	8
668	Egg,spanish omelet,salted 2 eggs,4 tbsp sauce	5.4 oz	330	8
1648	Omelet,spanish 2 eggs,4 tbsp sauce	5.4 oz	330	8
1681	Turkey pot pie,frz,commercial 1 8 oz pie	8.0 oz	450	8
1686	Whitefish,baked,stuffed,no salt 1 piece (3 × 3 × 1 inch)	3.5 oz	220	8
1963	Vegetable beef soup,w water 1 cup	8.6 oz	80	8
1649	Omelet w ham 2 eggs, 1/3 oz ham	4.8 oz	330	8
1669	Spaghetti,meatballs+tomato sauc 1 cup	8.7 oz	330	6
2108	Tomato paste,canned 1/4 cup or 4 tbsp	2.3 oz	50	6
1588	Cheese fondue 1 cup	6.2 oz	460	6
1622	Lasagna w beef 1 cup	8.5 oz	420	6
1642	Macaroni,beef+cheese+tom sauce 1 cup	8.0 oz	250	6
475	Oat cereal,inst,fort,ckd,w salt 1 packet	6.2 oz	100	6
1589	Cheese manicotti w sauce 1 cup	8.5 oz	280	6
1674	Tamale pie 1 cup	8.0 oz	180	6
349	Tomato juice 1 6-oz glass	6.5 oz	40	6
1097	Pizza H,thick,pepperoni 1/4 of 13 in pizza	5.3 oz	450	6
1274	Plantain(baking banana),raw 1/2 of 2 in diax11 in frt	4.6 oz	160	6
1998	Broccoli,fresh spears,ckd,drnd 1/2 cup of 1/2 in pieces	2.8 oz	20	6
1155	Apricots,cnd,sol+liq,w juice 3 halves + 13/4 tbsp liq	3.0 oz	40	6
1164	Apricots,frozen,sweetened 1/2 cup	3.0 oz	80	6
1331	Vegetable juice cocktail,cnd 1/2 cup	4.3 oz	20	6
1696	Lettuce and spinach,french drsg 1 cup,2 tbsp m/fat drsg	3.5 oz	180	6

Menu Items with Maximum Quantity of Vitamin C

No.	Name/Portion Size		KCAL	NUTRI-UNITS C
1228	Guavas,raw,whole,common 1 medium	3.2 oz	50	55
1581	Broccoli cheese casserole 1 cup	8.5 oz	330	41
1200	Currants,black or european,raw 1/2 cup	2.4 oz	40	40
1256	Peaches,frozen,sliced,swt,vit c 1/2 cup	4.4 oz	120	39
1266	Persimmons,raw,native 2 1/2 in dia × 3 in high	5.9 oz	210	37
2061	Peppers,hot,red,raw,pod-no seed 1 oz,2 tbsp	1.0 oz	20	34
1245	Papayas,raw 1/2 of 3.5 in diam fruit	5.4 oz	60	31
2064	Peppers,sweet,red,mature,raw 1/2 cup sleced	1.4 oz	10	27
482	Orange 1 orange 2 5/8 in diam	4.6 oz	60	25
92	Kiwi fruit,raw 1 medium	2.7 oz	50	25
1230	Kiwi fruit 1 medium	2.7 oz	50	25
1650	Peppers stuffed w beef 1 med pepper	6.5 oz	310	25
348	Orange juice 1 6-oz glass	6.6 oz	80	24
1243	Oranges,peeled,all varieties 2 5/8 in diam orange	4.6 oz	60	23
1956	Tomato soup,w milk 1 cup	8.8 oz	160	23
106	Screwdriver 1 7 oz glass	7.5 oz	180	22
1304	Apricot nectar,cnd,+ vit c 1/2 cup	4.4 oz	70	17
2062	Peppers,swt,green,immature,raw 1/2 cup sliced	1.4 oz	10	17
1317	Orange juic,fz,conc,unswt,dilut 1/2 cup	4.4 oz	60	16
1221	Grapefruit,raw,pink or red 1/2 of 4-in diam fruit	4.5 oz	40	16
1321	Pineapple juice,cnd,+ vit c 1/2 cup	4.4 oz	70	16
2002	Brussels sprout,frsh/fz,ckd,drn 1/2 cup,4 medium	2.7 oz	30	16
1308	Grapefruit jc,raw,red,pink,whte 1/2 cup	4.3 oz	50	16
1222	Grapefruit,raw,white 1/2 of 4-in diam fruit	4.8 oz	50	15
1306	Cranberry juice cocktail 1/2 cup	4.5 oz	70	15
1715	Lobster salad w tomato slices 1/2 cup sal,1 med tomato	8.8 oz	280	15
1645	Manicotti 1 cup	8.7 oz	340	15
2040	Kohlrabi,boiled,drained 1/2 cup	2.9 oz	20	15
429	King vitamin 1 oz (3/4 cup)	1.0 oz	110	15
1316	Orange juice,cnd,unsweetened 1/2 cup	4.4 oz	50	14
1296	Strawberries,raw 1/2 cup, whole or halves	2.6 oz	20	14
1232	Lemons,raw,peeled 1 med 2 1/8 in diam lemon	2.8 oz	20	14

1957	Tomato soup,w water 1 cup	8.6 oz	90	22
2001	Broccoli w cheese sauce 1/2 cup + 2 tbsp sauce	3.5 oz	90	22
169	Orange instant breakfast drink 1/2 cup	4.4 oz	60	22
2059	Peppers,hot,immature,green,raw 1 oz,2 tbsp	1.0 oz	10	22
2063	Peppers,swt,green,boiled,drnd 1/2 cup strips	2.4 oz	10	22
2014	Cauliflower,raw 1 cup sliced florets	3.2 oz	20	21
1315	Orange juice,raw,all varieties 1/2 cup	4.4 oz	60	21
2000	Broccoli cheese casserole 1/2 cup	4.2 oz	170	20
433	Most 1 oz (1/2 cup)	1.0 oz	90	20
442	Product 19 1 oz (1 cup)	1.0 oz	110	20
460	Total 1 oz (7/8 cup)	1.0 oz	100	20
1181	Cantaloupe,raw 1/4 cup	4.8 oz	50	19
1732	Peppers,hot,red,raw 1 tbsp	.5 oz	10	18
1324	Prune juice,bottled,+ vit c 1/2 cup	4.5 oz	100	18
1302	Apple juice,cnd or bottld+vit c 1/2 cup	4.4 oz	60	18
338	Instant breakfast, dry 1 serving	1.2 oz	120	18
1298	Strawberries,frozen,sliced,swtn 1/2 cup	4.5 oz	120	18
1326	Tangerine juice,raw 1/2 cup	4.4 oz	50	13
1958	Tomato soup,lo sodium 1 scant cup	7.9 oz	110	13
2016	Cauliflwr+broccol mix,boild,drd 1/2 cup+1 tsp butter	2.6 oz	70	13
1224	Grapefruit segments,cnd,syrup 1/2 cup	4.4 oz	90	13
2079	Potatoes,tator bars 3 oz	3.0 oz	170	13
95	Orange,raw Half of 2.6 in orange	2.3 oz	30	12
1229	Honeydew melon,raw 1/10 of 6 3/4 in dia meln	5.3 oz	50	12
1999	Broccoli,fz,choppd,boiled,drnd 1/2 cup	3.2 oz	30	12
1223	Grapefruit segments,cnd,art swt 1/2 cup	4.3 oz	40	12
1328	Tangerine jc,fz,conc,swt,dil 1/2 cup	4.4 oz	70	12
1730	Peppers,hot green,raw 1 tbsp	.5 oz	10	12
2015	Cauliflower,boiled,drained 1/2 cup	2.2 oz	20	12
1325	Tangelo juice,raw 1/2 cup	4.4 oz	50	11
1331	Vegetable juice cocktail,cnd 1/2 cup	4.3 oz	20	11
2115	Vegetable juice cocktail,canned 1/2 cup	4.3 oz	20	11
107	Tequilla sunrise 1 5.5 oz glass	6.1 oz	190	11
481	Grapefruit 1/2 gpft (3 1/2 in diam)	3.4 oz	30	11

continued

Menu Items with Maximum Quantity of Vitamin C *(continued)*

No.	Name/Portion Size		KCAL	NUTRI-UNITS C
1610	Eggplant parmigiana 1 cup	7.8 oz	410	11
1602	Chop suey,home prepared 1 cup	8.8 oz	300	11
1307	Cranberry juic cocktail w vit c 1/2 cup	4.5 oz	90	11
2099	Sweet potatoes,cnd,dietary pack 1/2 cup solids+liquids	4.2 oz	110	11
1397	Liver,calf,fried 1 sl (6 × 2 × .5 in)	3.0 oz	220	11
1998	Broccoli,fresh spears,ckd,drnd 1/2 cup of 1/2 in pieces	2.8 oz	20	10
968	Strawberry pie m/w lard 1/6 of 9 in diam pie	4.4 oz	250	10
969	Strawberry pie m/w veg fat 1/6 of 9 in diam pie	4.4 oz	250	10
162	Cranberry jc cocktail w vit c 1/2 cup or 4 oz	4.3 oz	90	10
1300	Watermelon,raw 2 cups, diced	11.3 oz	100	10
1453	Oysters,cnd,sol+liq w salt 1 can,3.6 oz	3.6 oz	80	10
165	Grape drink, canned, w vit c 1 8-oz cup	8.8 oz	140	10
1310	Grape juice,fz,swt,dilut,vit c 1/2 cup	4.4 oz	60	10
1628	Chicken w veg. w vermicelli 12.7 oz	12.7 oz	260	10
1631	Fish divan filet 12.4 oz	12.4 oz	270	10
1662	Ratatouille 5 oz	5.0 oz	80	10
748	Strawbr shortck+1 tbsp whip top 3×4 in pc+0.4 cup berries	4.3 oz	290	8
844	Strawberry shortcake w whp top 3×4 in ck/.4 cup berries	4.3 oz	290	8
861	Super donut 2 oz donut	2.0 oz	250	8
2103	Tomatoes,ripe,boiled 1/2 cup	4.2 oz	30	8
1274	Plantain(baking banana),raw 1/2 of 2 in dia×11 in frt	4.6 oz	160	8
1297	Strawberries,cnd,sol+liq, water 1/2 cup	4.2 oz	30	8
2101	Tomatoes,green,raw 1/2 of 3-in diam tomato	3.6 oz	20	8
1504	Ham,cured,extra lean,canned 1 slice (4 × 2.3 × .5 in)	3.0 oz	120	8
2109	Tomato puree,canned 1/4 cup or 4 tbsp	2.3 oz	30	8
1241	Mangos,raw 1/2 cup, diced or sliced	2.9 oz	50	8
1182	Casaba melon,raw 1/10 of 6 3/4 in dia meln	4.9 oz	40	8
1231	Kumquats,raw 3 medium	2.1 oz	40	8
1071	McDonalds chicken mcnuggets 1 serving, 20 pc	13.1 oz	900	7
1329	Tomato juice,canned,salted 1/2 cup	4.3 oz	20	7
1669	Spaghetti,meatballs+tomato sauc 1 cup	8.7 oz	330	7
2106	Tomato juice,canned 1/2 cup	4.3 oz	20	7

349	Tomato juice 1 6-oz glass	6.5 oz	40	10
1052	Arby's potato cakes 1 serving, 2 cakes	5.8 oz	300	10
1706	Fresh fruit w mayo + whip cream 1 cup on let,2 tbsp drsg	6.2 oz	160	9
1201	Currants,red or white,raw 1/2 cup	2.4 oz	40	9
1068	Kentucky Fr Chick,orig dinner 2 pc,pot,gravy,slaw,roll	15.0 oz	830	9
1327	Tangerine juice,cnd,sweetened 1/2 cup	4.4 oz	60	9
1718	Tomato stuffed w tuna salad 1/3 c tuna,2–1/2 in tomat	6.0 oz	100	9
192	Ovaltine mix,dry 1 serving package	.7 oz	80	9
347	Ovaltine mix, dry 1 serving package	.7 oz	80	9
1062	KFC extra crispy dinner 2 pc,pot,gravy,slaw,roll	15.4 oz	950	9
2108	Tomato paste,canned 1/4 cup or 4 tbsp	2.3 oz	50	9
2053	Peas,edible,podded,ckd,drnd 2 oz	2.0 oz	20	9
1299	Tangerines,raw 2 3/8 in diam med fruit	3.0 oz	40	9
991	Strawberries,frozen,sweetened 1/4 cup	2.2 oz	60	9
1685	Veal parmigiana 1 cup	7.9 oz	340	9
1759	Pepper,sweet green 1/4 cup sliced	.7 oz	10	9
380	Super donut,fortified 2 oz	2.0 oz	250	8
1104	McDonalds chicken salad oriental 1 serving,9.9 oz	9.9 oz	150	7
1623	Chicken chow mein w rice 11.3 oz	11.1 oz	250	7
2110	Tomato puree,canned,lo sodium 1/4 cup or 4 tbsp	2.3 oz	30	7
1971	Asparagus,cnd,green,drained 1/2 cup (1.5–2 in pieces)	4.2 oz	20	7
2065	Potatoes,baked in skin,w skin 2.3 in diam × 4.7 in	5.5 oz	168	7
1218	Gooseberries,raw 1/2 cup	2.6 oz	30	7
1291	Raspberries,red,frozen,sweetnd 1/2 cup	4.4 oz	130	7
1589	Cheese manicotti w sauce 1 cup	8.5 oz	280	7
1668	Shrimp creole on rice 1/2 cup on 1/2 cup rice	8.8 oz	270	7
2004	Cabbage,cooked 1/2 cup wedges	3.0 oz	20	7
99	Bloody mary 1 5 oz glass	5.2 oz	120	7
2105	Tomatoes,ripe,cnd,lo sod,sol+lq 1/2 cup	4.2 oz	20	7
170	Orange+apricot jc drink,cnd 1/2 cup	4.4 oz	60	7
171	Pineapl+grapefrt jc drink,cnd 1/2 cup	4.4 oz	70	7
172	Pineapl+orange jc drink,cnd 1/2 cup	4.4 oz	70	7
1524	Pork liver,fried 1 sl (6.5 × 2.5 × .4 in)	3.0 oz	140	7
2005	Cabbage,red,raw 1/2 cup shredded/sliced	1.2 oz	10	7

Menu Items with Maximum Quantity of Thiamin

No.	Name/Portion Size		KCAL	NUTRI-UNITS THI
1113	Arbys ham+cheese sandwich 1 serving, 8.25 oz	8.7 oz	480	21
433	Most 1 oz (1/2 cup)	1.0 oz	90	20
442	Product 19 1 oz (1 cup)	1.0 oz	110	20
460	Total 1 oz (7/8 cup)	1.0 oz	100	20
1112	Arbys super roast beef sandwich 1 serving, 9.5 oz	10.3 oz	620	19
429	King vitamin 1 oz (3/4 cup)	1.0 oz	110	16
1102	Pizza H,super,supreme 1/4 of 13 in pizza	7.1 oz	590	16
1111	Arbys beef and cheddar sandwich 1 serving, 6 oz	6.3 oz	480	15
1094	Pizza H,thin,super,supreme 1/4 of 13 in pizza	6.3 oz	520	14
1633	Lasagna, zucchini 11 oz	10.9 oz	270	14
1587	Canneloni 1 cup	8.8 oz	430	14
1099	Pizza H,thick,pork w mushroom 1/4 of 13 in pizza	5.3 oz	430	12
1100	Pizza H,thick,super,pork w mush 1/4 of 13 in pizza	6.0 oz	500	12
1101	Pizza H,thick,supreme 1/4 of 13 in pizza	6.0 oz	480	12
1504	Ham,cured,extra lean,canned 1 slice (4 × 2.3 × .5 in)	3.0 oz	120	12
1022	McDonalds sausage mcmuffin+egg 1 serving, 5.8 oz	5.8 oz	520	11

No.	Name/Portion Size		KCAL	NUTRI-UNITS THI
1503	Ham,fresh,lean only,roasted 1 slice (4 × 2.3 × .5 in)	3.0 oz	190	9
1512	Pork butt,lean only,rst 1 pc (2.5 × 2.5 × .8 in)	3.0 oz	190	9
1506	Ham,cured,extra lean,roasted 1 slice (4 × 2.3 × .5 in)	3.0 oz	120	9
1014	Jack in Box pancakes 1 serving, 8.2 oz	8.2 oz	630	8
1507	Ham,cured,roasted 1 slice (4 × 2.3 × .5 in)	3.0 oz	150	8
862	Banana split w soft serve 1 banana split	13.5 oz	540	8
1030	Dairy Queen banana split 1 serving, 13.5 oz	13.5 oz	540	8
1508	Ham,cured,country style,bkd 1 slice (4 × 2.3 × .5 in)	3.0 oz	330	8
1520	Pork picnic,cured,lean only,rst .6 cup chopped	3.0 oz	140	8
1664	Ravioli,meat 1 cup	8.6 oz	600	8
431	Life 1 oz (2/3 cup)	1.0 oz	100	8
1515	Pork loin roast,lean + fat 1 sl (2.5 × 2.5 × .8 in)	3.0 oz	270	8
1090	Pizza H,thin,suprstyle,pepproni 1/4 of 13 in pizza	5.3 oz	430	8
1092	Pizza H,thin,super,pork w mushr 1/4 of 13 in pizza	5.3 oz	450	8
1502	Ham,fresh,lean + fat,roasted 1 slice (4 × 2.3 × .5 in)	3.0 oz	230	8
1511	Pork butt,lean + fat,rst 1 pc (2.5 × 2.5 × .8 in)	3.0 oz	230	8

1096	Pizza H,thick,superstyle,cheese 1/4 of 13 in pizza	6.0 oz	450	11
1098	Pizza H,thick,suprstyl,pepproni 1/4 of 13 in pizza	6.0 oz	490	11
1097	Pizza H,thick,pepperoni 1/4 of 13 in pizza	5.3 oz	450	11
1138	Wendy's triple burger w cheese 1 serving, 14 oz	14.1 oz	1040	11
1114	Arbys sub (no dressing) 1 serving, 9.5 oz	10.1 oz	480	11
1119	Burger King,whopper 1 serving, 10 oz	10.0 oz	610	10
1095	Pizza H,thick,cheese 1/4 of 13 in pizza	5.3 oz	390	10
444	Puffed rice,fortified 1 oz (2 cups)	1.0 oz	110	10
1010	Jack in Box scrambled eggs 1 serving, 9.4 oz	9.4 oz	390	9
1021	McDonalds sausage mcmuffin 1 serving, 4.1 oz	4.1 oz	430	9
1505	Ham,cured,regular, canned 1 slice (4 × 2.3 × .5 in)	3.0 oz	190	9
1516	Pork loin roast,lean only 1 sl (2.5 × 2.5 × .8 in)	3.0 oz	200	9
1093	Pizza H,thin,supreme 1/4 of 13 in pizza	5.3 oz	400	9
1078	Taco Bell bean burrito 1 serving, 6.7 oz	6.7 oz	360	9
192	Ovaltine mix,dry 1 serving package	.7 oz	80	9
347	Ovaltine mix, dry 1 serving package	.7 oz	80	9
1513	Pork chop,loin,lean + fat,brl 1 chop,1/3 lb	2.8 oz	270	9
1784	Barbequed pork on bun 3.5 oz barb, 1.6 oz bun	5.0 oz	370	8
1017	McDonalds biscuit+sausage 1 serving, 4.3 oz	4.3 oz	470	7
1514	Pork chop,loin,lean only,brl 1 chop,trimmed	2.0 oz	140	7
1831	Pita bread 1 2.5 oz loaf	2.5 oz	200	7
475	Oat cereal,inst,fort,ckd,w salt 1 packet	6.2 oz	100	7
1018	McDonalds biscuit+sausage,egg 1 serving, 6.2 oz	6.2 oz	590	7
1091	Pizza H,thin,pork w mushroom 1/4 of 13 in pizza	4.6 oz	380	7
494	Ham,fried,lean only 1 sl (4 × 2.3 × 1/4 in)	1.5 oz	110	7
1088	Pizza H,thin,superstyle,cheese 1/4 of 13 in pizza	5.3 oz	410	7
1519	Pork picnic,cured,lean + fat,rst 1 pc (2.5 × 2.5 × .8 in)	3.0 oz	240	7
1663	Ravioli,cheese 1 cup	8.6 oz	580	7
1518	Pork picnic,lean only,sim 1 pc (2.5 × 2.5 × .8 in)	3.0 oz	210	7
446	Quisp 1 oz (1.2 cup)	1.0 oz	120	7
1489	Raccoon,roasted 3 oz	3.0 oz	220	7
395	Captain crunch 1 oz (3/4 cup)	1.0 oz	120	7
1103	McDonalds chef salad 1 serving,9.6 oz	9.6 oz	220	7
1510	Ham,light cure,lean only,bkd 1 slice (4 × 2.3 × .5 in)	3.0 oz	160	7

continued

Menu Items with Maximum Quantity of Thiamin *(continued)*

No.	Name/Portion Size		KCAL	NUTRI-UNITS THI
1082	Taco Bell combination burrito 1 serving, 6.7 oz	6.7 oz	380	7
1136	Wendy's double burger w cheese 1 serving, 11.5 oz	11.5 oz	800	7
397	Captn crunch p-nut buttr cereal 1 oz (3/4 cup)	1.0 oz	120	6
396	Captain crunch crunchberries 1 oz (3/4 cup)	1.0 oz	120	6
465	Wheat germ 1/4 cup (4 tablespoons)	1.0 oz	110	6
1123	J in b jumbo burger w cheese 1 serving,8.7 oz	8.7 oz	570	6
1137	Wendy's triple burger 1 serving, 12 oz	12.7 oz	840	6
1087	Pizza Hut pizza,thin,cheese 1/4 of 13 in pizza	4.6 oz	340	6
1089	Pizza H,thin,pepperoni 1/4 of 13 in pizza	4.6 oz	370	6
1517	Pork picnic,lean + fat,sim 1 pc (2.5 × 2.5 × .8 in)	3.0 oz	290	6
1081	Taco Bell burrito supreme 1 serving, 8.7 oz	8.7 oz	420	6
869	Hot fudge brownie w soft serve 1 serving	9.4 oz	560	6
1084	Taco Bell pintos n cheese 1 serving, 4.5 oz	4.5 oz	190	6
1108	Arbys chicken breast sandwich 1 serving, 7.25 oz	7.2 oz	550	6
1135	Wendy's double burger 1 serving, 10 oz	10.1 oz	670	6
1542	Bratwurst,cooked 1 3 oz link	3.0 oz	260	6

No.	Name/Portion Size		KCAL	NUTRI-UNITS THI
405	Corn flakes 1 oz (1 to 1.3 cup)	1.0 oz	110	5
407	Corny snaps 1 oz (1 cup)	1.0 oz	120	5
408	Count chocula 1 oz (1 cup)	1.0 oz	110	5
440	Pep wheat flakes 1 oz (1 cup)	1.0 oz	110	5
441	Post toasties 1 oz (1 1/4 cup)	1.0 oz	110	5
1071	McDonalds chicken mcnuggets 1 serving, 20 pc	13.1 oz	900	5
1617	Ham croquette 2 (1 in diam × 3 in)	4.6 oz	330	5
389	All bran 1 oz (1/2 cup)	1.0 oz	70	5
390	Alpha bits 1 oz (1 cup)	1.0 oz	110	5
391	Apple jacks 1 oz (1 cup)	1.0 oz	110	5
392	Bran buds 1 oz (1/3 cup)	1.0 oz	70	5
393	Bran chex 1 oz (1/2 cup)	1.0 oz	90	5
394	Bran flakes,40 percent 1 oz (2/3 cup)	1.0 oz	90	5
398	Cheerios 1 oz (1 1/4 cup)	1.0 oz	110	5
399	Cocoa krispies 1 oz (1 cup)	1.0 oz	110	5
400	Cocoa pebbles,rice 1 oz (.8 cup)	1.0 oz	110	5

1109	Arbys roast beef sandwich	1 serving, 5 oz	5.3 oz	350	6
1522	Pork and gravy,canned	3 oz serving	3.0 oz	220	6
1645	Manicotti	1 cup	8.7 oz	340	6
1814	Hot dog,large,on bun	1 serving,6.4 oz	6.4 oz	520	6
1009	Jack in Box breakfast jack	1 serving, 4.3 oz	4.3 oz	380	6
1012	J in b omelette,ham and cheese	1 serving, 6 oz	6.1 oz	430	5
1086	Taco Bell tostada	1 serving, 5.5 oz	5.5 oz	240	5
1509	Ham,light cure,lean + fat,bkd	1 slice (4 × 2.3 × .5 in)	3.0 oz	250	5
1079	Taco Bell beef burrito	1 serving, 6.5 oz	6.5 oz	400	5
1083	Taco Bell enchirito	1 serving, 7.5 oz	7.5 oz	380	5
1523	Pork w juice,canned,salted	3 oz serving	3.0 oz	190	5
297	Wild rice,raw	1/2 cup	3.0 oz	300	5
1134	Wendy's single burger w cheese	1 serving, 8.5 oz	8.5 oz	580	5
1806	Ham sandwich w butter,mayo,let	2 oz ham,1 tsp but + mayo	5.0 oz	320	5
1809	Hamburger,super	1 hamburger,8.9 oz	8.9 oz	560	5
329	Tahini,sesame butter	2 tablespoons	1.1 oz	180	5
401	Cocoa pops	1 oz	1.0 oz	110	5
402	Cookie crisp	1 oz (1 cup)	1.0 oz	110	5
404	Corn chex	1 oz (1 cup)	1.0 oz	110	5
410	CW Post family cereal	1 oz (1/4 cup)	1.0 oz	130	5
411	Crispy wheats n raisins	1 oz (2/3 cup)	1.0 oz	100	5
412	CW Post family cereal w raisins	1 oz (1/4 cup)	1.0 oz	120	5
413	Fortified oat flakes	1 oz (2/3 cup)	1.0 oz	100	5
414	Froot loops	1 oz (1 cup)	1.0 oz	110	5
415	Frosted miniwheats	1 oz (4 pieces)	1.0 oz	100	5
416	Frosted rice	1 oz (0.8 cup)	1.0 oz	110	5
417	Fruity pebbles	1 oz (7/8 cup)	1.0 oz	110	5
418	Golden grahams	1 oz (3/4 cup)	1.0 oz	110	5
421	Grapenuts	1 oz (1/4 cup)	1.0 oz	100	5
422	Grapenut flakes	1 oz (7/8 cup)	1.0 oz	100	5
425	Honeybran	1 oz (0.8 cup)	1.0 oz	100	5
426	Honeycomb	1 oz (1 1/3 cup)	1.0 oz	110	5
427	Honeynut cheerios	1 oz (7/8 cup)	1.0 oz	110	5
428	Honey nut cornflakes	1 oz (1 cup)	1.0 oz	110	5

Menu Items with Maximum Quantity of Riboflavin

No.	Name/Portion Size		KCAL	NUTRI-UNITS RIB
1397	Liver,calf,fried 1 sl (6 × 2 × .5 in)	3.0 oz	220	42
1396	Liver,beef,fried 1 sl (6 × 2 × .5 in)	3.0 oz	180	41
1395	Kidneys,simmered 1/2 cup	2.5 oz	100	33
1524	Pork liver,fried 1 sl (6.5 × 2.5 × .4 in)	3.0 oz	140	22
1576	Beef liver,onion gravy 1 pc (6.5 × 2.5 × 1/4 in)	3.5 oz	140	20
433	Most 1 oz (1/2 cup)	1.0 oz	90	20
442	Product 19 1 oz (1 cup)	1.0 oz	110	20
460	Total 1 oz (7/8 cup)	1.0 oz	100	20
429	King vitamin 1 oz (3/4 cup)	1.0 oz	110	17
1394	Heart,cooked 3 oz	3.0 oz	150	15
1428	Fried giblets 3 oz	3.0 oz	240	15
1429	Fried liver 1/2 cup	2.5 oz	110	14
1095	Pizza H,thick,cheese 1/4 of 13 in pizza	5.3 oz	390	14
1112	Arbys super roast beef sandwich 1 serving, 9.5 oz	10.3 oz	620	14
1113	Arbys ham+cheese sandwich 1 serving, 8.25 oz	8.7 oz	480	12
1102	Pizza H,super,supreme 1/4 of 13 in pizza	7.1 oz	590	11
1099	Pizza H,thick,pork w mushroom 1/4 of 13 in pizza	5.3 oz	430	8
196	Shake, vanilla 1 10-oz serving	10.2 oz	320	8
1007	McDonalds vanilla shake 1 serving, 10.2 oz	10.2 oz	320	8
1097	Pizza H,thick,pepperoni 1/4 of 13 in pizza	5.3 oz	450	8
1137	Wendy's triple burger 1 serving, 12 oz	12.7 oz	840	8
431	Life 1 oz (2/3 cup)	1.0 oz	100	8
684	Condensed milk,sweetened,canned 1/2 cup	5.4 oz	490	7
1587	Canneloni 1 cup	8.8 oz	430	7
1003	Jack in Box strawberry shake 1 serving, 11.6 oz	11.6 oz	380	7
862	Banana split w soft serve 1 banana split	13.5 oz	540	7
1030	Dairy Queen banana split 1 serving, 13.5 oz	13.5 oz	540	7
1002	Jack in Box chocolate shake 1 serving, 11 oz	11.2 oz	370	7
1008	Wendy's frosty 1 serving, 8.8 oz	8.8 oz	390	7
1088	Pizza H,thin,superstyle,cheese 1/4 of 13 in pizza	5.3 oz	410	7
1092	Pizza H,thin,super,pork w mushr 1/4 of 13 in pizza	5.3 oz	450	7
1019	McDonalds egg mcmuffin 1 serving, 4.7 oz	4.7 oz	310	7

1114	Arbys sub (no dressing) 1 serving, 9.5 oz	10.1 oz	480	11
1138	Wendy's triple burger w cheese 1 serving, 14 oz	14.1 oz	1040	10
183	Malt, chocolate, large 1 21-oz serving	20.7 oz	840	9
999	Dairy Queen choclate malt,large 1 large, 20.7 oz	20.7 oz	840	9
1101	Pizza H,thick,supreme 1/4 of 13 in pizza	6.0 oz	480	9
192	Ovaltine mix,dry 1 serving package	.7 oz	80	9
347	Ovaltine mix, dry 1 serving package	.7 oz	80	9
1013	J in b omelette,ranchero 1 serving, 6.9 oz	6.9 oz	410	9
1136	Wendy's double burger w cheese 1 serving, 11.5 oz	11.5 oz	800	9
1111	Arbys beef and cheddar sandwich 1 serving, 6 oz	6.3 oz	480	9
446	Quisp 1 oz (1.2 cup)	1.0 oz	120	8
1012	J in b omelette,ham and cheese 1 serving, 6 oz	6.1 oz	430	8
1011	J in b omelette,double cheese 1 serving, 5.8 oz	5.9 oz	420	8
1094	Pizza H,thin,super,supreme 1/4 of 13 in pizza	6.3 oz	520	8
1096	Pizza H,thick,superstyle,cheese 1/4 of 13 in pizza	6.0 oz	450	8
1098	Pizza H,thick,suprstyl,pepproni 1/4 of 13 in pizza	6.0 oz	490	8
1100	Pizza H,thick,super,pork w mush 1/4 of 13 in pizza	6.0 oz	500	8
1588	Cheese fondue 1 cup	6.2 oz	460	7
1135	Wendy's double burger 1 serving, 10 oz	10.1 oz	670	7
397	Captn crunch p-nut buttr cereal 1 oz (3/4 cup)	1.0 oz	120	7
1010	Jack in Box scrambled eggs 1 serving, 9.4 oz	9.4 oz	390	7
1614	Fz dinner,chicken,potato+veg 11 oz	11.0 oz	540	7
1071	McDonalds chicken mcnuggets 1 serving, 20 pc	13.1 oz	900	7
182	Malt, chocolate, medium 1 15-oz serving	14.7 oz	600	6
395	Captain crunch 1 oz (3/4 cup)	1.0 oz	120	6
403	Corn bran 1 oz (1 cup)	1.0 oz	100	6
998	Dairy Queen choclate malt,med 1 medium, 14.7 oz	14.7 oz	600	6
297	Wild rice,raw 1/2 cup	3.0 oz	300	6
396	Captain crunch crunchberries 1 oz (3/4 cup)	1.0 oz	120	6
696	Yogurt,skim w nfdm,plain 8 oz container	8.0 oz	130	6
919	Yogurt,plain,skim milk w nfdm 1 8-oz container	8.0 oz	130	6
1062	KFC extra crispy dinner 2 pc,pot,gravy,slaw,roll	15.4 oz	950	6
186	Milk, malted, beverage 1 8-oz glass	8.3 oz	210	6
1645	Manicotti 1 cup	8.7 oz	340	6

continued

Menu Items with Maximum Quantity of Riboflavin *(continued)*

No.	Name/Portion Size		KCAL	NUTRI-UNITS RIB
1068	Kentucky Fr Chick,orig dinner 2 pc,pot,gravy,slaw,roll	15.0 oz	830	6
1087	Pizza Hut pizza,thin,cheese 1/4 of 13 in pizza	4.6 oz	340	6
1091	Pizza H,thin,pork w mushroom 1/4 of 13 in pizza	4.6 oz	380	6
1093	Pizza H,thin,supreme 1/4 of 13 in pizza	5.3 oz	400	6
1795	Chili dog w bun 1.5 oz dog,1/2 c chili	8.3 oz	510	6
178	Cocoa,made from mix + skim milk 1 8-oz cup	9.3 oz	160	6
444	Puffed rice,fortified 1 oz (2 cups)	1.0 oz	110	6
1581	Broccoli cheese casserole 1 cup	8.5 oz	330	6
1022	McDonalds sausage mcmuffin+egg 1 serving, 5.8 oz	5.8 oz	520	6
1108	Arbys chicken breast sandwich 1 serving, 7.25 oz	7.2 oz	550	6
695	Yogurt,lo fat,plain 8 oz container	8.0 oz	140	6
917	Yogurt,plain,part skim milk 1 8-oz container	8.0 oz	140	6
1018	McDonalds biscuit+sausage,egg 1 serving, 6.2 oz	6.2 oz	590	6
1009	Jack in Box breakfast jack 1 serving, 4.3 oz	4.3 oz	380	6
1109	Arbys roast beef sandwich 1 serving, 5 oz	5.3 oz	350	6
1490	Venison,raw 3.5 oz	3.5 oz	130	6
1814	Hot dog,large,on bun 1 serving,6.4 oz	6.4 oz	520	5
1949	Oyster stew,home prp,2 pts milk 1 cup	8.5 oz	230	5
1950	Oyster stew,home prp,3 pts milk 1 cup	8.5 oz	210	5
188	Milk, 1 percent fat, a+d fort 1 8-oz glass	8.7 oz	110	5
189	Milk, 2 percent fat, a+d fort 1 8-oz glass	8.7 oz	130	5
341	Milk,1 percent fat,a+d fort 1 8-oz glass	8.7 oz	110	5
343	Milk,2 percent fat,a+d fort 1 8-oz glass	8.7 oz	130	5
691	Part skim milk,1 percent fat 1 cup	8.7 oz	110	5
692	Part skim milk,2 percent fat 1 cup	8.7 oz	130	5
866	Cone,soft serve,large 1 cone	7.5 oz	340	5
869	Hot fudge brownie w soft serve 1 serving	9.4 oz	560	5
879	Parfait,soft serve 1 parfait	10.0 oz	460	5
1016	McDonalds biscuit+bacon,egg,chee 1 serving, 5.1 oz	5.1 oz	480	5
1034	Dairy Queen cone,large 1 serving, 7.5 oz	7.5 oz	340	5
1044	Dairy Queen parfait 1 serving, 10 oz	10.0 oz	460	5
1089	Pizza H,thin,pepperoni 1/4 of 13 in pizza	4.6 oz	370	5

179	Egg nog, non-alcoholic 1 8-oz glass	8.7 oz	340	6
336	Egg nog,non alcoholic 1 8-oz glass	8.7 oz	340	6
1004	Jack in Box vanilla shake 1 serving, 11 oz	11.1 oz	340	6
1037	DQ choc dipped cone,large 1 cone, 8.3 oz	8.3 oz	450	6
1609	Dried beef,creamed 1 cup	8.6 oz	380	6
701	Yogurt,lo fat,van,coffee,lemon 8 oz container	8.0 oz	190	5
195	Shake, strawberry 1 10-oz serving	10.3 oz	350	5
1006	McDonalds strawberry shake 1 serving, 10.3 oz	10.3 oz	350	5
1014	Jack in Box pancakes 1 serving, 8.2 oz	8.2 oz	630	5
1079	Taco Bell beef burrito 1 serving, 6.5 oz	6.5 oz	400	5
1081	Taco Bell burrito supreme 1 serving, 8.7 oz	8.7 oz	420	5
1489	Raccoon,roasted 3 oz	3.0 oz	220	5
194	Shake,chocolate 1 10-oz serving	10.2 oz	370	5
1005	McDonalds chocolate shake 1 serving, 10.2 oz	10.2 oz	360	5
1090	Pizza H,thin,suprstyle,pepproni 1/4 of 13 in pizza	5.3 oz	430	5
1134	Wendy's single burger w cheese 1 serving, 8.5 oz	8.5 oz	580	5
1615	Fz dinner,meat loaf,potato+peas 11 oz	11.0 oz	410	5
1529	Braunschweiger 1 sl (3 1/8 dia × 1/8 in)	1.0 oz	100	5
1845	Braunschweiger 1 sl (3.1 in diam × 1/4)	1.0 oz	100	5
389	All bran 1 oz (1/2 cup)	1.0 oz	70	5
390	Alpha bits 1 oz (1 cup)	1.0 oz	110	5
391	Apple jacks 1 oz (1 cup)	1.0 oz	110	5
392	Bran buds 1 oz (1/3 cup)	1.0 oz	70	5
394	Bran flakes,40 percent 1 oz (2/3 cup)	1.0 oz	90	5
398	Cheerios 1 oz (1 1/4 cup)	1.0 oz	110	5
399	Cocoa krispies 1 oz (1 cup)	1.0 oz	110	5
400	Cocoa pebbles,rice 1 oz (.8 cup)	1.0 oz	110	5
401	Cocoa pops 1 oz	1.0 oz	110	5
402	Cookie crisp 1 oz (1 cup)	1.0 oz	110	5
405	Corn flakes 1 oz (1 to 1.3 cup)	1.0 oz	110	5
408	Count chocula 1 oz (1 cup)	1.0 oz	110	5
410	CW Post family cereal 1 oz (1/4 cup)	1.0 oz	130	5
411	Crispy wheats n raisins 1 oz (2/3 cup)	1.0 oz	100	5
412	CW Post family cereal w raisins 1 oz (1/4 cup)	1.0 oz	120	5

Menu Items with Maximum Quantity of Vitamin B_6

No.	Name/Portion Size		KCAL	NUTRI-UNITS B6
433	Most 1 oz (1/2 cup)	1.0 oz	90	20
442	Product 19 1 oz (1 cup)	1.0 oz	110	20
460	Total 1 oz (7/8 cup)	1.0 oz	100	20
429	King vitamin 1 oz (3/4 cup)	1.0 oz	110	16
1939	Green pea soup,lo sodium 1 scant cup	7.9 oz	150	16
1071	McDonalds chicken mcnuggets 1 serving, 20 pc	13.1 oz	900	14
1061	Kentucky Fried,orig,3 pieces 3 pieces, 7.5 oz	7.6 oz	360	13
1604	Chow mein,no noodles 1 cup	8.8 oz	260	13
1396	Liver,beef,fried 1 sl (6 × 2 × .5 in)	3.0 oz	180	12
1479	Tuna,broil/bake,no salt 1 steak,6.7 × 2.5 × 1 in	4.5 oz	170	12
1801	Fish burger w cheese,chili sce 2 oz fish,1 oz cheese,bun	5.3 oz	430	11
1124	J in b moby jack sandwich 1 serving,5 oz	5.0 oz	460	11
1062	KFC extra crispy dinner 2 pc,pot,gravy,slaw,roll	15.4 oz	950	11
1664	Ravioli,meat 1 cup	8.6 oz	600	10
1068	Kentucky Fr Chick,orig dinner 2 pc,pot,gravy,slaw,roll	15.0 oz	830	10
1463	Sardines,canned,drained 8 fish (3 × 1 × .5 in)	3.5 oz	180	7
1472	Swordfish,broiled 1 piece (4.5 × 2 × 1 in)	4.9 oz	240	7
87	Banana 1 banana (9 in long)	4.2 oz	110	7
480	Banana 8 3/4 × 1 3/8 inch	4.2 oz	110	7
1166	Bananas,raw 1 medium or 4/5 cup slicd	4.2 oz	110	7
1473	Trout,rainbow,broiled 3.5 oz serving	3.5 oz	200	7
1601	Chili con carne w/o beans 1 cup	8.8 oz	500	7
403	Corn bran 1 oz (1 cup)	1.0 oz	100	7
1611	Enchiladas,beef and cheese 2 small	8.9 oz	380	7
1614	Fz dinner,chicken,potato+veg 11 oz	11.0 oz	540	7
862	Banana split w soft serve 1 banana split	13.5 oz	540	7
1030	Dairy Queen banana split 1 serving, 13.5 oz	13.5 oz	540	7
1070	McDonalds chicken mcnuggets 1 serving, 9 pc	5.9 oz	400	7
1569	Beans and franks,canned 1 cup	9.0 oz	370	6
1615	Fz dinner,meat loaf,potato+peas 11 oz	11.0 oz	410	6

1639	Spagetti w beef,mushrooms 11.5 oz	11.4 oz	280	10
1650	Peppers stuffed w beef 1 med pepper	6.5 oz	310	10
1414	Broiler,one half,broiled 1 half broiler	6.2 oz	390	9
1799	Fish burger 3 oz breaded fish on bun	4.3 oz	330	9
1682	Turkey pot pie,biscuit topping 1 cup	8.3 oz	400	9
1802	Fish burger w cheese,tartar sce 2 oz fish, .5 oz ch, bun	4.1 oz	370	9
446	Quisp 1 oz (1.2 cup)	1.0 oz	120	9
397	Captn crunch p-nut buttr cereal 1 oz (3/4 cup)	1.0 oz	120	8
1397	Liver,calf,fried 1 sl (6 × 2 × .5 in)	3.0 oz	220	8
395	Captain crunch 1 oz (3/4 cup)	1.0 oz	120	8
1785	Barbequed turkey on bun 3 oz barb on 2 oz bun	5.3 oz	290	8
396	Captain crunch crunchberries 1 oz (3/4 cup)	1.0 oz	120	7
475	Oat cereal,inst,fort,ckd,w salt 1 packet	6.2 oz	100	7
1597	Chicken pot pie 1/3 of 9 in diam pie	8.2 oz	550	7
1450	Mackerel,broiled w butter 1 fillet,8.5 × 2.5 ×.5 in	3.7 oz	250	7
1670	Spaghetti,meat sauce+cheese 1 cup	8.1 oz	350	7
1079	Taco Bell beef burrito 1 serving, 6.5 oz	6.5 oz	400	7

1078	Taco Bell bean burrito 1 serving, 6.7 oz	6.7 oz	360	6
1401	Batter dipped breast 1/2 breast	4.9 oz	360	6
1582	Burrito,bean 1 tortilla, 1/2 cup beans	5.9 oz	340	6
1462	Salmon,smoked 3 oz jar or can	3.0 oz	150	6
1562	Turkey roll,salted 3 oz slice	3.0 oz	120	6
1583	Burrito,beef,medium 8 in tort,1/3 cup filling	5.4 oz	390	6
1788	Burrito,beef,in sauce 3 1/2 oz filling on tort	5.4 oz	390	6
1137	Wendy's triple burger 1 serving, 12 oz	12.7 oz	840	6
1672	Taco,beef+beans+cheese+lettuce 6-in tort, 4 oz filling	5.3 oz	340	6
1407	Broiled breast,w skin 1/2 breast	3.5 oz	190	6
1572	Beef meatloaf 2 slices (4 × 3 × 1/2 in)	6.4 oz	320	6
1113	Arbys ham+cheese sandwich 1 serving, 8.25 oz	8.7 oz	480	5
1482	Duck,wild,breast 3 oz	3.0 oz	110	5
1584	Burrito,beef+beans+chili 8 in tort,1/3 cup filling	5.4 oz	360	5
1431	Bass,baked,stuffed 1 pc w 1/3 cup stuffing	7.2 oz	530	5
1568	Blacksea bass,bkd,stuft,no salt 1 pc (3.5 × 4.5 × 1.5 in)	7.2 oz	530	5
1083	Taco Bell enchirito 1 serving, 7.5 oz	7.5 oz	380	5

continued

Menu Items with Maximum Quantity of Vitamin B_6 *(continued)*

No.	Name/Portion Size		KCAL	NUTRI-UNITS B6
1372	Porterhouse steak,lean+fat,brl Yield from 1/2 lb w bone	5.3 oz	450	5
1408	Broiled breast,no skin 1/2 breast	3.0 oz	140	5
1428	Fried giblets 3 oz	3.0 oz	240	5
1599	Chicken potpie w biscuit top 1 cup	8.4 oz	350	5
1633	Lasagna, zucchini 11 oz	10.9 oz	270	5
1421	Roast,light meat,no skin 1 pc (2.5 × 4 × .4 in)	3.0 oz	150	5
1680	Turkey pot pie,home prepared 1/3 of 9 in pie	8.2 oz	550	5
389	All bran 1 oz (1/2 cup)	1.0 oz	70	5
390	Alpha bits 1 oz (1 cup)	1.0 oz	110	5
391	Apple jacks 1 oz (1 cup)	1.0 oz	110	5
392	Bran buds 1 oz (1/3 cup)	1.0 oz	70	5
393	Bran chex 1 oz (1/2 cup)	1.0 oz	90	5
394	Bran flakes,40 percent 1 oz (2/3 cup)	1.0 oz	90	5
398	Cheerios 1 oz (1 1/4 cup)	1.0 oz	110	5
399	Cocoa krispies 1 oz (1 cup)	1.0 oz	110	5

No.	Name/Portion Size		KCAL	NUTRI-UNITS B6
422	Grapenut flakes 1 oz (7/8 cup)	1.0 oz	100	5
425	Honeybran 1 oz (0.8 cup)	1.0 oz	100	5
426	Honeycomb 1 oz (1 1/3 cup)	1.0 oz	110	5
427	Honeynut cheerios 1 oz (7/8 cup)	1.0 oz	110	5
428	Honey nut cornflakes 1 oz (1 cup)	1.0 oz	110	5
430	Kix 1 oz (1 cup)	1.0 oz	110	5
432	Lucky charm 1 oz	1.0 oz	110	5
434	Mueslix 1 oz (1/2 cup)	1.0 oz	140	5
435	Nutri-grain barley 1 oz (2/3 cup)	1.0 oz	100	5
436	Nutri-grain corn 1 oz (2/3 cup)	1.0 oz	110	5
437	Nutri-grain rye 1 oz (2/3 cup)	1.0 oz	100	5
438	Nutri-grain wheat 1 oz (2/3 cup)	1.0 oz	100	5
440	Pep wheat flakes 1 oz (1 cup)	1.0 oz	110	5
441	Post toasties 1 oz (1 1/4 cup)	1.0 oz	110	5
449	Rice chex 1 oz (1 1/8 cup)	1.0 oz	110	5

400	Cocoa pebbles,rice 1 oz (.8 cup)	1.0 oz	110	5
401	Cocoa pops 1 oz	1.0 oz	110	5
402	Cookie crisp 1 oz (1 cup)	1.0 oz	110	5
404	Corn chex 1 oz (1 cup)	1.0 oz	110	5
405	Corn flakes 1 oz (1 to 1.3 cup)	1.0 oz	110	5
407	Corny snaps 1 oz (1 cup)	1.0 oz	120	5
408	Count chocula 1 oz (1 cup)	1.0 oz	110	5
410	CW Post family cereal 1 oz (1/4 cup)	1.0 oz	130	5
411	Crispy wheats n raisins 1 oz (2/3 cup)	1.0 oz	100	5
412	CW Post family cereal w raisins 1 oz (1/4 cup)	1.0 oz	120	5
413	Fortified oat flakes 1 oz (2/3 cup)	1.0 oz	100	5
414	Froot loops 1 oz (1 cup)	1.0 oz	110	5
415	Frosted miniwheats 1 oz (4 pieces)	1.0 oz	100	5
416	Frosted rice 1 oz (0.8 cup)	1.0 oz	110	5
417	Fruity pebbles 1 oz (7/8 cup)	1.0 oz	110	5
418	Golden grahams 1 oz (3/4 cup)	1.0 oz	110	5
421	Grapenuts 1 oz (1/4 cup)	1.0 oz	100	5
450	Rice krispies 1 oz (1 cup)	1.0 oz	110	5
451	Special K 1 oz (0.7 cup)	1.0 oz	110	5
452	Sugar smacks 1 oz (1 cup)	1.0 oz	100	5
453	Sugar corn pops 1 oz (1 cup)	1.0 oz	110	5
454	Sugar frosted flakes 1 oz (1.3 cup)	1.0 oz	110	5
456	Super sugar crisp 1 oz (0.8 cup)	1.0 oz	110	5
457	Trix 1 oz (1 cup)	1.0 oz	110	5
458	Team 1 oz (2/3 cup)	1.0 oz	110	5
459	Tasteeos 1 oz (1 cup)	1.0 oz	110	5
461	Waffelos 1 oz (1cup)	1.0 oz	110	5
462	Wheaties 1 oz (1 cup)	1.0 oz	100	5
463	Wheat chex 1 oz (2/3 cup)	1.0 oz	100	5
1004	Jack in Box vanilla shake 1 serving, 11 oz	11.1 oz	340	5
1598	Chicken pot pie,commercial 1 8 oz pie	7.9 oz	490	5
1681	Turkey pot pie,frz,commercial 1 8 oz pie	8.0 oz	450	5
879	Parfait,soft serve 1 parfait	10.0 oz	460	5

Menu Items with Maximum Quantity of Calcium

No.	Name/Portion Size		KCAL	NUTRI-UNITS CA
1096	Pizza H,thick,superstyle,cheese 1/4 of 13 in pizza	6.0 oz	450	19
1357	Tofu,soybean curd 1 pc (2.5 × 2.8 × 1 in)	4.2 oz	170	16
1088	Pizza H,thin,superstyle,cheese 1/4 of 13 in pizza	5.3 oz	410	16
183	Malt, chocolate, large 1 21-oz serving	20.7 oz	840	12
999	Dairy Queen choclate malt,large 1 large, 20.7 oz	20.7 oz	840	12
1095	Pizza H,thick,cheese 1/4 of 13 in pizza	5.3 oz	390	12
1588	Cheese fondue 1 cup	6.2 oz	460	11
1090	Pizza H,thin,suprstyle,pepproni 1/4 of 13 in pizza	5.3 oz	430	11
1094	Pizza H,thin,super,supreme 1/4 of 13 in pizza	6.3 oz	520	11
1100	Pizza H,thick,super,pork w mush 1/4 of 13 in pizza	6.0 oz	500	11
1101	Pizza H,thick,supreme 1/4 of 13 in pizza	6.0 oz	480	11
1102	Pizza H,super,supreme 1/4 of 13 in pizza	7.1 oz	590	11
1611	Enchiladas,beef and cheese 2 small	8.9 oz	380	10
182	Malt, chocolate, medium 1 15-oz serving	14.7 oz	600	10
998	Dairy Queen choclate malt,med 1 medium, 14.7 oz	14.7 oz	600	10
1087	Pizza Hut pizza,thin,cheese 1/4 of 13 in pizza	4.6 oz	340	10
701	Yogurt,lo fat,van,coffee,lemon 8 oz container	8.0 oz	190	8
994	Burger King shake,vanilla 1 medium, 14 oz	14.0 oz	330	8
687	Evaporated skim milk,cnd,unswt 1/2 cup	4.5 oz	100	7
1138	Wendy's triple burger w cheese 1 serving, 14 oz	14.1 oz	1040	7
1111	Arbys beef and cheddar sandwich 1 serving, 6 oz	6.3 oz	480	7
1643	Macaroni w cheese,homesyyle 1 cup	7.1 oz	430	7
862	Banana split w soft serve 1 banana split	13.5 oz	540	7
1002	Jack in Box chocolate shake 1 serving, 11 oz	11.2 oz	370	7
1003	Jack in Box strawberry shake 1 serving, 11.6 oz	11.6 oz	380	7
1004	Jack in Box vanilla shake 1 serving, 11 oz	11.1 oz	340	7
1030	Dairy Queen banana split 1 serving, 13.5 oz	13.5 oz	540	7
178	Cocoa,made from mix + skim milk 1 8-oz cup	9.3 oz	160	7
196	Shake, vanilla 1 10-oz serving	10.2 oz	320	7
700	Yogurt,fruit,part skim milk 8 oz container	8.0 oz	230	7
1007	McDonalds vanilla shake 1 serving, 10.2 oz	10.2 oz	320	7
194	Shake,chocolate 1 10-oz serving	10.2 oz	370	7

1098	Pizza H,thick,suprstyl,pepproni 1/4 of 13 in pizza	6.0 oz	490	10
1097	Pizza H,thick,pepperoni 1/4 of 13 in pizza	5.3 oz	450	10
1113	Arbys ham+cheese sandwich 1 serving, 8.25 oz	8.7 oz	480	10
1645	Manicotti 1 cup	8.7 oz	340	10
1114	Arbys sub (no dressing) 1 serving, 9.5 oz	10.1 oz	480	9
696	Yogurt,skim w nfdm,plain 8 oz container	8.0 oz	130	9
919	Yogurt,plain,skim milk w nfdm 1 8-oz container	8.0 oz	130	9
1663	Ravioli,cheese 1 cup	8.6 oz	580	9
684	Condensed milk,sweetened,canned 1/2 cup	5.4 oz	490	9
1790	Cheese sandwich,grilled 2 oz cheese	4.2 oz	410	9
1581	Broccoli cheese casserole 1 cup	8.5 oz	330	9
1621	Lasagna,cheese 1 cup	8.1 oz	320	9
695	Yogurt,lo fat,plain 8 oz container	8.0 oz	140	8
917	Yogurt,plain,part skim milk 1 8-oz container	8.0 oz	140	8
1089	Pizza H,thin,pepperoni 1/4 of 13 in pizza	4.6 oz	370	8
1093	Pizza H,thin,supreme 1/4 of 13 in pizza	5.3 oz	400	8
1099	Pizza H,thick,pork w mushroom 1/4 of 13 in pizza	5.3 oz	430	8
195	Shake, strawberry 1 10-oz serving	10.3 oz	350	7
1005	McDonalds chocolate shake 1 serving, 10.2 oz	10.2 oz	360	7
1006	McDonalds strawberry shake 1 serving, 10.3 oz	10.3 oz	350	7
649	Ricotta,part skim 1/2 cup	4.4 oz	170	7
686	Evaporated milk,canned 1/2 cup	4.5 oz	170	7
688	Goat milk 1 cup	8.6 oz	170	7
1670	Spaghetti,meat sauce+cheese 1 cup	8.1 oz	350	7
179	Egg nog, non-alcoholic 1 8-oz glass	8.7 oz	340	6
336	Egg nog,non alcoholic 1 8-oz glass	8.7 oz	340	6
186	Milk, malted, beverage 1 8-oz glass	8.3 oz	210	6
188	Milk, 1 percent fat, a+d fort 1 8-oz glass	8.7 oz	110	6
189	Milk, 2 percent fat, a+d fort 1 8-oz glass	8.7 oz	130	6
341	Milk,1 percent fat,a+d fort 1 8-oz glass	8.7 oz	110	6
343	Milk,2 percent fat,a+d fort 1 8-oz glass	8.7 oz	130	6
691	Part skim milk,1 percent fat 1 cup	8.7 oz	110	6
692	Part skim milk,2 percent fat 1 cup	8.7 oz	130	6
918	Yogurt,part skim,fruit flavors 1 8-oz container	8.0 oz	230	6

continued

Menu Items with Maximum Quantity of Calcium *(continued)*

No.	Name/Portion Size		KCAL	NUTRI-UNITS CA
1795	Chili dog w bun 1.5 oz dog,1/2 c chili	8.3 oz	510	6
1587	Canneloni 1 cup	8.8 oz	430	6
1633	Lasagna, zucchini 11 oz	10.9 oz	270	6
690	Skim milk 1 cup	8.7 oz	90	6
1622	Lasagna w beef 1 cup	8.5 oz	420	6
181	Malt, chocolate, small 1 8-oz serving	8.5 oz	340	6
187	Milk, skim 1 8-oz glass	8.6 oz	90	6
339	Milk,skim 1 8-oz glass	8.6 oz	90	6
866	Cone,soft serve,large 1 cone	7.5 oz	340	6
879	Parfait,soft serve 1 parfait	10.0 oz	460	6
996	Dairy Queen freeze 1 serving, 14 oz	14.0 oz	520	6
997	Dairy Queen choclate malt,small 1 small, 8.5 oz	8.5 oz	340	6
1001	Dairy Queen misty freeze 1 serving, 14.5 oz	14.5 oz	500	6
1034	Dairy Queen cone,large 1 serving, 7.5 oz	7.5 oz	340	6
1037	DQ choc dipped cone,large 1 cone, 8.3 oz	8.3 oz	450	6
1040	DQ chocolate sundae,large 1 serving, 8.7 oz	8.7 oz	400	6
337	Hot chocolate or cocoa 1 8-oz cup	8.8 oz	210	6
683	Chocolate milk,whole 1 cup	8.8 oz	210	6
1013	J in b omelette,ranchero 1 serving, 6.9 oz	6.9 oz	410	6
1950	Oyster stew,home prp,3 pts milk 1 cup	8.5 oz	210	6
685	Dried milk,non fat,a+d fort. 1/3 cup (dry)	.8 oz	80	6
697	Yogurt,whole milk,plain 8 oz container	8.0 oz	140	6
920	Yogurt,plain,whole milk 1 8-oz container	8.0 oz	140	6
1011	J in b omelette,double cheese 1 serving, 5.8 oz	5.9 oz	420	6
1457	Salmon,chum,cnd,sol+liq,no salt 1/2 cup	3.9 oz	150	6
1949	Oyster stew,home prp,2 pts milk 1 cup	8.5 oz	230	6
650	Swiss cheese 1 oz (2 × 2 × 1/2 in)	1.0 oz	110	5
1008	Wendy's frosty 1 serving, 8.8 oz	8.8 oz	390	5
1458	Salmon,coho,cnd,sol+liq,w salt 1/2 cup	3.9 oz	170	5
1851	Cheese,swiss 1 sl (4 in sq × 1/8 in)	1.0 oz	110	5
177	Cocoa or hot choc w whole milk 1 8-oz cup	8.8 oz	240	5
1012	J in b omelette,ham and cheese 1 serving, 6 oz	6.1 oz	430	5

1044	Dairy Queen parfait 1 serving, 10 oz	10.0 oz	460	6
1626	Cannelloni,cheese 9.1 oz	9.1 oz	270	6
693	Whole milk 1 cup	8.7 oz	150	6
869	Hot fudge brownie w soft serve 1 serving	9.4 oz	560	6
190	Milk, whole, 3.5 percent fat 1 8-oz glass	8.6 oz	150	6
345	Milk,whole,3.5 percent fat 1 8-oz glass	8.6 oz	150	6
1590	Cheese rarebit,no toast 1/2 cup	4.1 oz	210	6
184	Milk, chocolate, 2 percent fat 1 8-oz glass	8.8 oz	180	6
333	Chocolate milk,2 percent fat 1 8-oz glass	8.8 oz	180	6
681	Buttermilk,cultured 1 cup	8.6 oz	100	6
682	Chocolate milk,2 percent fat 1 cup	8.8 oz	180	6
1461	Salmon,red,cnd,sol+liq w salt 1/2 cup	3.9 oz	190	6
1589	Cheese manicotti w sauce 1 cup	8.5 oz	280	6
176	Buttermilk, cultured 1 8-oz glass	8.5 oz	100	6
185	Milk,chocolate,3.5 percent fat 1 8-oz glass	8.8 oz	210	6
330	Buttermilk,cultured 1 8-oz glass	8.5 oz	100	6
334	Chocolate milk,3.5 percent fat 1 8-oz glass	8.8 oz	210	6

1083	Taco Bell enchirito 1 serving, 7.5 oz	7.5 oz	380	5
648	Ricotta 1/2 cup	4.4 oz	220	5
1010	Jack in Box scrambled eggs 1 serving, 9.4 oz	9.4 oz	390	5
1609	Dried beef,creamed 1 cup	8.6 oz	380	5
1677	Tostada,beans+cheese+lett+sauce 1 tortilla,5 oz filling	6.3 oz	220	5
1797	Corned beef and cheese on rye 1 oz each	4.1 oz	300	5
1130	McD quarter pounder w cheese 1 serving, 6.8 oz	6.8 oz	520	5
1793	Cheeseburger,quarter pounder 1 burger	6.8 oz	520	5
191	Milk, whole, low sodium 1 cup	8.6 oz	150	5
694	Whole milk, low sodium 1 cup	8.6 oz	150	5
1123	J in b jumbo burger w cheese 1 serving,8.7 oz	8.7 oz	570	5
1140	Clam chowder(potato base) 1 serving, 8 oz	8.8 oz	220	5
460	Total 1 oz (7/8 cup)	1.0 oz	100	5
1712	Chef salad,bolog,chees,egg,drsg 1 oz each,3 c let,4 tb dr	8.6 oz	580	5
1801	Fish burger w cheese,chili sce 2 oz fish,1 oz cheese,bun	5.3 oz	430	5
1809	Hamburger,super 1 hamburger,8.9 oz	8.9 oz	560	5
646	Parmesan 1/4 cup grated	.7 oz	80	5

Menu Items with Maximum Quantity of Iron

No.	Name/Portion Size		KCAL	NUTRI-UNITS IRN
433	Most 1 oz (1/2 cup)	1.0 oz	90	20
442	Product 19 1 oz (1 cup)	1.0 oz	110	20
460	Total 1 oz (7/8 cup)	1.0 oz	100	20
429	King vitamin 1 oz (3/4 cup)	1.0 oz	110	19
1524	Pork liver,fried 1 sl (6.5 × 2.5 × .4 in)	3.0 oz	140	17
447	Raisin bran,iron fort. 1 oz (1/2 cup)	1.0 oz	90	14
1357	Tofu,soybean curd 1 pc (2.5 × 2.8 × 1 in)	4.2 oz	170	14
1397	Liver,calf,fried 1 sl (6 × 2 × .5 in)	3.0 oz	220	13
1138	Wendy's triple burger w cheese 1 serving, 14 oz	14.1 oz	1040	12
1137	Wendy's triple burger 1 serving, 12 oz	12.7 oz	840	12
1136	Wendy's double burger w cheese 1 serving, 11.5 oz	11.5 oz	800	12
403	Corn bran 1 oz (1 cup)	1.0 oz	100	11
471	Cream of wheat,reg,ckd w salt 3/4 cup	6.6 oz	120	10
444	Puffed rice,fortified 1 oz (2 cups)	1.0 oz	110	10
1112	Arbys super roast beef sandwich 1 serving, 9.5 oz	10.3 oz	620	10
1428	Fried giblets 3 oz	3.0 oz	240	10

No.	Name/Portion Size		KCAL	NUTRI-UNITS IRN
446	Quisp 1 oz (1.2 cup)	1.0 oz	120	7
1571	Beans w pork in sweet sauce 1 cup	9.0 oz	380	7
1453	Oysters,cnd,sol+liq w salt 1 can,3.6 oz	3.6 oz	80	6
1094	Pizza H,thin,super,supreme 1/4 of 13 in pizza	6.3 oz	520	6
1099	Pizza H,thick,pork w mushroom 1/4 of 13 in pizza	5.3 oz	430	6
1101	Pizza H,thick,supreme 1/4 of 13 in pizza	6.0 oz	480	6
1134	Wendy's single burger w cheese 1 serving, 8.5 oz	8.5 oz	580	6
1133	Wendy's single burger 1 serving, 7 oz	7.1 oz	470	6
1396	Liver,beef,fried 1 sl (6 × 2 × .5 in)	3.0 oz	180	6
183	Malt, chocolate, large 1 21-oz serving	20.7 oz	840	6
999	Dairy Queen choclate malt,large 1 large, 20.7 oz	20.7 oz	840	6
1324	Prune juice,bottled,+ vit c 1/2 cup	4.5 oz	100	6
1395	Kidneys,simmered 1/2 cup	2.5 oz	100	6
1010	Jack in Box scrambled eggs 1 serving, 9.4 oz	9.4 oz	390	6
1569	Beans and franks,canned 1 cup	9.0 oz	370	5
1602	Chop suey,home prepared 1 cup	8.8 oz	300	5

1135	Wendy's double burger 1 serving, 10 oz	10.1 oz	670	9
413	Fortified oat flakes 1 oz (2/3 cup)	1.0 oz	100	9
422	Grapenut flakes 1 oz (7/8 cup)	1.0 oz	100	9
430	Kix 1 oz (1 cup)	1.0 oz	110	9
395	Captain crunch 1 oz (3/4 cup)	1.0 oz	120	8
431	Life 1 oz (2/3 cup)	1.0 oz	100	8
397	Captn crunch p-nut buttr cereal 1 oz (3/4 cup)	1.0 oz	120	8
396	Captain crunch crunchberries 1 oz (3/4 cup)	1.0 oz	120	8
1114	Arbys sub (no dressing) 1 serving, 9.5 oz	10.1 oz	480	8
1103	McDonalds chef salad 1 serving,9.6 oz	9.6 oz	220	7
1394	Heart,cooked 3 oz	3.0 oz	150	7
475	Oat cereal,inst,fort,ckd,w salt 1 packet	6.2 oz	100	7
1092	Pizza H,thin,super,pork w mushr 1/4 of 13 in pizza	5.3 oz	450	7
1100	Pizza H,thick,super,pork w mush 1/4 of 13 in pizza	6.0 oz	500	7
1102	Pizza H,super,supreme 1/4 of 13 in pizza	7.1 oz	590	7
1119	Burger King,whopper 1 serving, 10 oz	10.0 oz	610	7
1429	Fried liver 1/2 cup	2.5 oz	110	7
1603	Chop suey,canned 1 cup	8.8 oz	160	5
1068	Kentucky Fr Chick,orig dinner 2 pc,pot,gravy,slaw,roll	15.0 oz	830	5
1091	Pizza H,thin,pork w mushroom 1/4 of 13 in pizza	4.6 oz	380	5
1130	McD quarter pounder w cheese 1 serving, 6.8 oz	6.8 oz	520	5
1570	Beans w pork in tomato sauce 1 cup	9.0 oz	310	5
1572	Beef meatloaf 2 slices (4 × 3 × 1/2 in)	6.4 oz	320	5
1793	Cheeseburger,quarter pounder 1 burger	6.8 oz	520	5
1949	Oyster stew,home prp,2 pts milk 1 cup	8.5 oz	230	5
338	Instant breakfast, dry 1 serving	1.2 oz	120	5
954	Pecan pie m/w lard 1/6 of 9 in diam pie	4.8 oz	570	5
955	Pecan pie m/w veg fat 1/6 of 9 in diam pie	4.8 oz	570	5
1093	Pizza H,thin,supreme 1/4 of 13 in pizza	5.3 oz	400	5
1095	Pizza H,thick,cheese 1/4 of 13 in pizza	5.3 oz	390	5
1097	Pizza H,thick,pepperoni 1/4 of 13 in pizza	5.3 oz	450	5
1587	Canneloni 1 cup	8.8 oz	430	5
1672	Taco,beef+beans+cheese+lettuce 6-in tort, 4 oz filling	5.3 oz	340	5
380	Super donut,fortified 2 oz	2.0 oz	250	5

continued

Menu Items with Maximum Quantity of Iron *(continued)*

No.	Name/Portion Size		KCAL	NUTRI-UNITS IRN
389	All bran 1 oz (1/2 cup)	1.0 oz	70	5
391	Apple jacks 1 oz (1 cup)	1.0 oz	110	5
392	Bran buds 1 oz (1/3 cup)	1.0 oz	70	5
393	Bran chex 1 oz (1/2 cup)	1.0 oz	90	5
394	Bran flakes,40 percent 1 oz (2/3 cup)	1.0 oz	90	5
398	Cheerios 1 oz (1 1/4 cup)	1.0 oz	110	5
402	Cookie crisp 1 oz (1 cup)	1.0 oz	110	5
410	CW Post family cereal 1 oz (1/4 cup)	1.0 oz	130	5
411	Crispy wheats n raisins 1 oz (2/3 cup)	1.0 oz	100	5
412	CW Post family cereal w raisins 1 oz (1/4 cup)	1.0 oz	120	5
414	Froot loops 1 oz (1 cup)	1.0 oz	110	5
418	Golden grahams 1 oz (3/4 cup)	1.0 oz	110	5
425	Honeybran 1 oz (0.8 cup)	1.0 oz	100	5
427	Honeynut cheerios 1 oz (7/8 cup)	1.0 oz	110	5
432	Lucky charm 1 oz	1.0 oz	110	5
434	Mueslix 1 oz (1/2 cup)	1.0 oz	140	5

No.	Name/Portion Size		KCAL	NUTRI-UNITS IRN
1618	Hamburger goulash 1 cup	7.9 oz	270	5
1108	Arbys chicken breast sandwich 1 serving, 7.25 oz	7.2 oz	550	5
1123	J in b jumbo burger w cheese 1 serving,8.7 oz	8.7 oz	570	5
1129	McDonalds quarter pounder 1 serving, 5.8 oz	5.8 oz	420	5
1615	Fz dinner,meat loaf,potato+peas 11 oz	11.0 oz	410	5
1808	Hamburger,quarter pound 1 hamburger,5.8 oz	5.8 oz	420	5
1820	Reuben:kraut,beef,cheese on rye 1.75 oz corned beef	6.2 oz	310	5
466	Wheat n raisin chex 1 oz (1/2 cup)	1.0 oz	100	4
1012	J in b omelette,ham and cheese 1 serving, 6 oz	6.1 oz	430	4
1372	Porterhouse steak,lean+fat,brl Yield from 1/2 lb w bone	5.3 oz	450	4
1576	Beef liver,onion gravy 1 pc (6.5 × 2.5 × 1/4 in)	3.5 oz	140	4
1584	Burrito,beef+beans+chili 8 in tort,1/3 cup filling	5.4 oz	360	4
1664	Ravioli,meat 1 cup	8.6 oz	600	4
1482	Duck,wild,breast 3 oz	3.0 oz	110	4
1583	Burrito,beef,medium 8 in tort,1/3 cup filling	5.4 oz	390	4
1650	Peppers stuffed w beef 1 med pepper	6.5 oz	310	4

451	Special K	1 oz (0.7 cup)	1.0 oz	110	5
457	Trix	1 oz (1 cup)	1.0 oz	110	5
459	Tasteeos	1 oz (1 cup)	1.0 oz	110	5
461	Waffelos	1 oz (1cup)	1.0 oz	110	5
462	Wheaties	1 oz (1 cup)	1.0 oz	100	5
463	Wheat chex	1 oz (2/3 cup)	1.0 oz	100	5
861	Super donut	2 oz donut	2.0 oz	250	5
1096	Pizza H,thick,superstyle,cheese	1/4 of 13 in pizza	6.0 oz	450	5
1139	Wendy's chili w beans	1 serving, 8 oz	8.8 oz	230	5
1354	Soybeans,cooked,no salt	1/2 cup	3.0 oz	150	5
1795	Chili dog w bun	1.5 oz dog,1/2 c chili	8.3 oz	510	5
1814	Hot dog,large,on bun	1 serving,6.4 oz	6.4 oz	520	5
1600	Chili con carne w beans	1 cup	9.0 oz	340	5
1809	Hamburger,super	1 hamburger,8.9 oz	8.9 oz	560	5
1266	Persimmons,raw,native	2 1/2 in dia × 3 in high	5.9 oz	210	5
1579	Beef stroganoff w rice	2/3 cup on 1/2 cup rice	9.9 oz	370	5
1606	Clam fritters,no salt	3 (2 in diam × 1 3/4 in)	4.2 oz	370	5
1717	Taco salad,beef	1 cup	5.3 oz	340	4
1788	Burrito,beef,in sauce	3 1/2 oz filling on tort	5.4 oz	390	4
1013	J in b omelette,ranchero	1 serving, 6.9 oz	6.9 oz	410	4
1349	Red beans,cooked w salt	1/2 cup	4.5 oz	160	4
1359	Canned roast beef w juice	1/2 cup	4.3 oz	240	4
1578	Beef potpie,home prepared	1/3 of 9 inch pie	7.4 oz	520	4
1586	Burrito,supreme	1 very large	7.9 oz	460	4
1614	Fz dinner,chicken,potato+veg	11 oz	11.0 oz	540	4
1125	McDonalds big mac	1 serving, 6.6 oz	6.6 oz	520	4
1163	Apricots,dehyd,sulf,ckd w sugar	1/2 cup	5.3 oz	190	4
1454	Oysters,fried, no salt	4 med,1.75 in diam × 1 in	1.6 oz	110	4
1585	Burrito,combination	1 large	6.2 oz	400	4
1633	Lasagna, zucchini	11 oz	10.9 oz	270	4
1669	Spaghetti,meatballs+tomato sauc	1 cup	8.7 oz	330	4
1821	Roast beef sandwich w let+pickl	3 oz beef on 1.5 oz bun	5.1 oz	400	4
297	Wild rice,raw	1/2 cup	3.0 oz	300	4
1011	J in b omelette,double cheese	1 serving, 5.8 oz	5.9 oz	420	4

Menu Items with Maximum Quantity of Zinc

No.	Name/Portion Size		KCAL	NUTRI-UNITS ZNC
1453	Oysters,cnd,sol+liq w salt 1 can,3.6 oz	3.6 oz	80	99
1454	Oysters,fried, no salt 4 med,1.75 in diam × 1 in	1.6 oz	110	96
1138	Wendy's triple burger w cheese 1 serving, 14 oz	14.1 oz	1040	19
1137	Wendy's triple burger 1 serving, 12 oz	12.7 oz	840	18
1948	Oyster stew,frozen,w water 1 cup	8.5 oz	60	14
1949	Oyster stew,home prp,2 pts milk 1 cup	8.5 oz	230	14
1950	Oyster stew,home prp,3 pts milk 1 cup	8.5 oz	210	14
1136	Wendy's double burger w cheese 1 serving, 11.5 oz	11.5 oz	800	14
1947	Oyster stew,frozen,w milk 1 cup	8.5 oz	130	14
1135	Wendy's double burger 1 serving, 10 oz	10.1 oz	670	12
1119	Burger King,whopper 1 serving, 10 oz	10.0 oz	610	10
1359	Canned roast beef w juice 1/2 cup	4.3 oz	240	10
1364	Chuck,lean only,braised 1 piece (4 × 2.3 × .5 in)	3.0 oz	200	10
1368	Chuck arm,lean only,braised 1 pc (2.5 × 2.5 × .8 in)	3.0 oz	200	10
1372	Porterhouse steak,lean+fat,brl Yield from 1/2 lb w bone	5.3 oz	450	9
1809	Hamburger,super 1 hamburger,8.9 oz	8.9 oz	560	9
1134	Wendy's single burger w cheese 1 serving, 8.5 oz	8.5 oz	580	7
1390	Ground beef, extra lean, broiled 1 patty (3 in diam × 6 in	3.0 oz	220	7
1639	Spagetti w beef,mushrooms 11.5 oz	11.4 oz	280	7
1388	Rump roast,lean + fat 1 pc (4.1 × 2.2 × .5 in)	3.0 oz	220	7
1646	Meatballs,mushrm gravy,no salt 3 oz meatballs,2 tbsp grv	4.1 oz	440	7
1428	Fried giblets 3 oz	3.0 oz	240	7
1382	Rib,eye,lean + fat, brl 1 piece (2 × 4 × .5 in)	3.0 oz	250	7
1397	Liver,calf,fried 1 sl (6 × 2 × .5 in)	3.0 oz	220	7
1129	McDonalds quarter pounder 1 serving, 5.8 oz	5.8 oz	420	7
1371	Flank steak,braised 1 pc (2.5 × 2.5 × .8 in)	3.0 oz	220	7
1808	Hamburger,quarter pound 1 hamburger,5.8 oz	5.8 oz	420	7
1618	Hamburger goulash 1 cup	7.9 oz	270	7
1378	Sirloin,roundbone,lean+fat,brl 1 piece (2 × 4 × .5 in)	3.0 oz	240	7
1647	Meatloaf,lean 2 sl (4 × 3 × 3/8 in)	4.9 oz	250	7
1133	Wendy's single burger 1 serving, 7 oz	7.1 oz	470	6
1377	Tenderloin, lean only, brl 1 piece (2.6 × 2.6 × .8 i	3.0 oz	180	6

1365	Chuck blade,lean + fat,braised 1 piece (4 × 2.3 × .5 in)	3.0 oz	330	9
1381	Short ribs,lean only,braised 1 serving,(2/3 lb raw)	3.0 oz	250	9
1572	Beef meatloaf 2 slices (4 × 3 × 1/2 in)	6.4 oz	320	9
1573	Beef and vegetable stew,no salt 1 cup	8.6 oz	220	8
1574	Beef and veg stew,salt added 1 cup	8.6 oz	220	8
1575	Beef and vegetable stew,canned 1 cup	8.6 oz	190	8
1389	Rump roast,lean only 1 pc (4.1 × 2.2 × .5 in)	3.0 oz	160	8
1383	Rib,eye, lean only, brl 1 piece (2 × 4 × .5 in)	3.0 oz	200	8
1385	Rib roast,whole,lean only,rst 1 sl (4.1 × 2.2 × .5 in)	3.0 oz	210	8
1367	Chuck arm,lean + fat,braised 1 pc (2.5 × 2.5 × .8 in)	3.0 oz	290	8
1130	McD quarter pounder w cheese 1 serving, 6.8 oz	6.8 oz	520	8
1363	Chuck,lean + fat,braised 1 piece (4 × 2.3 × .5 in)	3.0 oz	300	8
1524	Pork liver,fried 1 sl (6.5 × 2.5 × .4 in)	3.0 oz	140	8
1793	Cheeseburger,quarter pounder 1 burger	6.8 oz	520	8
1062	KFC extra crispy dinner 2 pc,pot,gravy,slaw,roll	15.4 oz	950	8
1379	Sirloin,roundbone,lean only,brl 1 piece (2 × 4 × .5 in)	3.0 oz	180	7
1068	Kentucky Fr Chick,orig dinner 2 pc,pot,gravy,slaw,roll	15.0 oz	830	7
465	Wheat germ 1/4 cup (4 tablespoons)	1.0 oz	110	6
1396	Liver,beef,fried 1 sl (6 × 2 × .5 in)	3.0 oz	180	6
1615	Fz dinner,meat loaf,potato+peas 11 oz	11.0 oz	410	6
1080	Taco Bell beefy tostada 1 serving, 6.5 oz	6.5 oz	320	6
1373	Porterhouse steak,lean only,brl 1 piece (3.5 × 2 × .8 in)	3.0 oz	190	6
1375	T-bone steak,lean only,brl 1 piece (3.5 × 2 × .8 in)	3.0 oz	180	6
1391	Ground beef,lean,broiled 1 patty,3 in diam × .6 in	3.0 oz	230	6
1676	Tostada,beefy 1 large	6.5 oz	290	6
1370	Club steak,lean only,broiled 1 piece (2 × 4 × .5 in)	3.0 oz	180	6
1392	Ground beef,regular,broiled 1 patty,3 in diam × .6 in	3.0 oz	250	6
1608	Crab imperial 1 cup	7.8 oz	320	6
1619	Hot turkey sandwich,pot+gravy 1 serving	12.0 oz	370	6
1123	J in b jumbo burger w cheese 1 serving,8.7 oz	8.7 oz	570	6
1384	Rib roast,whole,lean + fat,rst 1 sl (4.1 × 2.2 × .5 in)	3.0 oz	330	6
1569	Beans and franks,canned 1 cup	9.0 oz	370	6
1570	Beans w pork in tomato sauce 1 cup	9.0 oz	310	6
1376	Tenderloin,lean + fat, brl 1 piece (2.6 × 2.6 × .8 i	3.0 oz	230	6

continued

Menu Items with Maximum Quantity of Zinc *(continued)*

No.	Name/Portion Size		KCAL	NUTRI-UNITS ZNC
1518	Pork picnic,lean only,sim 1 pc (2.5 × 2.5 × .8 in)	3.0 oz	210	6
1579	Beef stroganoff w rice 2/3 cup on 1/2 cup rice	9.9 oz	370	6
1819	Pizzaburger on bun 2 oz bf,.3 oz ch,1 tb sce	5.1 oz	410	6
1380	Short ribs,lean + fat,braised 1 serving (2/3 lb raw)	3.0 oz	400	6
1600	Chili con carne w beans 1 cup	9.0 oz	340	6
1607	Crab,deviled 1 cup	8.5 oz	450	6
1071	McDonalds chicken mcnuggets 1 serving, 20 pc	13.1 oz	900	5
1601	Chili con carne w/o beans 1 cup	8.8 oz	500	5
1717	Taco salad,beef 1 cup	5.3 oz	340	5
1387	Round steak,lean only,brl 1 pc (4.1 × 2.2 × .5 in)	3.0 oz	170	5
1633	Lasagna, zucchini 11 oz	10.9 oz	270	5
1125	McDonalds big mac 1 serving, 6.6 oz	6.6 oz	520	5
1362	Corned beef,cooked 3 oz	3.0 oz	210	5
1369	Club steak,lean + fat,broiled 1 piece (2 × 4 × .5 in)	3.0 oz	240	5
1521	Pork spareribs,braised 3 oz serving	3.0 oz	340	5
438	Nutri-grain wheat 1 oz (2/3 cup)	1.0 oz	100	5
451	Special K 1 oz (0.7 cup)	1.0 oz	110	5
1139	Wendy's chili w beans 1 serving, 8 oz	8.8 oz	230	5
1496	Lamb,leg,lean only,roasted 2 slices (4 × 2 × .3 in)	3.0 oz	160	5
1498	Lamb,shoulder,lean only,roasted 3 sl (2.5 × 2.5 × .25 in)	3.0 oz	170	5
1595	Chicken fried steak w gravy 2 oz steak,1/3 cup gravy	5.6 oz	290	5
1111	Arbys beef and cheddar sandwich 1 serving, 6 oz	6.3 oz	480	5
1131	Taco Bell bellbeefer 1 serving, 4.3 oz	4.3 oz	220	5
464	Wheat germ w brown sugar+honey 1 oz (1/4 cup)	1.0 oz	110	5
1386	Round steak,lean + fat,brl 1 pc (4.1 × 2.2 × .5 in)	3.0 oz	230	5
1517	Pork picnic,lean + fat,sim 1 pc (2.5 × 2.5 × .8 in)	3.0 oz	290	5
1439	Crab,steamed 1/2 cup	2.8 oz	70	5
1510	Ham,light cure,lean only,bkd 1 slice (4 × 2.3 × .5 in)	3.0 oz	160	5
1449	Lobster,cooked 1 cup	5.3 oz	140	4
1616	Fz dinner,turkey,potato+peas 11 oz	11.0 oz	350	4

1650	Peppers stuffed w beef 1 med pepper	6.5 oz	310	5
1670	Spaghetti,meat sauce+cheese 1 cup	8.1 oz	350	5
1821	Roast beef sandwich w let+pickl 3 oz beef on 1.5 oz bun	5.1 oz	400	5
1374	T-bone steak,lean + fat,brl 1 piece (3.5 × 2 × .8 in)	3.0 oz	280	5
183	Malt, chocolate, large 1 21-oz serving	20.7 oz	840	5
999	Dairy Queen choclate malt,large 1 large, 20.7 oz	20.7 oz	840	5
1559	Roast turkey,dark meat 4 pc (2 1/2×1 5/8×1/4 in)	3.0 oz	160	5
1580	Beef w mashed potatoes,gravy 3 oz beef,1/2 cup potato	7.4 oz	300	5
389	All bran 1 oz (1/2 cup)	1.0 oz	70	5
391	Apple jacks 1 oz (1 cup)	1.0 oz	110	5
392	Bran buds 1 oz (1/3 cup)	1.0 oz	70	5
394	Bran flakes,40 percent 1 oz (2/3 cup)	1.0 oz	90	5
414	Froot loops 1 oz (1 cup)	1.0 oz	110	5
434	Mueslix 1 oz (1/2 cup)	1.0 oz	140	5
435	Nutri-grain barley 1 oz (2/3 cup)	1.0 oz	100	5
436	Nutri-grain corn 1 oz (2/3 cup)	1.0 oz	110	5
437	Nutri-grain rye 1 oz (2/3 cup)	1.0 oz	100	5
1558	Canned turkey,salted 1/2 cup	3.5 oz	160	4
1587	Canneloni 1 cup	8.8 oz	430	4
1645	Manicotti 1 cup	8.7 oz	340	4
1679	Turkey and noodles 1 cup	8.3 oz	300	4
403	Corn bran 1 oz (1 cup)	1.0 oz	100	4
1484	Goose,domestic,flesh only,rstd 3 slices (3.5×3×.3 in)	3.5 oz	240	4
1563	Veal chop,broiled or braised 1 pc (2 1/2 in sq × 3/4)	3.0 oz	200	4
1614	Fz dinner,chicken,potato+veg 11 oz	11.0 oz	540	4
1623	Chicken chow mein w rice 11.3 oz	11.1 oz	250	4
1664	Ravioli,meat 1 cup	8.6 oz	600	4
1083	Taco Bell enchirito 1 serving, 7.5 oz	7.5 oz	380	4
1118	Burger King,hamburger 1 serving, 3.7 oz	3.7 oz	250	4
1564	Veal chuck,braised or pot roast 1 pc (2 1/2 in sq × 3/4)	3.0 oz	200	4
1567	Veal patty 1 patty (3 in dia × 3/4)	3.0 oz	200	4
1589	Cheese manicotti w sauce 1 cup	8.5 oz	280	4
1622	Lasagna w beef 1 cup	8.5 oz	420	4
1828	Turkey sandwich w gravy 1.6 oz turkey,1/2 c gravy	8.5 oz	280	4

Menu Items with Maximum Quantity of Potassium

No.	Name/Portion Size		KCAL	NUTRI-UNITS POT
183	Malt, chocolate, large 1 21-oz serving	20.7 oz	840	6
999	Dairy Queen choclate malt,large 1 large, 20.7 oz	20.7 oz	840	6
1163	Apricots,dehyd,sulf,ckd w sugar 1/2 cup	5.3 oz	190	6
1057	Wendys french fries,salted 1 serving, 4.2 oz	4.2 oz	330	5
1162	Apricots,dehyd,sulfured,unckd 1/2 cup	1.8 oz	160	5
1055	Dairy Queen french fr,salted 1 serving, 4.0 oz	4.0 oz	320	5
862	Banana split w soft serve 1 banana split	13.5 oz	540	5
1030	Dairy Queen banana split 1 serving, 13.5 oz	13.5 oz	540	5
2065	Potatoes,baked in skin,w skin 2.3 in diam × 4.7 in	5.5 oz	168	5
1631	Fish divan filet 12.4 oz	12.4 oz	270	4
1632	Fish jardiniere filet 11.2 oz	11.3 oz	280	4
182	Malt, chocolate, medium 1 15-oz serving	14.7 oz	600	4
998	Dairy Queen choclate malt,med 1 medium, 14.7 oz	14.7 oz	600	4
1001	Dairy Queen misty freeze 1 serving, 14.5 oz	14.5 oz	500	4
1052	Arby's potato cakes 1 serving, 2 cakes	5.8 oz	300	4
1112	Arbys super roast beef sandwich 1 serving, 9.5 oz	10.3 oz	620	4
1569	Beans and franks,canned 1 cup	9.0 oz	370	4
1669	Spaghetti,meatballs+tomato sauc 1 cup	8.7 oz	330	4
1715	Lobster salad w tomato slices 1/2 cup sal,1 med tomato	8.8 oz	280	4
1992	Beet greens,boiled,drained 1/2 cup	2.6 oz	20	4
1002	Jack in Box chocolate shake 1 serving, 11 oz	11.2 oz	370	3
1630	Fish florentine 9 oz	9.0 oz	240	3
1639	Spagetti w beef,mushrooms 11.5 oz	11.4 oz	280	3
191	Milk, whole, low sodium 1 cup	8.6 oz	150	3
694	Whole milk, low sodium 1 cup	8.6 oz	150	3
1160	Apricots,dried,ckd w/o sugar 1/2 cup fruit + liquid	4.4 oz	110	3
1332	Adzuki beans,ckd,w salt 1/2 cup	4.1 oz	150	3
1573	Beef and vegetable stew,no salt 1 cup	8.6 oz	220	3
1574	Beef and veg stew,salt added 1 cup	8.6 oz	220	3
1633	Lasagna, zucchini 11 oz	10.9 oz	270	3
1159	Apricots,dried,ckd w sugar 1/2 cup fruit + liquid	4.8 oz	150	3
1209	Figs,dried,uncooked 1/2 cup,chopped	3.0 oz	220	3

1000	Dairy Queen misty float 1 serving, 14.3 oz	14.3 oz	440	4
180	Ice cream float 1 14-oz serving	14.0 oz	330	4
995	Dairy Queen float 1 serving, 14 oz	14.0 oz	330	4
996	Dairy Queen freeze 1 serving, 14 oz	14.0 oz	520	4
1618	Hamburger goulash 1 cup	7.9 oz	270	4
1472	Swordfish,broiled 1 piece (4.5 × 2 × 1 in)	4.9 oz	240	4
1071	McDonalds chicken mcnuggets 1 serving, 20 pc	13.1 oz	900	4
1165	Avocados,raw,commercial variety 1/2 of 3.1 in avocado	4.0 oz	180	4
1572	Beef meatloaf 2 slices (4 × 3 × 1/2 in)	6.4 oz	320	4
1638	Salisbury steak,veg 9.5 oz	9.5 oz	270	4
1645	Manicotti 1 cup	8.7 oz	340	4
194	Shake,chocolate 1 10-oz serving	10.2 oz	370	4
1005	McDonalds chocolate shake 1 serving, 10.2 oz	10.2 oz	360	4
1053	Burger King french fr,no salt 1 serving, small,3.75 oz	3.7 oz	210	4
1119	Burger King,whopper 1 serving, 10 oz	10.0 oz	610	4
1274	Plantain(baking banana),raw 1/2 of 2 in dia×11 in frt	4.6 oz	160	4
1447	Halibut,broiled or baked 1 fillet 6.5 × 2.5 ×.6 in	4.4 oz	210	4

1580	Beef w mashed potatoes,gravy 3 oz beef,1/2 cup potato	7.4 oz	300	3
1600	Chili con carne w beans 1 cup	9.0 oz	340	3
1642	Macaroni,beef+cheese+tom sauce 1 cup	8.0 oz	250	3
1656	Pollack,creamed 1 cup	8.8 oz	320	3
1670	Spaghetti,meat sauce+cheese 1 cup	8.1 oz	350	3
2108	Tomato paste,canned 1/4 cup or 4 tbsp	2.3 oz	50	3
696	Yogurt,skim w nfdm,plain 8 oz container	8.0 oz	130	3
919	Yogurt,plain,skim milk w nfdm 1 8-oz container	8.0 oz	130	3
1139	Wendy's chili w beans 1 serving, 8 oz	8.8 oz	230	3
1601	Chili con carne w/o beans 1 cup	8.8 oz	500	3
684	Condensed milk,sweetened,canned 1/2 cup	5.4 oz	490	3
1003	Jack in Box strawberry shake 1 serving, 11.6 oz	11.6 oz	380	3
1054	Dairy Queen french fr,salted 1 serving, 2.5 oz	2.5 oz	200	3
1056	McDonalds french fries,salted 1 serving, 2.4 oz	2.4 oz	210	3
1108	Arbys chicken breast sandwich 1 serving, 7.25 oz	7.2 oz	550	3
1456	Salmon,broil/bake,no salt 1 steak, 6.7 × 2.5 × 1 in	4.5 oz	230	3
1579	Beef stroganoff w rice 2/3 cup on 1/2 cup rice	9.9 oz	370	3

continued

Menu Items with Maximum Quantity of Potassium *(continued)*

No.	Name/Portion Size		KCAL	NUTRI-UNITS POT
1581	Broccoli cheese casserole 1 cup	8.5 oz	330	3
1619	Hot turkey sandwich,pot+gravy 1 serving	12.0 oz	370	3
1640	Stuffed cabbage w meat 10.8 oz	10.8 oz	210	3
1809	Hamburger,super 1 hamburger,8.9 oz	8.9 oz	560	3
195	Shake, strawberry 1 10-oz serving	10.3 oz	350	3
879	Parfait,soft serve 1 parfait	10.0 oz	460	3
1004	Jack in Box vanilla shake 1 serving, 11 oz	11.1 oz	340	3
1006	McDonalds strawberry shake 1 serving, 10.3 oz	10.3 oz	350	3
1044	Dairy Queen parfait 1 serving, 10 oz	10.0 oz	460	3
1061	Kentucky Fried,orig,3 pieces 3 pieces, 7.5 oz	7.6 oz	360	3
1138	Wendy's triple burger w cheese 1 serving, 14 oz	14.1 oz	1040	3
1570	Beans w pork in tomato sauce 1 cup	9.0 oz	310	3
1571	Beans w pork in sweet sauce 1 cup	9.0 oz	380	3
1616	Fz dinner,turkey,potato+peas 11 oz	11.0 oz	350	3
71	Soy nuts no salt 1/3 cup	1.3 oz	160	3
72	Soy nuts with salt 1/3 cup	1.3 oz	160	3
883	Sundae,deluxe,soft serve 1 sundae	9.5 oz	570	3
1007	McDonalds vanilla shake 1 serving, 10.2 oz	10.2 oz	320	3
1042	Dairy Queen fiesta sundae 1 serving, 9.5 oz	9.5 oz	570	3
1068	Kentucky Fr Chick,orig dinner 2 pc,pot,gravy,slaw,roll	15.0 oz	830	3
1114	Arbys sub (no dressing) 1 serving, 9.5 oz	10.1 oz	480	3
1137	Wendy's triple burger 1 serving, 12 oz	12.7 oz	840	3
1455	Rockfish,oven steamed 1 fillet, 7 × 3.5 × .6 in	4.1 oz	120	3
1610	Eggplant parmigiana 1 cup	7.8 oz	410	3
1622	Lasagna w beef 1 cup	8.5 oz	420	3
1100	Pizza H,thick,super,pork w mush 1/4 of 13 in pizza	6.0 oz	500	3
1343	Hummus 1/3 cup	2.9 oz	270	3
1351	Refried beans,canned 1/2 cup	4.4 oz	140	3
1595	Chicken fried steak w gravy 2 oz steak,1/3 cup gravy	5.6 oz	290	3
1620	Hummus 1/3 cup	2.9 oz	270	3
1682	Turkey pot pie,biscuit topping 1 cup	8.3 oz	400	3
1795	Chili dog w bun 1.5 oz dog,1/2 c chili	8.3 oz	510	3

695	Yogurt,lo fat,plain 8 oz container	8.0 oz	140	3
917	Yogurt,plain,part skim milk 1 8-oz container	8.0 oz	140	3
994	Burger King shake,vanilla 1 medium, 14 oz	14.0 oz	330	3
1062	KFC extra crispy dinner 2 pc,pot,gravy,slaw,roll	15.4 oz	950	3
1266	Persimmons,raw,native 2 1/2 in dia × 3 in high	5.9 oz	210	3
1283	Prunes,dried,uncooked,pitted 5 large prunes	1.8 oz	170	3
1349	Red beans,cooked w salt 1/2 cup	4.5 oz	160	3
1372	Porterhouse steak,lean+fat,brl Yield from 1/2 lb w bone	5.3 oz	450	3
1431	Bass,baked,stuffed 1 pc w 1/3 cup stuffing	7.2 oz	530	3
1568	Blacksea bass,bkd,stuft,no salt 1 pc (3.5 × 4.5 × 1.5 in)	7.2 oz	530	3
1647	Meatloaf,lean 2 sl (4 × 3 × 3/8 in)	4.9 oz	250	3
1678	Turkey a la king 1/2 cup on 1 sl toast	5.7 oz	210	3
193	Soybean milk, fluid 1 cup	9.3 oz	90	3
196	Shake, vanilla 1 10-oz serving	10.2 oz	320	3
688	Goat milk 1 cup	8.6 oz	170	3
701	Yogurt,lo fat,van,coffee,lemon 8 oz container	8.0 oz	190	3
869	Hot fudge brownie w soft serve 1 serving	9.4 oz	560	3
1986	Beans,lima,fresh/fz,boiled,drnd 1/2 cup	3.0 oz	110	3
2075	Potaotes,scallop/au grat+cheese 1/2 cup	4.3 oz	160	3
87	Banana 1 banana (9 in long)	4.2 oz	110	3
178	Cocoa,made from mix + skim milk 1 8-oz cup	9.3 oz	160	3
186	Milk, malted, beverage 1 8-oz glass	8.3 oz	210	3
392	Bran buds 1 oz (1/3 cup)	1.0 oz	70	3
480	Banana 8 3/4 × 1 3/8 inch	4.2 oz	110	3
1037	DQ choc dipped cone,large 1 cone, 8.3 oz	8.3 oz	450	3
1040	DQ chocolate sundae,large 1 serving, 8.7 oz	8.7 oz	400	3
1075	Fish,batter fried 2 pieces, 4.8 oz	4.8 oz	370	3
1102	Pizza H,super,supreme 1/4 of 13 in pizza	7.1 oz	590	3
1111	Arbys beef and cheddar sandwich 1 serving, 6 oz	6.3 oz	480	3
1166	Bananas,raw 1 medium or 4/5 cup slicd	4.2 oz	110	3
1258	Pears,dried,sulf,unckd 5 halves	3.1 oz	230	3
1346	Lima beans,cooked,no salt 1/2 cup	3.3 oz	110	3
1465	Scallops,steamed 6 scallops,(.5 oz each)	3.5 oz	110	3
1604	Chow mein,no noodles 1 cup	8.8 oz	260	3

Menu Items with Maximum Quantity of Dietary Fiber

No.	Name/Portion Size		KCAL	NUTRI-UNITS FIB
1570	Beans w pork in tomato sauce 1 cup	9.0 oz	310	19
1571	Beans w pork in sweet sauce 1 cup	9.0 oz	380	19
1569	Beans and franks,canned 1 cup	9.0 oz	370	18
1209	Figs,dried,uncooked 1/2 cup,chopped	3.0 oz	220	15
1863	Refried beans 1/2 cup	4.6 oz	200	14
1651	Pinto beans+cheese,no salt 3/5 cup	5.6 oz	170	13
1084	Taco Bell pintos n cheese 1 serving, 4.5 oz	4.5 oz	190	13
1081	Taco Bell burrito supreme 1 serving, 8.7 oz	8.7 oz	420	12
1586	Burrito,supreme 1 very large	7.9 oz	460	12
1332	Adzuki beans,ckd,w salt 1/2 cup	4.1 oz	150	11
1333	Baked beans 1/2 cup	4.5 oz	120	11
1334	Baked beans,canned,w/franks 1/2 cup	4.5 oz	180	11
1335	Baked beans,cnd,pork+sweet sce 1/2 cup	4.4 oz	140	11
1336	Baked beans,cnd,pork+tom sce 1/2 cup	4.4 oz	120	11
1337	Baked beans, homemade w salt 1/2 cup	4.4 oz	190	11
1338	Black beans,ckd,no salt 1/2 cup	3.0 oz	110	11

No.	Name/Portion Size		KCAL	NUTRI-UNITS FIB
1600	Chili con carne w beans 1 cup	9.0 oz	340	10
1585	Burrito,combination 1 large	6.2 oz	400	9
1139	Wendy's chili w beans 1 serving, 8 oz	8.8 oz	230	9
1291	Raspberries,red,frozen,sweetnd 1/2 cup	4.4 oz	130	9
1674	Tamale pie 1 cup	8.0 oz	180	9
1788	Burrito,beef,in sauce 3 1/2 oz filling on tort	5.4 oz	390	9
2091	Spinach,canned,lo sod,drained 1/2 cup	3.6 oz	30	9
595	Peanut butter 1/2 cup	4.2 oz	710	9
563	Wheat bran + sugar and vit,dry 1/4 cup	1.1 oz	80	9
1079	Taco Bell beef burrito 1 serving, 6.5 oz	6.5 oz	400	9
1203	Dried fruit,mixed 2 oz (approx 1/2 c)	1.9 oz	130	9
1258	Pears,dried,sulf,unckd 5 halves	3.1 oz	230	9
1289	Raspberrys,blk,cnd,sol+liq,watr 1/2 cup	4.2 oz	60	9
1290	Raspberrys,red,cnd,sol+liq,watr 1/2 cup	4.2 oz	40	9
1339	Black bean soup,cnd,dil,salted 1 cup	8.7 oz	120	9
1720	Tuna apple salad 1 cup	4.2 oz	230	9

1342	Garbanzo beans,chickpeas,ckd ½ cup,salted	2.9 oz	130	11
1346	Lima beans,mature,ckd,nosalt ½ cup	3.3 oz	110	11
1347	Pinto beans,ckd,no salt ½ cup	3.0 oz	120	11
1078	Taco Bell bean burrito 1 serving, 6.7 oz	6.7 oz	360	11
1582	Burrito,bean 1 tortilla, ½ cup beans	5.9 oz	340	11
594	Coconut,dried,sweetned,shredded ½ cup	1.7 oz	260	10
1348	Red beans,canned,no salt ½ cup	4.5 oz	120	10
1349	Red beans,cooked w salt ½ cup	4.5 oz	160	10
1583	Burrito,beef,medium 8 in tort,⅓ cup filling	5.4 oz	390	10
1584	Burrito,beef+beans+chili 8 in tort,⅓ cup filling	5.4 oz	360	10
1789	Burrito,beef and bean 1 burrito	4.6 oz	300	10
70	Pumpkin or squash kernels 3 tablespoons	1.0 oz	130	10
1910	Black bean soup,cnd,w water 1 cup	8.7 oz	120	10
1283	Prunes,dried,uncooked,pitted 5 large prunes	1.8 oz	170	10
1351	Refried beans,canned ½ cup	4.4 oz	140	10
1350	Navy,white beans,ckd,no salt ½ cup	3.3 oz	110	10
1082	Taco Bell combination burrito 1 serving, 6.7 oz	6.7 oz	380	10
389	All bran 1 oz (½ cup)	1.0 oz	70	8
1987	Beans,lima,canned,drained ½ cup	3.0 oz	80	8
1988	Beans,lima,canned.lo sod,draind ½ cup	3.0 oz	80	8
425	Honeybran 1 oz (0.8 cup)	1.0 oz	100	8
392	Bran buds 1 oz (⅓ cup)	1.0 oz	70	8
1274	Plantain(baking banana),raw ½ of 2 in dia×11 in frt	4.6 oz	160	8
439	Oat bran, dry ⅓ cup dry	1.0 oz	120	8
1083	Taco Bell enchirito 1 serving, 7.5 oz	7.5 oz	380	8
1716	Taco salad,beans + beef 1 cup	5.3 oz	200	7
1603	Chop suey,canned 1 cup	8.8 oz	160	7
1265	Pears,dried,sulf,ckd w sugar ½ cup, sol + liq	4.9 oz	200	7
1138	Wendy's triple burger w cheese 1 serving, 14 oz	14.1 oz	1040	7
1162	Apricots,dehyd,sulfured,unckd ½ cup	1.8 oz	160	7
2085	Soybeans,immature seeds,ckd ½ cup	2.6 oz	90	7
1080	Taco Bell beefy tostada 1 serving, 6.5 oz	6.5 oz	320	7
1163	Apricots,dehyd,sulf,ckd w sugar ½ cup	5.3 oz	190	7
1282	Prunes,dehy,ckd,sol+liq,w sugar ¼ cup	2.5 oz	80	7

continued

Menu Items with Maximum Quantity of Dietary Fiber *(continued)*

No.	Name/Portion Size		KCAL	NUTRI-UNITS FIB
1143	Apples,dehyd,sulfured,unckd 1/2 cup	1.8 oz	170	7
1938	Green pea soup/ham,fz, water 1 cup	8.6 oz	180	7
1955	Split pea soup,w water 1 cup	8.6 oz	180	6
1264	Pears,dried,sulfrd,ckd w/o sugr 1/2 cup,sol+liq	4.5 oz	160	6
1677	Tostada,beans+cheese+lett+sauce 1 tortilla,5 oz filling	6.3 oz	220	6
1137	Wendy's triple burger 1 serving, 12 oz	12.7 oz	840	6
1195	Coconut meat,fresh 2 × 2 × 1/2 in piece	1.6 oz	160	6
555	Graham cracker crumbs,sugr coat 1 cup,not packed	3.0 oz	350	6
403	Corn bran 1 oz (1 cup)	1.0 oz	100	6
1123	J in b jumbo burger w cheese 1 serving,8.7 oz	8.7 oz	570	6
1200	Currants,black or european,raw 1/2 cup	2.4 oz	40	6
433	Most 1 oz (1/2 cup)	1.0 oz	90	6
447	Raisin bran,iron fort. 1 oz (1/2 cup)	1.0 oz	90	6
2020	Chard,swiss,boiled,drained 1/2 cup	3.0 oz	20	5
596	Raisins 1/2 cup	2.5 oz	220	5
245	Spoon bread 1/2 cup	4.2 oz	230	5
394	Bran flakes,40 percent 1 oz (2/3 cup)	1.0 oz	90	5
1119	Burger King,whopper 1 serving, 10 oz	10.0 oz	610	5
1135	Wendy's double burger 1 serving, 10 oz	10.1 oz	670	5
1145	Apples,dried,sulfured,unckd 1/2 cup	1.5 oz	100	5
1288	Raspberries,red,raw 1/2 cup	2.3 oz	40	5
1639	Spagetti w beef,mushrooms 11.5 oz	11.4 oz	280	5
1235	Loganberries,raw 1/2 cup	2.5 oz	50	5
1352	Split peas,cooked,no salt 1/2 cup	3.5 oz	120	5
1633	Lasagna, zucchini 11 oz	10.9 oz	270	5
329	Tahini,sesame butter 2 tablespoons	1.1 oz	180	5

568	Whole wheat flour 1/2 cup	2.1 oz	200	6
1136	Wendy's double burger w cheese 1 serving, 11.5 oz	11.5 oz	800	6
1236	Loganbrries,cnd,sol+liq,art swt 1/2 cup	3.5 oz	40	6
1237	Loganberries,cnd,sol+liq, juice 1/2 cup	3.5 oz	50	6
1238	Loganbrries,cnd,sol+liq,lit syr 1/2 cup	3.5 oz	70	6
1239	Loganbrries,cnd,sol+liq,hvy syr 1/2 cup	3.5 oz	90	6
1240	Loganbrrys,cnd,sol+liq,xhvy syr 1/2 cup	3.5 oz	110	6
1997	Blackeye/cowpeas,young pods,ckd 3 oz,scant cup	3.0 oz	30	6
393	Bran chex 1 oz (1/2 cup)	1.0 oz	90	5
1717	Taco salad,beef 1 cup	5.3 oz	340	5
1287	Raspberries,black,raw 1/2 cup	2.5 oz	30	5
1996	Blackeye/cowpea,immat seeds,ckd 1/2 cup	2.9 oz	90	5
476	Oatmeal,ckd w salt 1 cup	8.5 oz	150	5
477	Oatmeal,ckd,no salt 1 cup	8.5 oz	150	5
1253	Peaches, dried, uncooked 1/4 cup	1.4 oz	100	5
1685	Veal parmigiana 1 cup	7.9 oz	340	5

445	Puffed wheat 1 oz (2 cups)	1.0 oz	100	5
560	Rye flour,medium 1 cup	3.1 oz	310	5
950	Mince pie m/w lard 1/6 of 9 in diam pie	5.5 oz	430	5
951	Mince pie m/w veg fat 1/6 of 9 in diam pie	5.5 oz	430	5
964	Raisin pie m/w lard 1/6 of 9 in diam pie	5.5 oz	420	5
965	Raisin pie m/w veg fat 1/6 of 9 in diam pie	5.5 oz	420	5
1167	Black/boysenberries,raw 1/2 cup	2.5 oz	40	5
1172	Blackberries,froz,unswt 1/2 cup	2.5 oz	50	5
1344	Lentils,cooked,no salt 1/2 cup	3.5 oz	120	5
1345	Lentil soup w ham 1 cup	8.7 oz	140	5
1602	Chop suey,home prepared 1 cup	8.8 oz	300	5
1610	Eggplant parmigiana 1 cup	7.8 oz	410	5
1809	Hamburger,super 1 hamburger,8.9 oz	8.9 oz	560	5
1986	Beans,lima,fresh/fz,boiled,drnd 1/2 cup	3.0 oz	110	5
1159	Apricots,dried,ckd w sugar 1/2 cup fruit + liquid	4.8 oz	150	4

Index of Food Items in Nutri-Unit Tables